ROCK HARD!

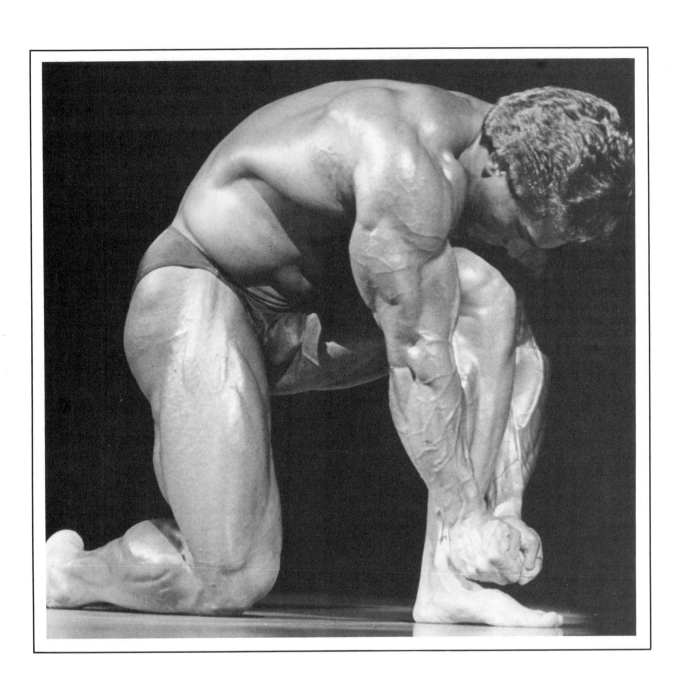

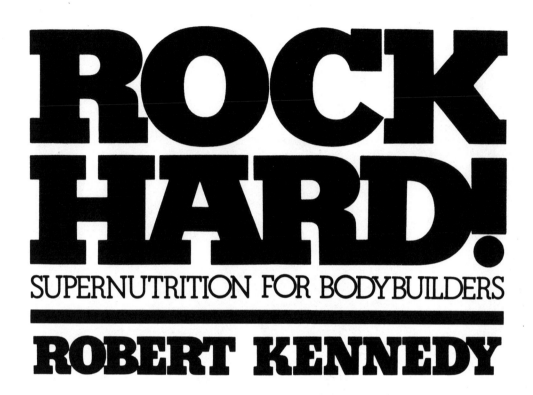

ROCK HARD!

SUPERNUTRITION FOR BODYBUILDERS

ROBERT KENNEDY

WARNER BOOKS

A Warner Communications Company

Library of Congress Cataloging-in-Publication Data

Kennedy, Robert, 1938–
  Rock hard !

  Includes index.
  1. Bodybuilders—Nutrition. 2. Bodybuilding
I. Title.
TX361.B64K46 1987   613.2'0247964   86-24624
ISBN 0-446-37044-4
ISBN 0-446-37045-2

Designed by Giorgetta Bell McRee

Contents

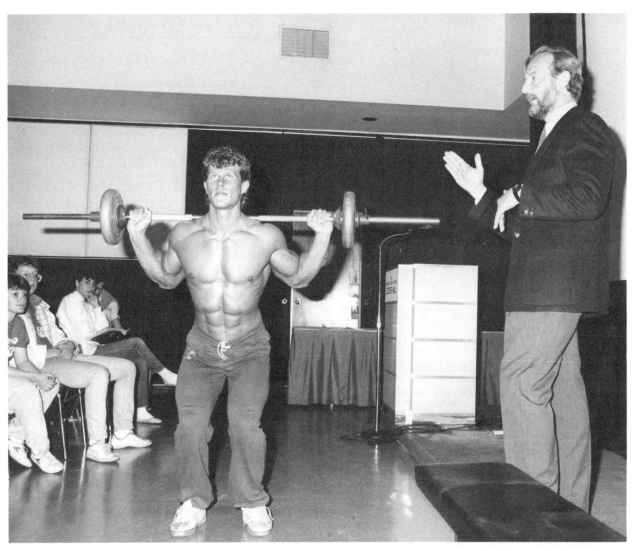

Author Bob Kennedy gives a seminar at the Canadian National Sports and Fitness Show. (Ray Tourville is the model.)

FACING PAGE: Joe Weider, the Master Blaster, with Juliette Bergman of Holland.

Acknowledgments

Tradition demands that I thank all the photographers who have helped with the visual part of this book. I am indeed indebted to them, but before I name them I would also like to give my thanks to the bodybuilders. Without these dedicated, single-minded individuals we would have no books or magazines at all. Remember, these guys and gals train all year round, and often there is little glory for them at the end of the road. They are indeed appreciated. Greatly.

I would also like to thank my wife, Lynda, who helped compile and test out the recipes in this book. I gained almost twenty pounds trying out the various recipes—over a hundred recipes in all!

My appreciation also to Ben and Joe Weider, who keep the sport alive and well through their magazines *Flex* and *Muscle and Fitness* and who keep bodybuilding a respected worldwide sport through the finely tuned organization of the International Federation of Bodybuilders (IFBB).

To World Gym and Gold's, the finest training centers on planet Earth, who kindly allow my photographers free rein at their fabulous California emporiums; to Ken Wheeler of Super Fitness, Toronto; Marsha and Eric Levine of Gold's, Toronto; Frank Grieco of Fitness Plus, Brampton; Jack Niehausen and Louis Miua of Gold's, Richmond Hill; Jim Parker of Olympic Gym, Brampton; and George Tsakiris of Fitness Heaven, Toronto...you have all helped me and I appreciate your kindness.

To Kathy McBride at Warner Books and my editor, Bob Oskam, your faith, confidence, and practical help is acknowledged with the warmest gratitude.

An additional word of appreciation to my staff members Steve Douglas, Val Phillips, Francis Farrugia, Trudy Boetto, Fay Fegan, and Nancy Marysh.

The photographers to whom I owe a debt of gratitude for their work are: Art Zeller, Bill Heimanson, Al Antuck, Roger Shelley, Bill Dobbins, Craig Dietz, Francis Renou, Denie Walters, Garry Bartlett, Doris Barrilleaux, Alan Leff, Bob Flippin, Steve Douglas, Norberto Torriente, Wayne Gallasch, Tapio Hautala, Chris Lund, John Balik, Mike Neveaux, Geoff Collins, Bob Gruskin, Stephen Downs, and Robert Nailon.

Special thanks also to Mike Read of Read Freelance Photograph for his exceptional custom processing work.

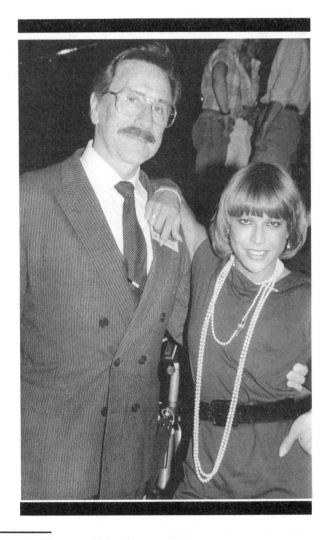

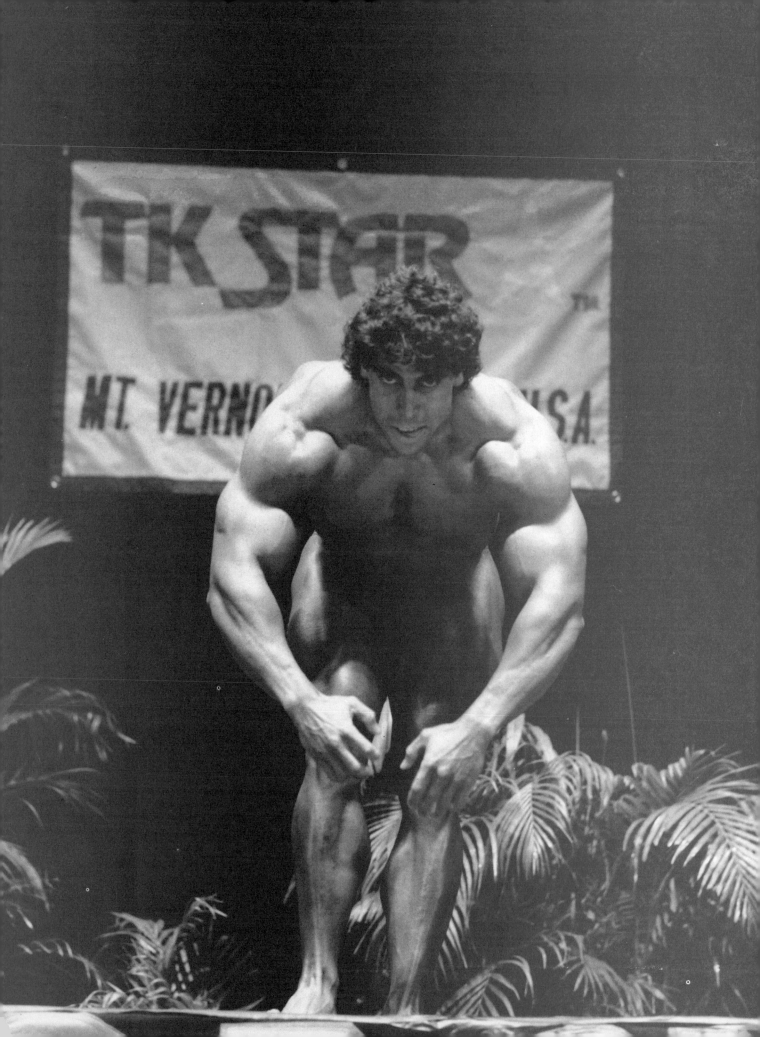

ROCK HARD!

Ed Kawak, Mr. Universe.

Everyone needs a diet that provides adequate amounts of energy (calories), protein, fat, carbohydrates, vitamins, minerals, and water, but for the bodybuilder this need goes deeper. A bodybuilder needs a nutritional plan to help bring about distinctive maximum-achievement goals:

- A bodybuilder needs to max out lean body mass and add strength quickly.
- On occasion a bodybuilder will need to lose fat while on his or her training program.
- At contest time bodybuilders need to reduce body fat temporarily to very low levels while maintaining muscle mass.

When the subject of nutrition is broached, the average bodybuilder rarely claims to be doing anything special where diet is concerned. But as questioning proceeds, one finds that bodybuilders hardly eat like the rest of us. They have discovered, many times through trial and error, that serious workouts tear down muscle and only superior nutrition can build it up again. For them ultimate nutrition depends on these elements: complex carbohydrates, protein, vitamins and minerals, and water.

Nutrition is a science, but it has only really started to be understood during the last quarter of a century. "It belongs," says bodybuilding expert Ellington Darden, Ph.D., "to the group of natural sciences that concern nature and the physical world. Natural sciences may be divided into those described as *pure*, such as mathematics, physics, chemistry and biology, and those described as *applied*, such as engineering, medicine, agriculture, geology...and nutrition."

The bodybuilder knows that nutrition is responsible to a great degree for success or failure. Poor or insufficient nutrition will halt or at the very least hold back progress. Optimum nutrition will feed your muscles 100 percent and steer you toward your goal, whether it is to win a bodybuilding contest...or simply to be the best you can be for everyday living.

Joe Bozich shows massive chest and shoulders in this pose.

1

BODYBUILDING NUTRITION

Eating for Ultimate Results

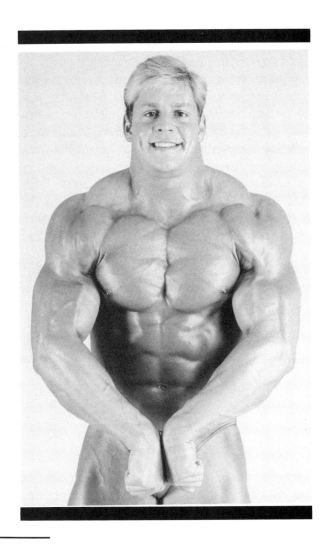

As Bill Reynolds, editor of *Muscle and Fitness* magazine, observes in his book *Supercut* (Contemporary Books), "Nutrition has been an inexact folk art for more than 2,500 years....It's interesting to note that proper nutrition has been considered an aid to athletic performance for nearly 3,000 years, at least since the first recorded classic Olympic Games in 776 B.C."

Before the modern era of enlightened scientific nutrition, the human race was constantly led down different paths of apparent lunacy with regard to diet. For example, at various times during history humans believed that eating the lungs of a deer improved endurance, that powdered rhino horns were the answer to failing virility, that eating bull testicles increased strength, that seafood added to intelligence...The list of nutritional superstitions was endless. Even today millions still consider rhino horn to contain the secrets of manhood, much to the sorrow of the poor rhino, and bull testicles are still marketed to strength enthusiasts (though invariably in desiccated form) via health food stores and through prolific muscle mag advertisements.

In all fairness to our ancestors, many of their viewpoints, while not precisely correct—we now know that eating the heart of a lion does not give us courage, as they believed—do have some broad, useful applications. Glandulars (heart, liver, kidneys, etc.) *are* generally extremely nutritious. Seafoods *do* benefit the brain. Bull testicles (orchis) *do* benefit the development of strength more than many other foods do. And, yes, chicken broth *does* help ward off colds and flu.

The public is still prone to fad diets. There is an ever changing fashion in foods, as there is in clothes, art, music, and architecture. Remember the vitamin C era, when whole books were devoted to the promotion of that particular vitamin? Then there was vitamin E, claimed to be a cure for heart disease and impotence, and used in creams to promote youthful hair and skin. And then it was B_{15}. There's always something new. It seems there's a "hot" or "in" nutrient for every new era.

Years ago bodybuilders believed totally in milk—this was back in the forties and fifties. In fact, it was considered impossible to build a great physique without drinking quarts of the stuff daily. I well remember reading a Charles Atlas course while in my early teens in England. There it was in bold print: "It is recommended that you drink four to six quarts of whole milk daily to get best muscle-building results." I couldn't believe my eyes. At the time milk was rationed and my allotment was one pint (half a quart) per week!

No wonder American bodybuilders at the time were way ahead of the rest of the world. Men like Jack Delinger (Mr. America) and John Grimek (Mr. Universe) were gorging on milk. Steve Reeves went one better and drank goat's milk. Ounce for ounce it delivered even more nutrition and protein than cow's milk.

After milk came the steak craze. Not just bodybuilders ate steaks. All athletes did. In fact, it was common for football, hockey, baseball, and other players to have a pregame steak to fight off the competition.

The next craze was introduced by Irvin Johnson, a Chicago gym owner who moved to California to make his fortune. When Irvin arrived in the sunny state, a fortune teller told him to change his name to Rheo H. Blair if he hoped to make it big. He obeyed and became one of the most successful nutritionists in California. Rheo's star pupil was Larry Scott, who won loads of titles, culminating with two IFBB Mr. Olympia titles, and then retired. Blair made sure that Scott took his new innovation, milk and egg protein powder, mixed with half milk and half cream and consumed in large quantities throughout the day. Even today, in middle age, Larry Scott swears by milk and egg protein if you want muscle mass to come your way. Frank Zane credits Scott as the first bodybuilder to use scientific nutrition and says that's why Scott was so far ahead of his time. Others to take Blair's protein included Don Howarth and Dave Draper.

When I visited Arnold Schwarzenegger during his early years of California training (around 1970), he trained at 10:30 A.M. at Gold's Gym every day, then drove back to his apartment in the Volkswagen that Joe Weider had leased for him and downed a full quart of mixed protein. I noticed the label. It was Blair's. When I asked Arnold about it, he told me that Rheo gave it to him for nothing, even though Arnold, because of his contract with Weider, was unable to endorse the product publicly.

Blair's diet regimen for bodybuilders was based on a very high-protein, low-carbohydrate formula, which today could be regarded as downright unhealthy. Even so, while Arnold was gorging himself on Blair's milk and egg protein, he became bigger than any other bodybuilder in the history of the sport. His chest was 59 inches, his waist 35, going steady with 28-inch thighs and 20-inch calves. He was also at his all-time smoothest.

After the milk and egg protein craze came egg mania. Vince Gironda pointed out that "eggs have the highest biological protein rating of all foods," which is true. He sneered at the cholesterol scare of the time, defying anyone to show that eating eggs actually increased one's cholesterol count, and wholeheartedly recommended eating dozens of eggs daily to help a bodybuilder gain muscles faster than ever. At the time his gym was turning out some pretty rugged guys, world-rated champions.

Amino acids were the next craze. I first heard of them being used by bodybuilders in Vince Gironda's writing way back in the middle fifties. However, it was Blair who was the first to market them directly to bodybuilders. I recall Arnold taking them when he went up against Sergio Oliva for his early Mr. Olympia titles. Frank Zane, too, was paying Blair $1.50 a pill for amino acids at the time he was winning his three Olympia titles (1977, 1978, 1979). Dozens of companies followed up in the hope of making big money, promoting amino acids as steroid replacements. Women also found them useful in maintaining mass and holding down body fat levels.

Since about 1960 there has been an increasing emphasis on lower and lower body fat levels. Today a bodybuilder has to be "cut to ribbons," "ripped," or "shredded" (take your choice) to win a top contest. Prior to 1960 all you needed was muscle mass to win a trophy.

Zane brought a new meaning to muscularity with his three Olympia wins. He beat men who outweighed him by fifty pounds or more. What he lacked in size he made up for with proportion and cuts. This ripped-up body style continues to dominate today.

In Zane's era the precompetition countdown regimen was first to follow a low-carbohydrate/high-fat/high-protein diet and then, as the con-

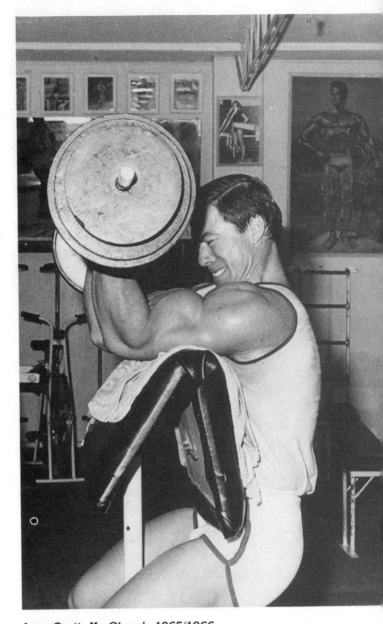

Larry Scott, Mr. Olympia 1965/1966.

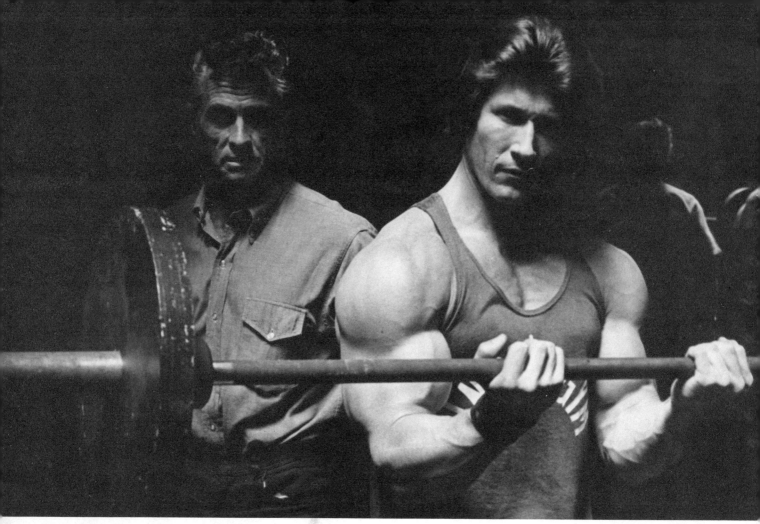

"Iron Man" Vince Gironda and Don Howorth.

test date approached, to replace this diet with an intake of only meat (or fish) and water. No carbohydrates at all were taken. Around 1974 competitive bodybuilders saw the light and started to avoid the meat-and-water diet for definition. They increasingly turned to a more balanced, less harsh diet, characteristically an intake of low fat, modest carbohydrate, and moderate protein. They got even more ripped following this method than they had on zero carbs. More important, they held on to more mass and had more training energy as the date of competition closed in.

"Bodybuilding success is 85 percent nutrition," says Vince Gironda, the Iron Guru and owner of Vince's Gym in North Hollywood. "People are often skeptical of my statement," he quips, "but I have known hundreds of bodybuilders who train hard yet never get anywhere because they don't eat properly. Let's face it, today millions of people train hard, but there are still only a few hundred champions. They are the ones who use ultimate nutrition to maximize their training."

No matter what our sex, age, condition, genetic potential, or ambitions, we all train to improve. To neglect taking advantage of ultimate nutrition is to forfeit from the outset at least half your chances of success.

Dr. Forrest Teunant surveyed a group of six- and seven-year-old children on the subject of basic health rules, including nutrition. He discovered that they were surprisingly aware of the rules of good nutrition...but often unwilling to follow those rules. Bodybuilders act pretty much the same way. When you have digested the contents of this book, remember that I wrote it to help *you,* the hard-training bodybuilder. Make sure you apply what you learn to your own situation. Follow the advice and become the best you can be!

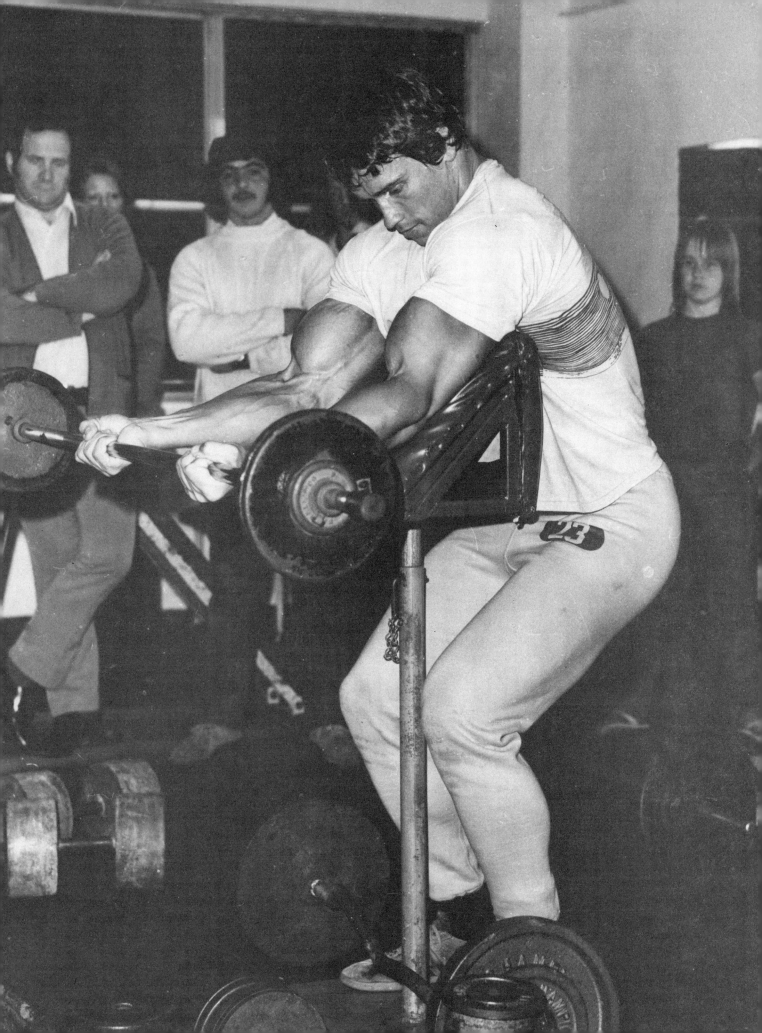

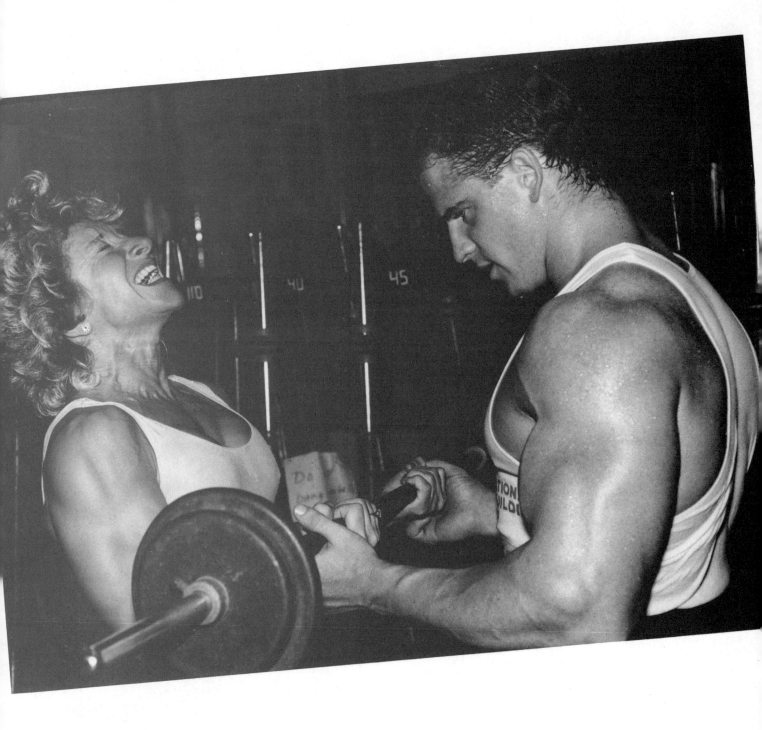

Kay Baxter and Tommy Terwilliger.

Can you believe it? The governments of our world, including those elected by the people, whose services we pay for through a never-ending system of crippling taxes, hardly look after our interests with any real concern or care. As the old Gilbert and Sullivan song says: "Things are seldom what they seem, skim milk masquerades as cream."

There are a great number of false faces confronting civilians in the supermarket today. Yes, the governments have their agencies, understaffed for the most part, to keep an eye on foods and drugs, but in America alone they allow at least 300 standard foods—things like ketchup, rye bread, and mayonnaise—to be sold *without* an ingredients list. Even when the law specifies that manufacturers must declare their ingredients, it is left to the customer to interpret the label.

Ideally, food should be eaten in its natural form—unchanged, uninterfered with…fresh food that is void of coloring, additives, chemicals, refinement, or enrichment. But what do we get? The exact opposite. Little wonder that those of us subjected to this madness suffer more illness, depression, and poor general health as a result.

For starters, let it be said that there is little doubt that traditional medical practice has ignored one of the four pillars of medicine: diet. Instead they have relied only on the other three: drugs, surgery, and psychotherapy. While most doctors are well versed in surgery and pharmacology when it comes to healing the sick, few have ever tried diet. In fact, doctors frequently know very little about nutrition.

Today literally billions of dollars are spent on curing the ills of mankind—cancer, heart disease, leukemia, diabetes, etc.—yet even the modestly intelligent among us know through an innate gut feeling that we are going about things the wrong way. Surely the "cure" has to come in the form of preventive medicine, namely, proper control of the environment and of the production of food for the world's population. New diseases and cancers spring up almost daily.

Lou Ferrigno, Mr. Universe.

2
FOOD PROBLEMS
Enough to Make You Sick

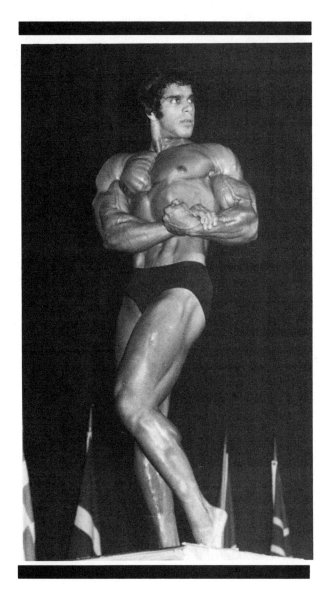

What hope is there that the billions poured into research will find a magic cure for them all? *Prevention has to be the answer.* Why go on kidding ourselves?

Processed foods are a departure from nature. Health food manufacturers are not allowed to make claims, while drug manufacturers bombard doctors and members of the medical community with expensive full-color advertisements in virtually every medical journal published. Bodybuilders, and everyone else, need whole foods, nourishment that contains the molecules of nutrients essential to developing and sustaining the highest quality of life. We have to train and gain. We need to be healthy. We cannot live on junk.

The International Federation of Bodybuilders (IFBB) technical committee put out a report, researched by Ben Weider, entitled "You Are What You Eat." Here is a quote from the introduction. "High quality nourishment is the foundation of inner strength and without it championship performance and robust health for athletes and non-athletes is impossible.

"Every sinew, every cell, every last bit of you comes from what you eat and the quality of your life and athletic achievement can be no better than the quality of that nourishment."

You've read those bread and cereal labels that make you wish you had a degree in chemistry so you could interpret them. You have a sugar- or salt-loaded product where the germ has been taken out of the wheat, where chemicals have been put in to make the product seem fresh, where bleach has been used to take out the natural hue so that the artificial coloring will take better...and a sprinkling of flour thrown in so that the manufacturers can claim the product is "vitamin enriched."

Hear what Dr. Richard A. Kunin has to say in his best-selling book *Mega Nutrition* (Plume): "Since the technology of canning foods and milling grains was developed in the mid 19th century, the trend has been for *processed* foods—nutritionally altered foods—to make up an increasingly greater part of the American diet. We are learning, unfortunately, that the more processed foods we eat, the fewer nutrients we receive. It's as simple as that."

Back in 1940, processed foods comprised only 10 percent of the American diet. In 1970, the proportion had risen to 50 percent, and in 1980 it was 60 percent. The trend is skyrocketing.

You may be wondering, How does a bodybuilder get good, wholesome nutrition, every item perfectly healthful and in just the right amount? The answer is, "You don't." No wonder Vince Gironda wants to take us back to "Stone Age nutrition." A balanced diet was real for our grandparents, whose food was mainly unprocessed. How can we ever know for sure where our food was grown or how much our meat has been degraded?

Bread, for example, has been with us for over 3,000 years. The Bible refers to it as the "staff of life." Today it barely supports life at all. One recent experiment found that rats fed only on white-flour bread died within six weeks, while a comparison group of rats fed only whole-wheat bread thrived indefinitely. No, rats are not human beings, and we don't try to survive on bread alone, but the point is obvious.

Remember the film *Network,* in which the character played by Peter Finch says, "I'm mad as hell and I'm not going to take it anymore"? Well that's how the current state of the westernized food industry makes me feel. Frankly, I have a sense of being cheated.

Most food derives its nutritional character from the soil it's grown in. Grains, fruits, vegetables, and meats grown *on* soil that has been depleted fail to supply optimum amounts of the protein, vitamins, minerals, and enzymes vital for proper growth and development. Soils become poor in quality because of overfarming and loss of arable top soil, but mainly due to the continuous *poisoning* of the land by insecticides and chemicals.

As soon as crops are harvested it is conservatively estimated that about 10 percent of their nutritional value has already been lost. The calories remain, but the micronutrients—numerous vitamins and minerals—are depleted. During the time it takes to transport them to a store, fruits and vegetables lose around another 10 percent of their micronutrient value. For lengthy storage in a grocery store, deduct another 10 percent. We are now left with a product approximately 70 percent of its original value. It has been said that a Mexican eating a carrot gets far more from the product than his American counterpart, simply

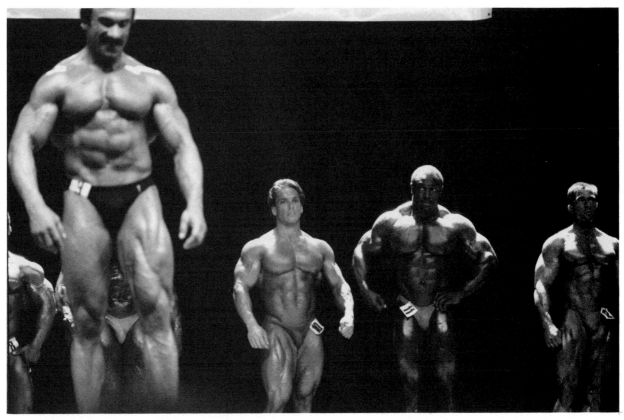

Comparing the physiques.

because Mexico, usually considered an agriculturally poor country, grows carrots everywhere, whereas the average American eats carrots that were grown hundreds of miles from his home.

So we're down to 70 percent. Take off 5 to 10 percent for defrosting frozen vegetables because most "fresh" items are picked green so that they ripen when they are on sale. Outer leaves and skin are often stripped from vegetables when they are washed causing additional vitamin and mineral loss—another 5 percent. So we are down to a 60 percent food item.

Now consider the way we usually prepare food for home eating—boiling, baking, overcooking. It all reduces goodness dramatically. One study showed that as much as 50 percent of the nutrients in vegetables are removed by the most usual methods of cooking. Items like spinach and broccoli are often cooked to death! Conservatively stated, we probably burn out of our meat and boil out of our vegetables some 20 percent of their original nutrients. We now have on our plates 40 percent of the micronutritional value the food had as it was originally grown or

raised. And make no mistake about it, we are talking about so-called fresh food.

What about the insecticides on your fruit that permeate through the skin? How about the spongy bread that feels as fresh as a newly baked loaf but in fact only *appears* so because of the added commercial chemicals and preservatives. It may well be weeks old; and you would never guess it. Then there are the additives—to make beets redder, peas greener, eggs yellower—and the *processing*—for items like that everlasting cheese spread that can endure for months in its package because it is riddled with chemical preservatives. Not only do these factors devitalize products, in many cases the items in question are robbed of goodness to such an extent that they are nutritionally bankrupt. They are worth zip.

Several food dyes have been linked to cancer and other illnesses. Some have been removed (after years of use, I might add) from the market by the FDA, but many that are suspect remain. I'm sure that if you had your say you wouldn't want unnaturally greener peas or redder beets, yet in order to sell us their products manufacturers are using up their dyes at a faster rate than ever before. Oceans of suspect color formulations are used in the production of jams, ketchups, soft drinks, candies, and a host of other foods that North Americans ingest daily. Yes, I'm as mad as hell, and you should be, too.

Remember the Johnny Carson joke? "Ladies and gentlemen. This is a very historical moment. According to the newspapers no new cause for cancer was discovered during the entire day." The audience roared with laughter, but the underlying sinisterism rumbles in one's mind for a lifetime.

Yes, there are problems with food. We have to live with most and circumvent what we can by eating the freshest and most natural that we can find. Try to get fresh-grown produce from your own garden or neighborhood—food that has not been tampered with. Prepare foods carefully. Do not overcook. Avoid, when possible, canned foods, cured and smoked foods, sugar-loaded empty-calorie junk foods. Cut down on the killers: sugar, salt (sodium), and fat. All three nourish disease.

The consumption of sugar has been on the rise for the last two centuries. Recently it has become a favorite ingredient of manufacturers because it is relatively cheap. Soft drinks often contain 90 percent sugar, ketchup 35 percent, canned vegetables 3 to 5 percent. Manufacturers use sugar to hook consumers on a product and to mask any bitter taste, whatever the food category. In North America refined sugar furnishes some 26 percent of total calories consumed. Unlike sugarcane, which is a complete food, table sugar furnishes *empty* calories with no nutritional value. Get your sugar from fruits and vegetables, even honey. Do not use refined table sugar, including brown sugar (white sugar dyed brown). Adjust your taste to enjoy less sweetness. It can be done, and you will be the better for it. And so will your muscles.

Table salt causes high blood pressure and, taken in excess, contributes to poor general health. Bodybuilders who train hard and sweat profusely may need more salt than the average person, particularly in hot or humid weather, but this does not mean you should cover your food with table salt before eating it. Ellington Darden,

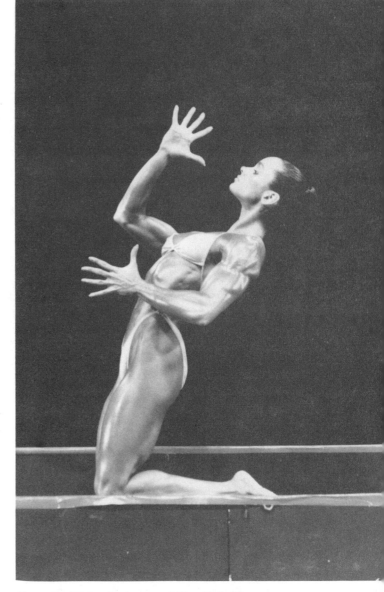

Dramatic Gladys Portugues of New York City.

Research Director for Nautilus Sports/Medical Industries and a practicing bodybuilder, has noted that an athlete/bodybuilder may lose as much as three to five grams of salt per liter of sweat. This can be replaced by the drinking of salt water.

Salt contains about 39 percent sodium. It is a needed ingredient in our diet, but most westernized people ingest far too much of it for good health.

People with a history of circulatory problems such as heart disease, swollen ankles, or high blood pressure must avoid excessive salt intake. As with sugar, it is a good rule to avoid processed salt altogether and rely on natural fruits and vegetables for your supplies.

Fat, once thought to be good for us, is now fast becoming a recognized enemy. Recent statistics on food consumption show that the overall diet in North America and Europe takes about 45 percent of its calories from fat, 40 percent from carbohydrates, and 15 from protein. We are eating far too much fat and not enough carbohydrates. Eating large quantities of land animals and land animal products, both high in fat, is making us ill. In reality no more than 25 percent of your daily calories should come from fat, with 20 percent from protein and the remaining 55 percent from carbohydrate.

And what about that comparatively new phenomenon, fake foods. The only sensible application for wholly fabricated foods, one would think, is for astronauts traveling through space. But no, simulated, fake foods are with us for consumption as normal everyday meals and, hell of all hells, they are proliferating by the day!

Refined flour, margarine, and sugar are just the starting points in the new commercial foods. The food industry is coming out with an array of fake foods; a whole new technology for replicating and replacing natural foods is advancing on us like some death-threatening radioactive cloud. It's scary.

To quote from Ben Weider's IFBB technical committee report on nutrition, "Simulated steak is made of crushed soy beans, extracted with hexane, a petroleum solvent. The remaining flour is extracted with industrial alcohol and hydro-

Franco Columbu looks on as "Sly" Stallone curls 85 pounds . . . for ten reps.

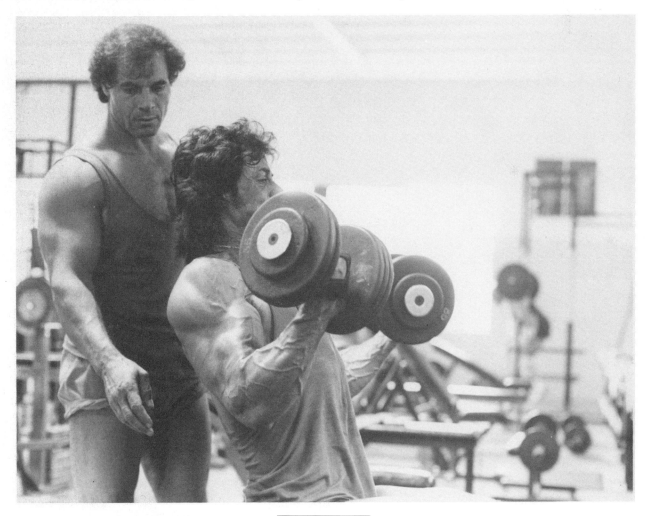

chloric acid and the residual protein is dissolved in lye. This is forced through a spineret into an acid bath, causing protein to precipitate in a fine thread which is wound up on a bobbin. The threads are cemented together to make a textured vegetable protein, which is dyed and flavored and textured to resemble bacon, turkey, hamburger, flounder, steak or sausage." Now, I ask you, do you still have an appetite?

Other fake foods—and I'll spare you the details of manufacture—include imitation sour cream, restructured French fries, fake cheese, artificial mashed potatoes, synthetic orange juice, and artificial powdered (you add water) tomatoes.

The problem is that you may not be able to tell whether you are eating fake foods or not. They are seldom identified. You'll almost certainly get them in packaged or boxed foods—TV dinners, for example. Most restaurants serve them up, as do institutional cafeterias. The additives in these foods run into the thousands. The average North American consumes about ten pounds a year of food additives, including synthetic dyes, flavors, acidulants, stabilizers, and emulsifiers. It's enough to make you sick.

I've been around bodybuilders a lot. I've trained with them. I've eaten with them. I have shared my knowledge on nutrition with both men and women competitors—when they have been on maintenance diets, during precontest preparation, and after bodybuilding events, when they can relax for a few days and eat anything that takes their fancy.

There is not one champion I know who doesn't consider nutrition to be the key to ultimate success in a bodybuilding contest. You cannot simply train and eat anything you want...and win!

It is true that in the early contests years ago this was done. Sergio Oliva was known to eat burgers and hot dogs and wash it all down with Coke! Reg Park would break in the middle of his workout for tea and biscuits. John Grimek would eat quarts of ice cream. And even Arnold Schwarzenegger would have a beer and a cigar after his workout. But as competition got keener, it is interesting to note that all four men tightened up their nutrition enormously. In the 1980s Oliva dieted hard for his Olympia attempts. Schwarzenegger broke new ground in calorie restriction and the use of free amino acids. Grimek cut out the ice cream. Reg Park threw out the biscuits... and the teapot.

Eating management is important. Not only must you be selective in what you eat, but there is a need to eat proper quantities. Even the order in which you eat your foods can have a bearing on their assimilation.

A bodybuilder cannot afford the luxury of eating for pure pleasure. At least not for long. That sounds a little harsh, doesn't it? What I mean to say is that a bodybuilder cannot afford to eat indiscriminately. For the most part, what you eat must contribute to your goal fulfillment. Norman Zale, a top American bodybuilding nutritionist, says, "Eating is fun and you should enjoy it, but you must plan; you must think. There are other factors apart from knowing what foods to eat."

Dave Hawk works his stupendous thighs on the hack machine.

3
EATING MANAGEMENT
Getting the Most Out of What You Eat

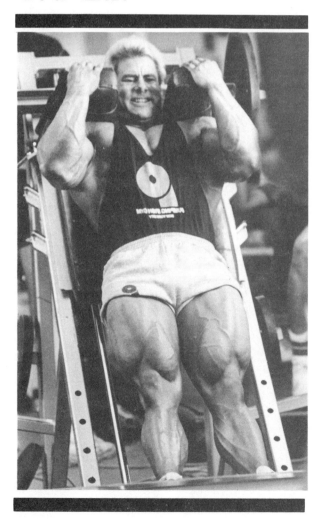

These other factors include:

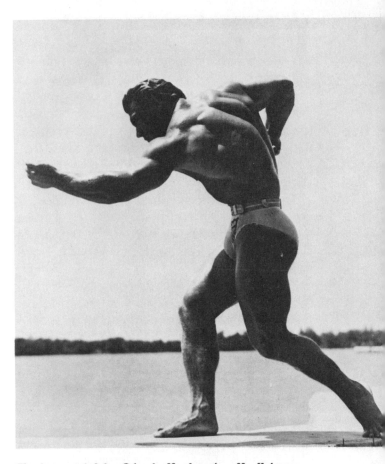

EAT IT RAW

Overcooking robs your food of vital nutrients. Meats, of course, should be cooked, but always with a view to keeping their nutrient value intact. Other foods—seeds, nuts, vegetables, fruits—can be eaten raw. Sometimes you may want to cook these items. That's fine, but don't cook out every last gram of goodness. Overheating can kill heat-sensitive vitamins and devalue certain proteins. There are in addition ingredients that we have not isolated (named) as yet, and these can be harmed by the cooking process, too—perhaps more than we even imagine.

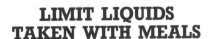

The immortal John Grimek: Mr. America, Mr. Universe.

FACING PAGE:
Sergio Oliva, "the Myth," Mr. Olympia 1967/1968/1969.

LIMIT LIQUIDS
TAKEN WITH MEALS

Drinking liquids with meals can dilute the stomach's hydrochloric acid concentration to a point where the digestive enzymes can't function at optimum level. Digestion suffers, especially with respect to muscle-building proteins, which will be excreted from the system instead of being efficiently assimilated.

DON'T EXERCISE
FOR AT LEAST TWO HOURS
AFTER A MEAL

Wait an even longer period if you have had a heavy meal. Working out is very strenuous, and a large meal often stretches your stomach in all

directions. The last thing you want is to subject it to more of the same. Additionally, both the digestive process and the training process require large supplies of blood. Your digestive system and your muscles should be allowed to perform their jobs without having to compete for energy resources with each other.

Neither should you eat immediately *after* a workout. Your breathing and heart rate should first return to normal, and it takes about an hour for hormones and the pumping effects of training to settle down. Don't force food on yourself at this time. It could confuse your system, and unwanted changes could occur in both the digestive system and the elimination process. Regardless of how a particular system responds, it's generally better not to force food on your body after a workout. Instead, warm down; take a seat and relax. After an hour your system will be eager for food. And the time will be right!

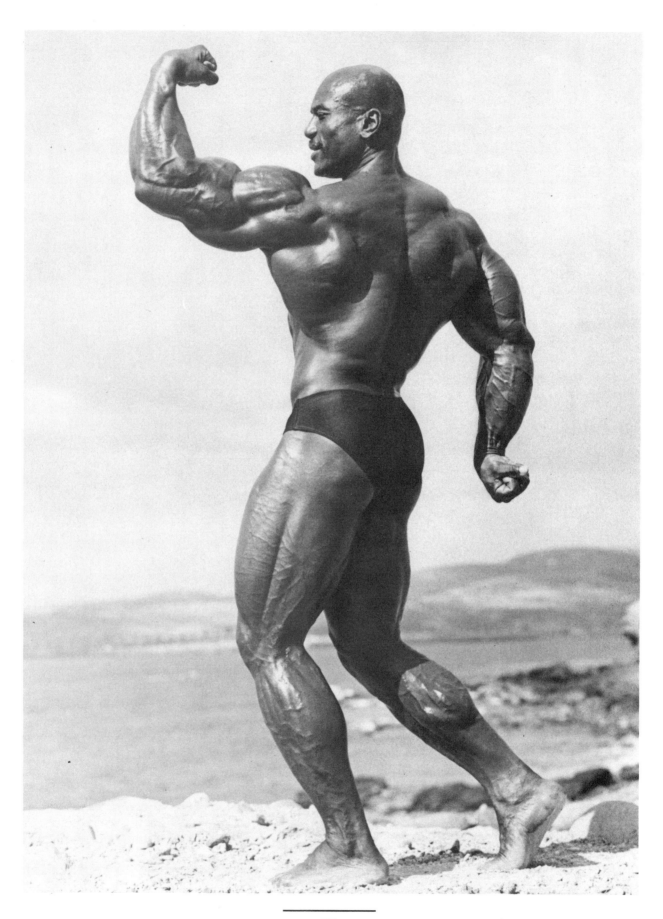

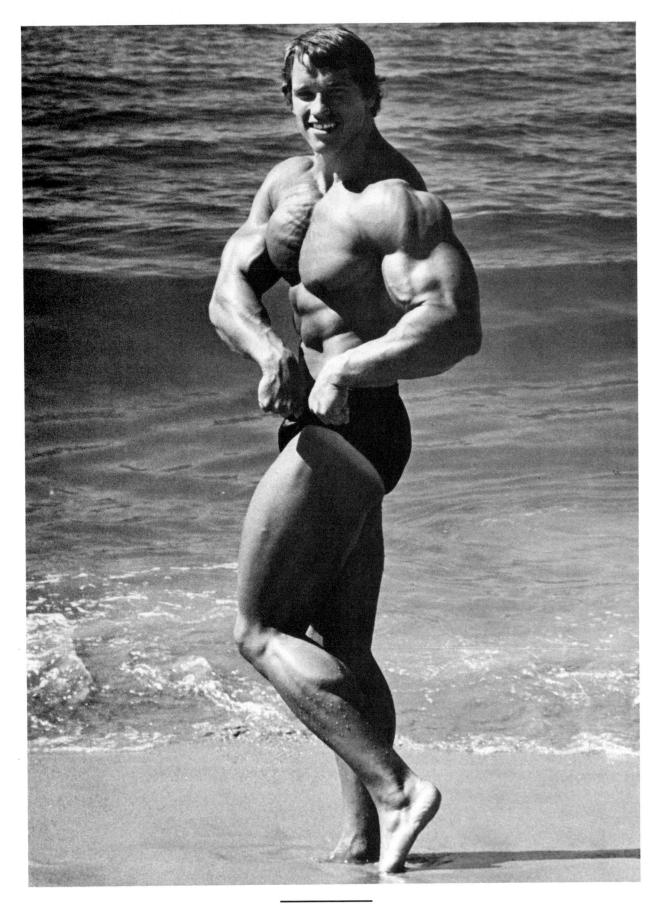

EAT SMALL PORTIONS

It is important not to stuff yourself with food, even when trying to gain weight. Your digestive system can generate only so many enzymes at one feeding. Overeating is the most frequent dietary sin committed by bodybuilders. You can liken overeating to overtraining. The system just cannot take it, and it will rebel. Learn to eat small portions and you will be doing your stomach a favor. You will be rewarded by perfect food assimilation, which is, after all, exactly what you need.

FACING PAGE: *The amazing Arnold at his all-time best.*

EAT SLOWLY

Learn to chew and spend more time masticating your food. You cannot expect to rush through a thirty-minute meal in just eight minutes! Body processes cannot be rushed. Bolt your food down and you will get indigestion, sometimes quite violent. You may even vomit. If your boss suddenly allows you only a short break for lunch, then do not rush your food to beat the clock. Rather, simply eat one item and finish the meal at a later time. The same applies to training. If you can only work out for half an hour instead of ninety minutes, then select your basic exercises and perform them properly. If you attempt to squeeze in every set and rep that is normally done, you will throw your system into unwanted shock.

Dave Hawk working lateral raises.

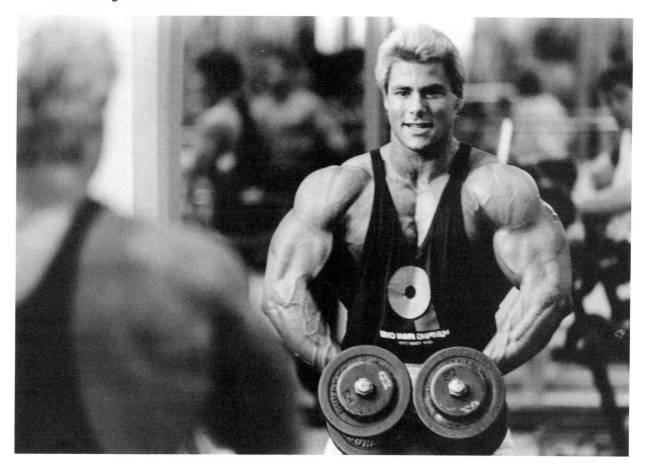

EAT IN THE RIGHT ORDER

According to Frank Zane (*Zane Nutrition,* Simon and Schuster), "The best time to eat fruit is just before breakfast, when the stomach is empty." At this time the fruit is quickly digested and passed through the colon. "Eaten after meals," says Zane, "fruit must wait for the meal to empty out of the stomach. By this time the fruit ferments and cause flatulence, distension of the stomach and digestive problems."

Norm Zale takes the other view. "First eat protein. Eat your meat, eggs, grains, seed food, vegetables and fruits in that order. This will ensure that your protein at least has a fighting chance, since its digestion will have begun before carbohydrates enter your stomach."

Actually, I believe small amounts of fruits can be eaten at the end of a meal, but if you are going to eat substantial amounts, then follow Zane's advice and make them the first meal of the day, or else have them on their own as a between-meal snack.

DON'T ADD JUNK

As I noted earlier, it's pretty hard to avoid junk food totally. No one in the western world has done it yet. But that doesn't mean you should give up trying. A quick way to ruin the goodness of a dish is to add calorie-rich gravies, dressings, or ketchup. Other so-called flavor enhancers like sodium chloride (salt), monosodium glutamate (MSG), pepper, mustard, caffeine, paprika, and sugar are bad news, too. Occasional use is okay, but as regulars in the diet? Not if you want to hit the big leagues.

Bodybuilding, through the use of progressive resistance exercise via free weights or specially designed machines, depends to a great degree on explosive, anaerobic activity that places unique demands on your muscles. Weight training can also be aerobic, if you use the circuit training method—supersets, trisets, or giant sets without significant rest—wherein the heartbeat is not given a chance to slow down. Research has demonstrated that you must engage in *continuous* lifting for at least twenty minutes for a progressive weight resistance workout to become aerobic.

Bodybuilders, especially in the beginning stages where they are trying to add muscle mass, frequently require more food than other athletes, but they do not need the large amounts of muscle glycogen that marathon runners rely on to complete long distance practices and races. In the past, weight trainers desiring fast results have relied upon protein overloading to build muscles. Some individuals were taking in excess of 300 grams of protein daily in order to grow muscles faster. Today we look upon this practice of the sixties as an error. Bodybuilders today get better results by increasing protein consumption only slightly above average requirements while dramatically increasing their consumption of complex carbohydrates.

No other athlete has to do what a bodybuilder does, namely, eat sufficient calories to get through a normal day of living, working, and training plus take in additional nutrition to allow muscle mass to *store* on the body. At the same time, calorie levels must *not* be so high that excessive fat is also stored. That detracts greatly from an athletic (well-muscled) appearance.

Dennis B. Weis, coauthor of *Mass!* (Contemporary Books) and an unparalleled expert in the field of bodybuilding, points out that "to maintain your present body weight (neither gaining nor losing weight) you must take in an average of 15 to 17 calories per pound of body weight daily. This is the basic requirement for your body to function correctly. This does not take into

French physique star Gerard Buinond performs alternate dumbbell curls.

4
ACTIVITY AND CALORIES
Your Requirements

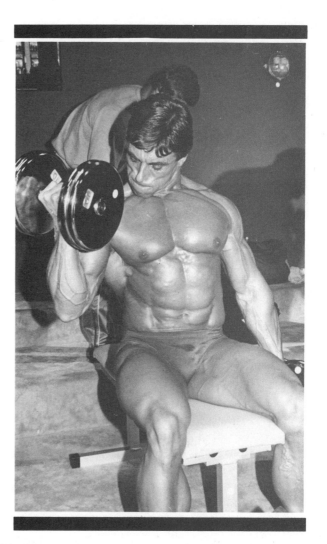

account your additional caloric requirements during your work day, recreational periods, or time spent in the gym working out. To compute energy expenditures for an average day (over and above the basic requirements) we must look at four different work categories, one of which will approximate your life-style and living pattern."

CALORIE COMPUTATION CHART

Bodyweight	Calories Required	Medium-Light Work	Medium Work	Medium-Heavy Work	Heavy Work
148 lbs.	2,500	150	300	525	750
152 lbs.	2,570	155	310	540	770
156 lbs.	2,640	160	320	555	790
160 lbs.	2,710	165	330	570	810
164 lbs.	2,780	170	340	585	830
168 lbs.	2,850	175	350	600	850
172 lbs.	2,920	180	360	615	870
176 lbs.	2,990	185	370	630	890
180 lbs.	3,060	190	380	645	910
184 lbs.	3,130	195	390	660	930
188 lbs.	3,200	200	400	675	950
192 lbs.	3,270	205	410	690	970
196 lbs.	3,340	210	420	705	990
200 lbs.	3,410	215	430	720	1,010
204 lbs.	3,480	220	440	735	1,030
208 lbs.	3,550	225	450	750	1,050
212 lbs.	3,620	230	460	765	1,070
216 lbs.	3,690	235	470	780	1,090
220 lbs.	3,760	240	480	795	1,110
224 lbs.	3,830	245	490	810	1,130
228 lbs.	3,900	250	500	825	1,150
232 lbs.	3,970	260	520	850	1,180

The calorie computation chart is not difficult to use. For example, if you weigh 188 pounds, the chart indicates that you should be taking in at least 3,200 calories per day. Let's assume that you would place yourself in the medium-light work category. A quick glance will show that you should be taking in an additional 200 calories over and above your daily minimum of 3,200. This will give you a total of 3,400 per day.

With regard to your weight training program, you burn up 1 calorie for every 100 pounds that you lift. The most efficient way to compute your calorie expenditure in a workout is by using the tonnage system.

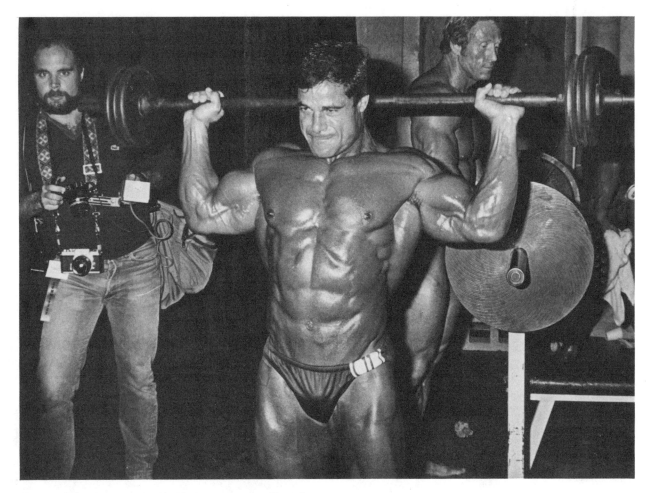

Franco pumps up his deltoids backstage at the Olympia.

Using the bench press as a typical example, let's assume that you can bench press 200 pounds for 8 reps. Eight times 200 pounds is 1,600 pounds for that particular set. You should add the total tonnage for each set of every exercise you perform. *For example:*

Bench Press

Set 1	200 × 8	=	1,600 lbs.
Set 2	210 × 6	=	1,260 lbs.
Set 3	210 × 6	=	1,260 lbs.
Set 4	190 × 10	=	1,900 lbs.
Set 5	180 × 10	=	1,800 lbs.
Set 6	180 × 6	=	1,080 lbs.
			8,900 lbs. total

The burning up of 1 calorie per 100 pounds lifted (or 10 calories for each 1,000 pounds) in the above example will record an expenditure of 90 calories on these six sets alone. Accordingly, you will understand how the calories pyramid as you add up the tonnage of your workouts.

Daily Calories Required

Body weight	188 lbs.	3,200
Category	Medium-light	200
Daily workout tonnage	8,900	90
		3,490 total calories

All of the above assumes you are an average person who fits all the indicated norms. But who

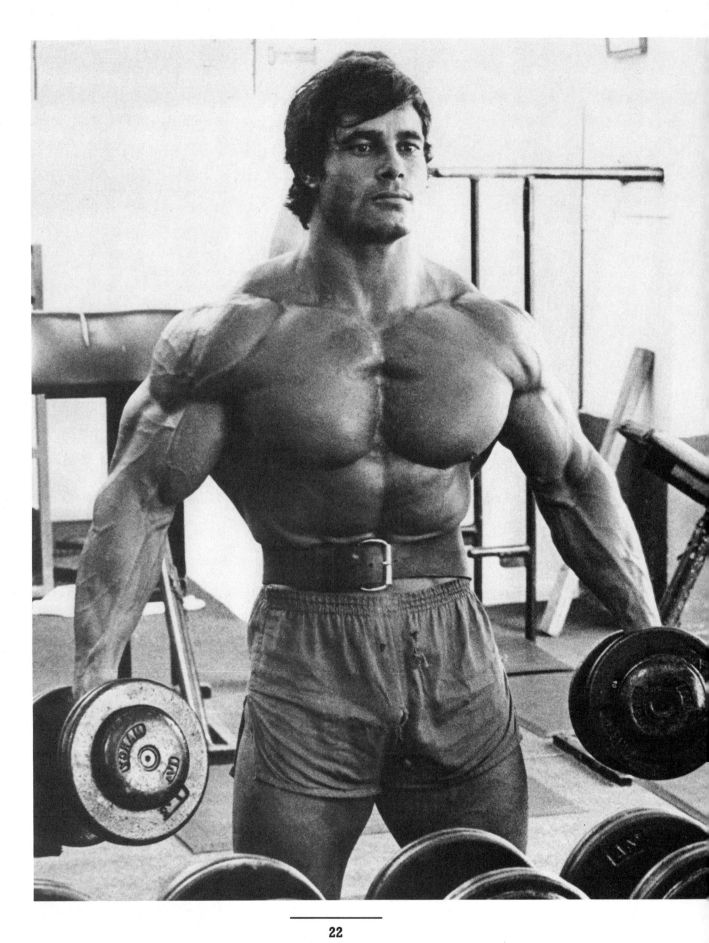

among us is totally average? You could drive yourself crazy trying to figure out your *exact* calorie requirements to lose weight, gain weight, or maintain weight. In fact, it can't be done with any degree of accuracy. I know that earlier on I indicated that nutrition is an exact science. Well it is, but only Mother Nature knows *all* the zillions of variables that can throw a wrench in the works. For example, it is accepted that one has to burn 3,500 calories to *lose* one pound of fat, or take in 3,500 calories over and above one's daily caloric needs to gain one pound in weight. But we all know people who eat like horses and yet do not gain any additional weight. Conversely, some people eat very little and yet fail to lose weight.

This phenomenon exists because of the varying physical makeup of individuals. Metabolic rates, the degree at which one's body burns up fuel, vary from person to person. To further compound the situation, there are additional factors that can make your metabolic rate change to burn energy either faster or slower. (I will deal with metabolism in more detail in chapter 5.)

While I do not think it practical to try to work out your calorie needs to the last digit (simply because you would spend a huge amount of time and still not get an accurate assessment), you should be aware that too few calories will hinder your gains, and too many will increase the likelihood of your becoming somewhat obese.

Monitoring your activity level will help you estimate calorie needs. Energy is required for all body functions and movement. The foods we eat provide the calories needed for this energy. The chart below indicates the approximate number of calories used per hour for various human activities and several sample body weights. Remember, the heavier you are, the more calories you will burn during any activity.

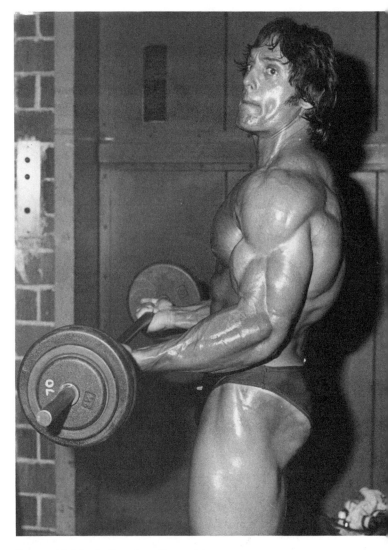

Super strict barbell curls performed by Mr. America Bob Birdsong.

Few can look as impressive as Franco Columbu (Mr. Olympia 1976/1981) in this semi-relaxed pose taken by master lensman Art Zeller.

ACTIVITY CHART

Type of Activity	Per Pound	Calories Burned Per Hour 125 lbs.	150 lbs.	175 lbs.
Sleeping	.6	75	90	105
Sitting	.67	83	100	117
Typing	.7	88	105	123
Eating	.8	100	120	140
Driving an automobile	.88	110	132	154
Dishwashing	.9	113	135	158
Standing	.93	117	140	163
Ironing	1.0	125	150	175
Sweeping with broom	1.1	138	165	193
Housework (regular)	1.3	162	195	227
Bicycling (5½ mph)	1.4	175	210	245
Walking (2½ mph)	1.4	175	210	245
Gardening	1.47	183	220	257
Cooking	1.6	200	240	280
Golf (without cart)	1.67	208	250	292
Dancing (regular)	1.67	208	250	292
Lawn mowing (power)	1.67	208	250	292
Bowling	1.8	225	270	315
Lawn mowing (hand)	1.9	237	285	332
Mopping floor	2.0	250	300	350
Skating (medium pace)	2.0	250	300	350
Sweeping with vacuum	2.2	275	330	385
Dancing (strenuous)	2.28	285	342	399
Badminton	2.33	292	350	408
Horseback riding (trotting)	2.33	292	350	408
Table tennis	2.4	300	360	420
Swimming (pleasure)	2.4	300	360	420
Wood chopping	2.67	333	400	467
Tennis (medium pace)	2.8	350	420	490
Skiing (medium pace)	3.2	400	480	560
Hill climbing (100 ft./hr.)	3.27	408	490	572
Trampoline jumping	4.0	500	600	700
Handball	4.0	500	600	700
Jogging (5½ mph)	4.33	542	650	758
Skipping rope (100 turns/min.)	4.7	587	705	822
Running (9 mph)	5.9	737	895	1,032

I'll say it later in this book, no doubt, but you should know now that a normal person desiring to add solid muscle to his or her frame will lessen the chances of doing so if he or she squanders energy by indulging in other sports, games, or pastimes in addition to bodybuilding workouts. If you want to gain, you cannot play tennis before your workout and go dancing afterward. Hold off on the extra activities, at least until you have achieved your target lean muscle objectives.

Chemically we humans are all very much alike, yet at the same time we differ from each other. Our basic metabolic rates (BMR) are one way in which we differ.

What is metabolic rate? It is the degree at which we burn up energy, the *speed* of the various body processes.

A car has a rate of idle, the speed at which the engine runs when the car is not moving, the tick-over speed. Some vehicles have a slow idle. Some fast. It is the same with humans.

We are all aware of the high-strung person (invariably skinny) who is always rushing around, who can't sit still or talk without wild hand waving. He or she is always on the go. This typifies the individual with a *fast* metabolism. People like this burn up energy like crazy. They seldom gain weight, often smoke incessantly (to calm their nerves?), and jabber and worry from morning till night. If they have to turn on the television, they'll walk around the room twice just to get to it.

On the other hand, the person with a lazy tick-over speed, the slow mover who relaxes almost to the point of passing out, who talks (and often thinks) slowly, can be categorized as having a slow metabolism. This person is almost slothful and quite often overweight. If this person has to turn off the television, you can bet your bottom dollar someone else is solicited for the job! Naturally fat people have *thrifty,* or efficient cells. This means that when they eat their body only uses a small amount of the food; the remaining calories go to the fat cells for storage.

Those who have a fast metabolism burn energy like it's going out of style. Even in a sedentary job they use up great amounts of energy just spinning their wheels. This high-revving metabolism (inefficient, wasteful use of energy) can actually be measured in the laboratory, because naturally thin people give off more heat as they do their daily work.

According to British bodybuilder Frank Richards, "The average skinny person trying to gain muscular body weight should concentrate on learn-

Rich Gaspari.

5
FACTS ABOUT METABOLISM
Adjusting Your BMR

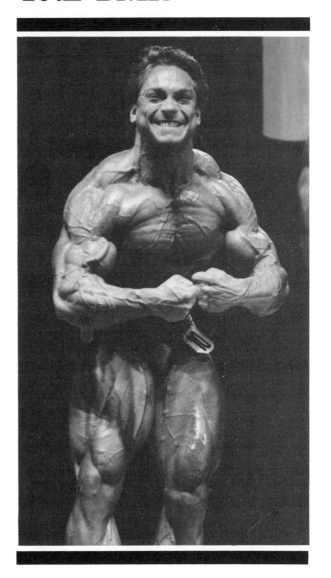

ing to relax so that their high-revving metabolic rate has a chance to slow down. In some cases this takes years. Certain extreme cases *never* succeed."

It is interesting to note that metabolism becomes less efficient after the age of twenty. Lean muscle tissue begins to decrease and existing fat cells increase in size. *In our sport, the person with a natural metabolism leaning toward the slow end of the scale tends to make faster progress that those with fast metabolic rates.* Actually, extremes, either high or low, are not conducive to success. If you suspect that you are either the slothful type or the hyper type, then you need to act accordingly to normalize your metabolic rate. Yes, it can be done. By combining certain training techniques with correct eating practices, you can take steps to control your metabolism. No doubt about it!

SLOW DOWN A HYPERACTIVE METABOLISM

To make perfect gains in bodybuilding one needs to possess a normal metabolic rate. If you have a fast, "hyper" type of metabolism that seems to be preventing you from gaining weight, then try the following:

1. Eat more than the usual three meals a day. Snack between meals on a variety of foods that you find satisfying. "The metabolism slows 8–10 percent during the evening (after 8:00 P.M.)," says Dennis Weis, author of *Mass!* (Contemporary Books). Therefore it is a good idea to eat late snacks if you have an overactive metabolism.

2. Increase your fat intake (dairy products) for a three-week period, three times a year. The metabolic cost is far higher to store carbohydrates as fat, so up your fat intake for short periods (unless you suffer from high cholesterol or other high-fat problems). Ask any Iowa pig farmer how he gets his pigs so big; he'll tell you it isn't by feeding them wheat; it's by feeding them fat.

3. Keep your house temperature comfortable but on the warm side—not super hot, and certainly not cold. Low temperatures speed up the metabolism.

4. Do not perform aerobic exercises such as walking, running, dancing, rope jumping, cross-country skiing, rowing, climbing, cycling; never exercise prior to half an hour after a meal or snack.

5. Keep to free weights in your bodybuilding. Rest completely between sets, and never start a second set of exercise before your breathing has returned to normal. Select only one exercise per body part, three to five sets of six to eight reps each movement. Train individual body parts only about twice weekly. The every-other-day split routine described later in this book is ideal for those with a fast BMR.

6. Relax whenever the opportunity arises. Never run when you can walk, stand when you can sit, or sit when you can lie down. Learn to relax completely after meals for as long as possible.

7. Tune out the worries of life. If you find yourself pacing the floor over problems or worrying about loved ones, politics, money, etc., make a determined effort to remove the cause of the problems. It does no good to harbor anxiety. Out of sight, out of mind. For example, if the evening news on television upsets you, don't watch it.

8. Walk slowly. Drive slowly. If you have to travel from one place to another, leave extra time so you can conserve energy rather than expend it carelessly hurrying. Stretch out and relax.

9. Do only one thing at a time. Never try to read while watching television. Do not attempt to work while talking on the phone or while eating. Doing more than one thing at a time confuses the brain and leaves you open for increased hyperactivity.

10. Take a high-dosage vitamin E pill daily. Scientific studies have shown that this contributes to lowering BMR.

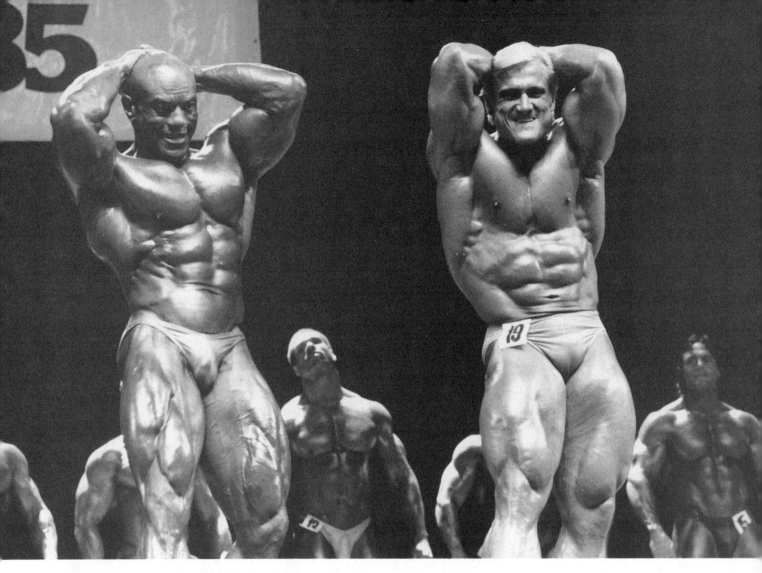

Sergio compares abdominals with Tom Platz.

SPEED UP A SLUGGISH METABOLISM

For those who are overweight and inclined toward laziness, the problem is probably a slow BMR. You need to "hyper" your metabolism so that you burn up more calories even while at rest. This process is known as dietary thermogenesis, "roasting" calories that would otherwise be stored as fat.

When you hyper your metabolism, your body is far more inclined to take on that muscular, shapely look, because you will shed fat. Both men and women improve their appearance (and appeal) enormously when surplus fat is discarded. Women, however, are at a slight physiological

disadvantage in respect to BMR in comparison to men, but BMR is not genetically determined once and for all. You *can* do something about it, whether you are a man or a woman.

To rev up your metabolism and drop unwanted pounds, follow these guidelines:

1. Increase your training frequency. Split your workout into two or three parts and train at least five days a week. In extreme cases you may want to split up your training routine even more and train twice daily. This will stimulate your metabolism even more. Extra calories will be burned and additional fat will be lost.

2. Do not cut calories drastically. Keep your diet natural by eating plenty of raw, wholesome fruits, vegetables, and grain, the complex

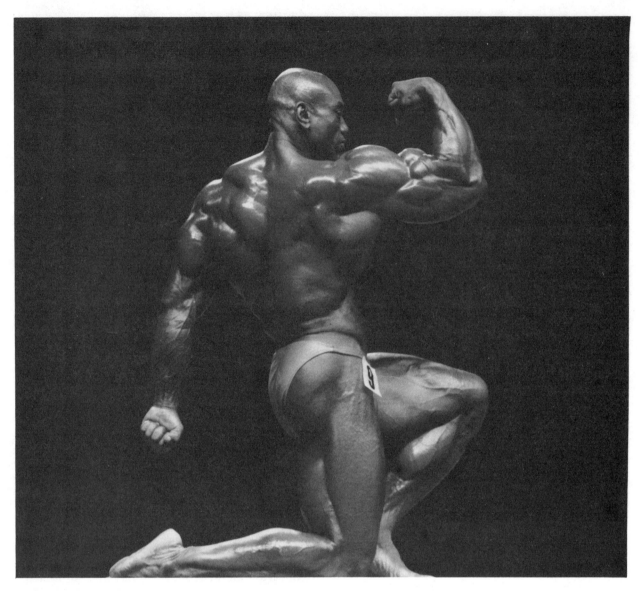

Sergio Oliva.

carbohydrates. Fat levels should be low. Even moderate caloric cutbacks can be construed by the slow metabolic type's body as a signal that starvation is at hand; consequently it stores more fat than ever.

3. Exercise in addition to your bodybuilding routine can fan the flames of a sluggish metabolism. The best exercises to get those metabolic fires stoked are aerobic exercises, done for thirty minutes three times a week. Jogging, aerobic dance, rowing, stair climbing, mountaineering, cross-country skiing, and swimming are ideal. Regular aerobic exercise increases metabolism all day long. "Those who are aerobically active burn increased numbers of calories even when not exercising," say researchers at the University of New Hampshire.

4. Avoid simple carbohydrates (candy, soft drinks, desserts, sugar, ice cream, and processed foods). They clog up the system and pander to the slow metabolism. Your diet should be

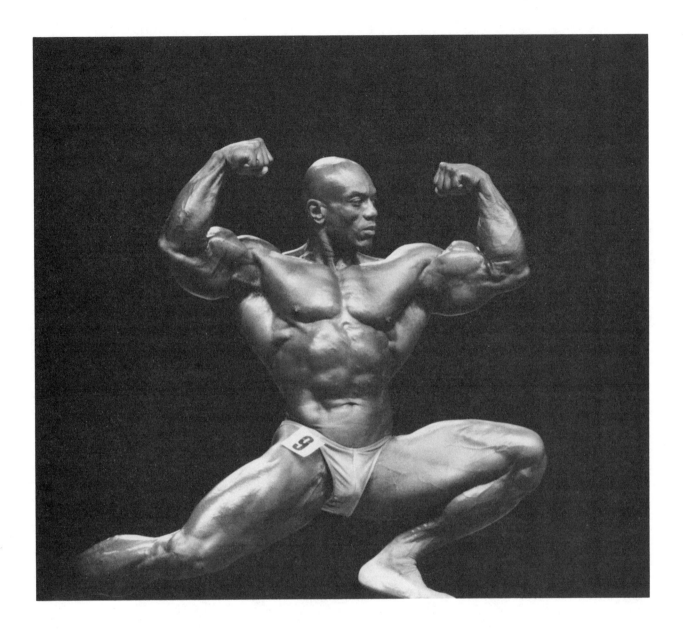

about two-thirds complex carbohydrates (fruits, vegetables, whole grains).

5. Go for a walk after all meals. This mild exercise increases dietary thermogenesis, using up calories before they have a chance to be stored as fat.

6. Keep up your progressive resistance, body-building workouts. One of the rewards of adding muscle mass to the frame is that muscle by its very existence increases metabolic rate. The more muscle you build, the more fat you burn. You are subtracting extra calories from your system every moment of the day and night. Muscle is active tissue. It burns calories around the clock.

7. According to *Prevention* magazine, extremes of heat or cold increase your metabolism by as much as 10 percent. Even a small deviation helps. "Set your thermostat at 68° in winter," says Dr. Peter Miller, director of the Hilton Head Health Institute, in South Carolina. "And set [it] at 79° in summer. You'll get used

to the temperatures and your metabolism will get a boost."

8. To compensate for a less efficient metabolism after the age of twenty, which makes us tend to lose muscle tissue, simply reduce your daily caloric intake by 2 percent for every ten-year segment past twenty—at age thirty deduct 2 percent; at forty deduct 4 percent, etc.

Once you perk up your metabolism you will feel more alert and alive. It will be your ally. But you've got to keep it revving by diet and exercise.

Sergio Oliva and Rich Gaspari.

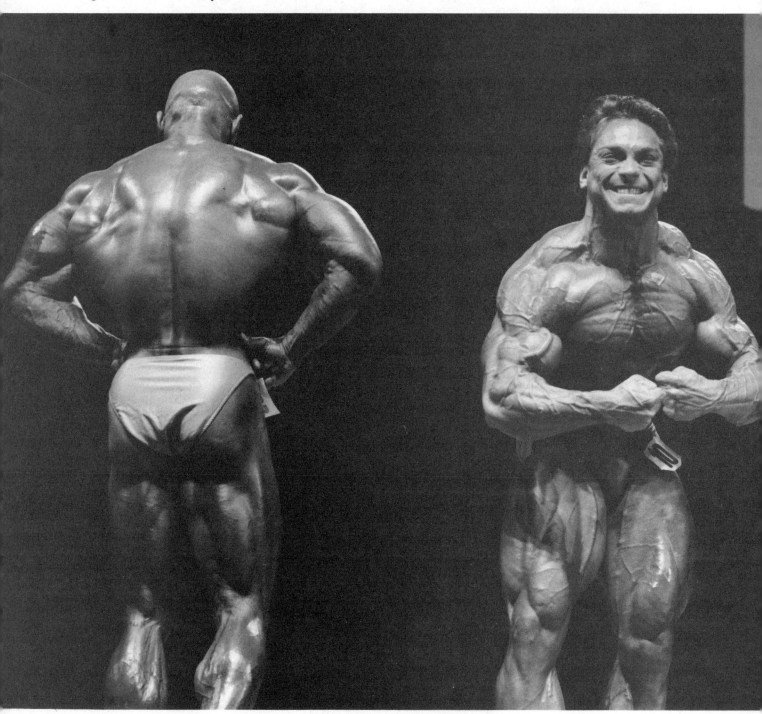

Despite its ups and downs as a nutritional priority for bodybuilders, protein can still be considered the most important ingredient in the diet, since it is protein that actually builds muscle tissue. Ben Weider, C.M., the president of the International Federation of Bodybuilders (IFBB) and a man with an enormous interest in scientific nutrition, states: "Protein is the great builder of all nature, from the tiniest micro-insect to the tallest tree." The term *protein* was formulated from the Greek word *protus,* meaning of first importance.

Although muscle tissue is 70 percent water, a full 20 percent is protein, so if you remove the water, you can easily see that the greatest building block remaining is protein. Clarence Bass, writing in his excellent book *Ripped 2* (Bass Enterprises), says, "Drinking water doesn't cause the muscles to become larger, and neither does consuming extra protein." Bass concedes that once he was a protein freak and consumed loads of it at one period, but now he feels that only a little extra is needed to build muscle size. Bodybuilding champion and physiology expert Mike Mentzer is of the same opinion.

The recommended daily allowance (RDA) for protein is set according to "positive nitrogen balance" studies. We are in positive nitrogen balance when we take in *more* protein than we lose. Vince Gironda says that in order to gain "we must always be in positive nitrogen balance, or else training time is totally wasted." We go into a negative nitrogen balance when we ingest less protein than we are using up; we are not getting enough to maintain muscle mass, let alone build more. In positive nitrogen balance we are ingesting more than is required for general maintenance. The most recent RDA for protein is set at 1 gram per 2.2 pounds of body weight—70 grams of protein per day for a 154-pound man.

Five years ago it was thought that an athlete did not require more protein than the average inactive man. This thinking has now changed. Athletes do require more protein, and bodybuilders

Holland's Berry DeMey.

6
PROTEIN
The Muscle Builder

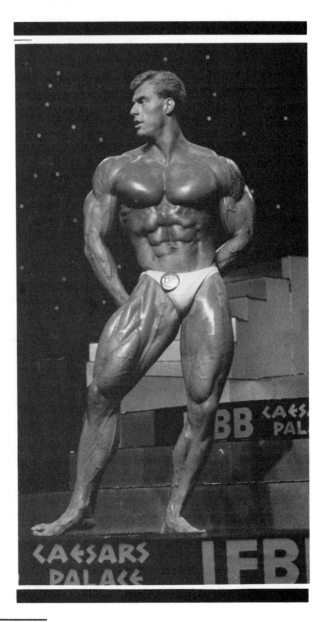

aiming to maintain or increase mass require even more than other athletes.

But don't make the mistake of stuffing yourself with protein—or any other foodstuff, fat or carbohydrate—when you are trying to gain muscle. Calories much beyond those necessary to maintain your body weight will almost always be added in the form of fat. Remember, too, that however much protein (or food generally) you eat, if you don't stimulate the muscle tissue with vigorous, progressive resistance training, then you will lose muscle rather than build it! "The bottom line," says Clarence Bass, "is if you deviate too far from your maintenance calorie requirements, up or down, you'll gain fat or lose muscle. A balanced diet, fairly high in protein, is best whether you are trying to gain or lose. Eat *slightly* less if you are trying to lose fat and *slightly* more when you wish to add muscle."

Boyer Coe reminds us that proteins "are among the most chemically complex of all organic compounds. The molecules of some proteins are the largest known and have an extremely high molecular weight."

Proteins are actually made up of amino acids, some forty of which have been discovered. Only twenty-three of them have been accepted as common "building blocks" of proteins, and only about twenty of those are found widely distributed in living organisms. No one protein has been found thus far that contains all of these, but casein of milk contains eighteen of them.

The so-called nonessential amino acids are those that your body can synthesize out of the other materials present in the food you eat. They are in fact just as important for proper maintenance and muscle building as those termed essential; the difference is they do not have to be in your diet.

Experiments have shown that rats kept on diets whose principal source of protein came from gelatin (lacking the essential amino acid

Danny Padilla and Mike Mentzer.

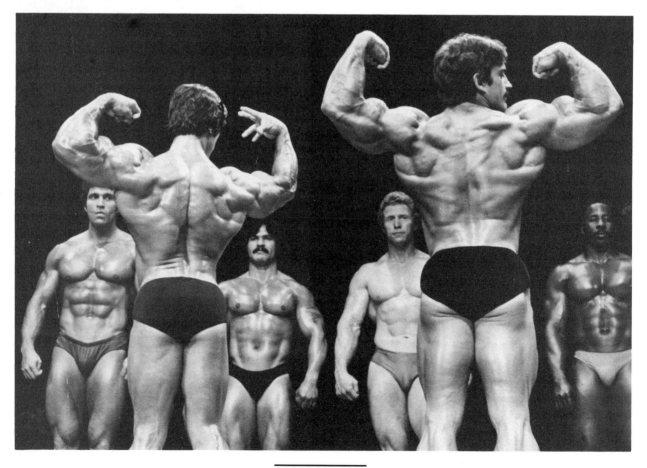

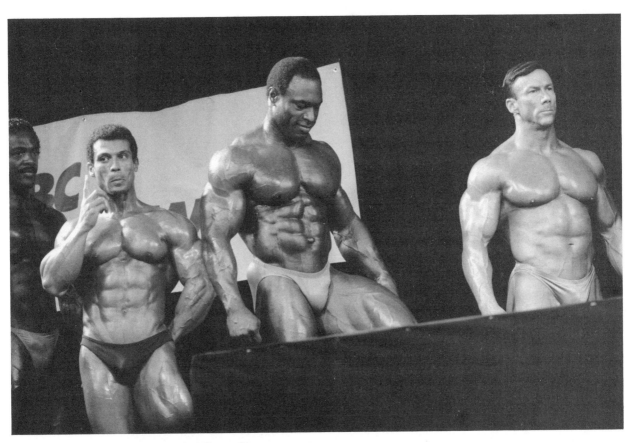

Mohamed Makkawy, Lee Haney, and Boyer Coe.

tryptophan) were able to maintain their protoplasm (the living matter in all cells and tissues) but could not grow bigger. Remember that the principal use of protein is to build and repair protoplasm and to form new living tissue. It is therefore strongly advised that each meal contain some amount of high-quality protein food and that this protein be obtained from a wide variety of available sources. The body needs this variety to do the best building job. Just as hundreds of thousands of words are made up from the twenty-six letters of the alphabet by combining different letters, thousands of proteins are made out of different combinations of amino acids. The protein in milk, for example, differs greatly from the protein in wheat, but both can pack muscle onto your frame.

All tissue is made up of protein, just as a house is built with bricks. In the same way that the house gets bigger as new bricks are added, so too will your body grow with added protein if the muscles are stressed both regularly and progressively.

The demands of exercise and time both require protein to be supplied throughout our lives, preferably via several daily meals. If insufficient protein is supplied in the diet, our muscles (stored proteins) will be used to fuel essential body functions such as breathing, circulation, etc. Your muscles will literally be robbed, and size loss will occur.

The secondary use for protein in the diet is to supply energy, but the liver can lay down only a limited amount of storage protein. Accordingly, excess protein that cannot find a use as building blocks, repair material, or energy reserves stored in the liver is turned into fat and glucose and stored as body fat on your body where it is least disturbed (usually the waist and hips). Yes, excess protein can make you fat!

Eggs and milk rank as the number one protein suppliers. Glandular meats such as liver, kidneys, and pancreas rank next, and muscle meats (roasts, steaks, and chops) are third in order of value. In general, proteins from animal sources such as milk, meat, fish, eggs, and cheese are superior to those found in vegetable sources (peas, corn, lima beans). Egg white and gelatin, however, each lack several essential amino acids. Proteins from nuts, soybeans, wheat and wheat germ, and cottonseed flour are complete proteins.

The best protein supplements are made from milk and egg proteins. However, don't be fooled. Egg albumin is very expensive, so most milk and egg protein powders have *very* little actual egg content. The milk protein content usually comes from calcium caseinate, which is 95 percent protein. According to Bill Reynolds, "A lot of so-called milk and egg protein powders contain a significant percentage of yeast or soya based protein, both of which are very inexpensive when compared to egg albumin and calcium caseinate. Thus the price may be lowered, but only because the ingredients are cheaper to obtain in the first place. These mixed products are considered to be of lesser bodybuilding value than pure milk and egg supplements."

Protein supplements are also available in tablet form and as liquid protein. Tablets were once very popular, but they taste dry and are awkward to eat. Also, tablets have to contain a binder (glue) to keep the particles together. This in itself is undesirable. They are also far more expensive than the traditional powders.

Liquid proteins have also lost their popularity. They have a very low protein efficiency ratio (P.E.R.) and invariably lack tryptophan, one of the essential amino acids. These liquid concoctions taste obnoxious, and with good reason: They are made from animal by-products that most civilized people would deem totally unsuitable for human consumption.

Desiccated liver is very high in protein and is often taken by serious bodybuilders. (Tim Belknap and Frank Richards have been known to take upward of 200 tablets daily when in serious training.) Be warned, however: As in any dietary habit, start with small dosages and build up gradually. A sudden dose of 200 desiccated liver tablets could give you an upset stomach and violent diarrhea for a week!

If you are looking for an economical protein supplement, you cannot do better than powdered milk. According to Bill Evans, Ph.D., a scientist at Tufts University, powdered milk is the "best

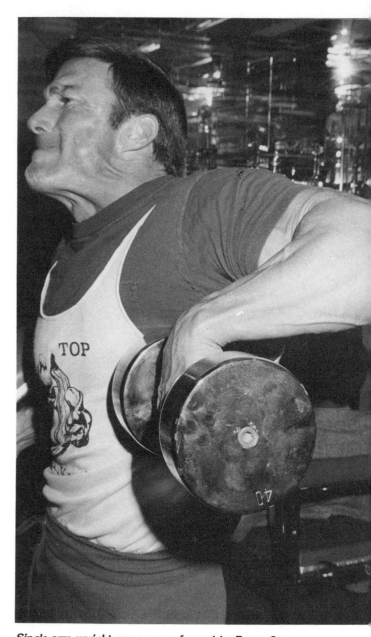

Single-arm upright rows, as performed by Boyer Coe.

protein buy, being high quality, containing an abundance of vitamins and minerals; [it] is easily digestible, contains a good deal of calcium and is inexpensive."

On no occasion should a health-conscious person's diet contain less than 12 percent protein. Normal people should make protein about 15 percent of their diets, and aspiring, hardworking bodybuilders should aim for a protein intake that is approximately 20 percent of their nutritional plan, or even more.

Armand Tanny, who has over fifty years as a heavy-training bodybuilder to his credit, states his opinion that the hard-training bodybuilder requires 50 percent more protein than the average active laborer. He cites an arbitrary figure of up to 150 grams per day. Tanny adds: "When a person starts to train or returns to training after a layoff, the body makes an increased demand for protein. The demand will level off at a certain point as long as the training intensity doesn't change. Among bodybuilders an increased demand for protein is noticeable within a day after one adds an extra exercise to a regular routine, or even substitutes one exercise for another. An unaccustomed demand made upon a muscle upgrades the protein requirements." No formal studies have confirmed these observations with respect to changes in routines and training regimes, but alert athletes, tuned in to their body feedback processes, are aware of the appetite demands for more protein when such changes in the routine are made.

A survey of Mr. Olympia contestants during the last few weeks of training showed that very

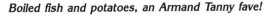

Boiled fish and potatoes, an Armand Tanny fave!

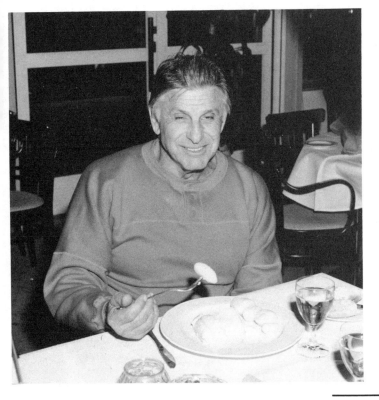

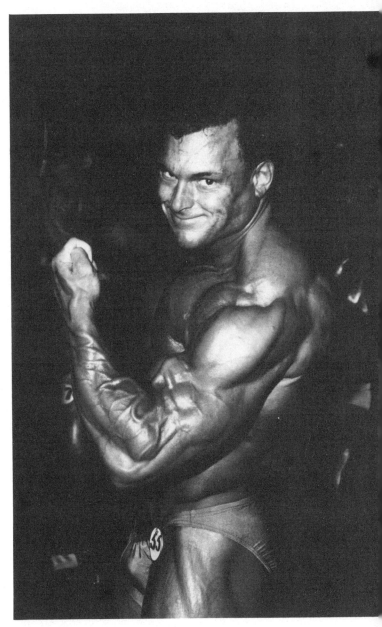

Tom Belknap, Mr. America.

little red meat was eaten at this time, mainly because of the high fat content of such meats. However, you can eat this type of meat with confidence when in a normal off-season training mode.

For the average bodybuilder a diet of meat, fish, fowl, eggs, dairy products, vegetables, fruits, legumes, seeds, grains, and a milk or egg protein drink once or twice daily will provide the protein and all-round nutrition required for supergrowth!

The egg, bless it, came under heavy fire in the 1970s as a result of the cholesterol scare, but it is in fact one of the most versatile and nutritious of foods, and definitely the best source of protein. All protein ratings are comparisons to the solitary egg. Let us not forget that our ancestors ate a high-cholesterol diet, and they had little heart disease even in old age.

Back in 1955 Harvard University studied the effect of exercise on blood cholesterol levels. Dr. G. V. Mann and his colleagues concluded that the blood cholesterol levels did not rise in healthy young medical students placed on extremely high-calorie diets with large amounts of saturated fats, as long as they exercised regularly and maintained body weight.

Joe Weider explains: "The bodybuilders like eggs for a number of reasons. An egg gives you about 6 or 7 grams of protein and only 80 calories. Whereas each egg contains 6 grams of fat, it also provides a great deal of lecithin, which is instrumental in breaking down cholesterol in the body."

You'll find loads of calcium in eggs (approximately 27 milligrams per egg), and they are high in vitamin A (585 I.U. per egg). Eggs are definitely a bodybuilding food. They also contain phosphorus, potassium, sodium, iron, riboflavin, thiamine, and niacin.

Tom Platz eats up to a dozen eggs daily. England's Frank Richards eats six to eight scrambled or poached eggs just for breakfast, and before the day is over he will have downed a full dozen more.

Veteran bodybuilder Vince Gironda is famous for his strong advocation of eggs. "It's quite simple really," says the Iron Guru. "Eggs are the best quality protein you can find. They feed your muscles more efficiently than any other food known. So I simply recommend that bodybuilders eat them copiously." This is not to say that Gironda recommends that you eat dozens of eggs every day for the rest of your life. He merely suggests that you add eggs to your diet (up to thirty-six a day) when you want to make a

Vince Gironda.

7
THE RETURN OF THE EGG
Quality Protein

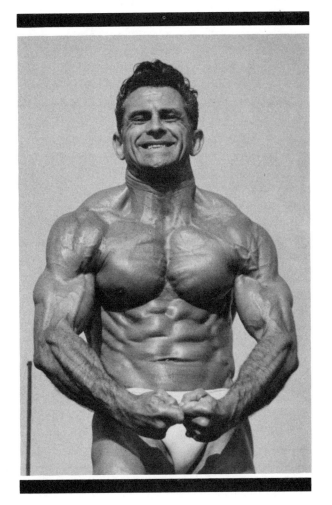

spurt in gains and get the job done. Needless to say, those who are not in good, robust health or have a predisposition to high blood cholesterol levels should *not* follow these recommendations. If such is the case, consult your doctor for the best dietary procedures.

Prehistoric man ate eggs, as did the ancient Egyptians. Louis XIII was renowned for being able to cook eggs a hundred different ways. Generally, you are best off either boiling or poaching them. That way you are not adding extra calories in the form of fat or oil.

HOW TO BOIL OR POACH AN EGG

Remember the expression "She couldn't boil an egg"? Well, sometimes boiling an egg can be difficult, especially when you want to get it dead right. First off, don't take it straight out of the refrigerator and pop it into boiling water. Room temperature eggs cook best. And take the pot off the burner before putting the egg in the water, then bring it back to the boil immediately. Some people like to start their eggs off in cold water and then bring it to the boil. Another good tip is to use a strainer (wire basket) inside the pot to keep the eggs from touching the bottom.

No, I'm not going to tell you how long to cook your eggs. You'll have to figure that out by trial and error yourself. But once you know, you'll know for life.

If you poach your eggs then use a traditional poacher, which has saucers to hold each egg individually. Always place the lid on the poacher, because much of an egg's nutritional value is lost when it is exposed to light. Only as a last resort plop a broken egg into boiling water. Do that and you'll drown the egg—and it'll taste worse than the water you cooked it in. Most people call this poaching an egg. I call it heresy.

Whereas boiling and poaching are superior, I do not mean to turn you completely away from scrambled eggs or omelettes. Both cooking techniques can be utilized from time to time for the

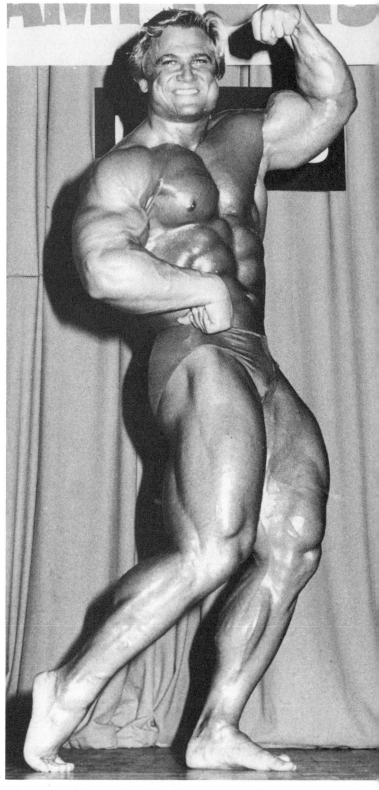

The Golden Eagle, Tom Platz.

sake of variety. Omelettes, in particular, can be prepared in scores of variations. You can include cheese and tomatoes, onions, green peppers, or mushrooms. You can include ham or seafood to add even more muscle-building protein to the meal. When scrambling or frying eggs, keep in mind that safflower oil is superior to butter or heavy fats.

THE PERFECT PROTEIN

Yes, at the height of its popularity, the egg was suddenly banished into a culinary Siberia. But now this original convenience food has been vindicated. Once again it is at the head of the list, as an almost perfect food. Remember, bodybuilders, the egg contains all the essential amino acids. Dr. Alexander MacNair wrote in the British medical journal, the *Lancet,* "It seems to be open season for eggs. I presume that the same simple souls who cannot comprehend a more complex explanation for a raised serum cholesterol than too much in the food, find it easiest to identify cholesterol with eggs. I see no reason to alter my view that, in healthy subjects of normal body weight, and taking adequate, regular, physical exercise, the number of eggs eaten as part of a varied diet has no significant effect on the serum cholesterol."

Eggs are a superior food. Their protein is almost entirely usable. However, one caution: Raw egg white contains avidin, a protein that destroys biotin, one of the B vitamins with growth factors. If you use *raw* eggs in shakes or blender-stirred protein mixes, then it is probably wise to take a biotin supplement. Otherwise, muscle fans, get crackin'.

"Fiber is useless!" Well, that is what was believed for many years, not only by bodybuilders but by the entire world community en masse. Only recently have we begun to realize that the "worthless" vegetable fiber removed almost completely from our diet by the advances of the Industrial Revolution during the last century (via the invention of high-speed rollers for milling white flour and the advent of the canning industry) is in fact vital for our health and well-being.

Yes, fiber, or roughage, as it is sometimes known, has until recently been completely overlooked as an essential part of diet. But today nutritional experts like Dr. Van Soest (Division of Nutritional Sciences, Cornell University) and Audrey Eyton, author of *The F-Plan Diet* (Bantam), tell us that increased intake of fiber can be beneficial to our health, although not because of its nutritional value. Dietary fiber *is* pretty useless as nourishment, because it is comprised of the indigestible portions of plants. The cell walls of plants contain substances that are tougher than the rest of the plant. This is the fiber. These substances hold the structure together and can be likened to the walls of a building that houses perishable goods.

The chemical makeup of fiber includes five main substances found in varying proportions in different plants:

- Cellulose—found especially in bran, grains, carrots
- Hemicellulose—found especially in eggplants, radishes, grains
- Pectins—found especially in apples, bananas, oranges, cabbage
- Gums—found especially in oatmeal
- Lignin—found especially in toasted whole grains, pears, seed husks

None can be digested by the human stomach, and therefore they have no direct nutritional value for the bodybuilder. But they have other values that can really help your success as a competitor. It is the very fact that these chemical

Deanna Panting, Canada.

8

FIBER
The Foodless Necessity

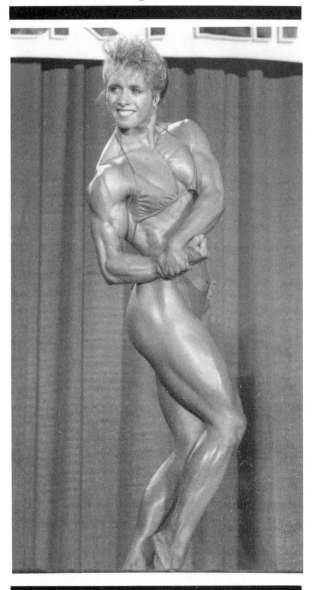

substances (fibers) are resistant to digestion that makes them vitally important in the working of your lower digestive tract.

As food moves through your system on its way to being evacuated, the fiber content promotes the wavelike contractions that keep materials traveling through the intestines. It is the fiber content that maintains the proper speed of elimination. It is the fiber content that dictates the consistency of your feces, an important consideration for health. A stool of waste matter should be neither too hard nor too liquid; rather it should be large, bulky, and soft. Naturally, there will be times when you suffer from overhard stools and other periods when you may suffer from diarrhea, but these should be the exception rather than the rule. There is no doubt that a high fiber diet will help regularize your digestion and elimination processes and help prevent, halt, or even reverse digestive tract disorders.

Many heavy squatters have found themselves susceptible to hemorrhoids. This is caused by straining while in the low squat position—you may need to use a new position that doesn't put such a heavy stress on the area—but it may also occur as a result of preweakening the area through straining during the act of elimination, an unnecessary occurrence if you eat sufficient fiber. Without wishing to belabor the point to bodybuilders—who, after all, are principally interested in bigger and better looking muscles and to hell with health and all that junk—allow me one partly repetitive statement: Many researchers feel that eating more fiber, because it improves the working of our intestines and the elimination process, may help offset diseases and conditions such as cancer of the bowel, hypercholesterolemia (high cholesterol), diabetes, obesity, gallbladder disease, varicose veins, appendicitis, hiatal hernia, irritable bowel syndrome (IBS), diverticular disease, constipation, hemorrhoids, and heart disease.

Bodybuilders and nonathletes must learn to "think fiber" for a while in order to change dietary habits to incorporate more fiber. Estimates are that most North Americans and Europeans would have to double or even triple their fiber intake to get an adequate level, largely because of the highly processed, low-fiber foods they tend to live on.

Ironically, when the average person thinks of fiber he or she understandably conjures up a vision of a food like celery, because of its appearance and stringy texture, yet curiously, the pea (known for its softness) contains almost four times more fiber than celery, weight for weight.

Rolf Muller, West Germany.

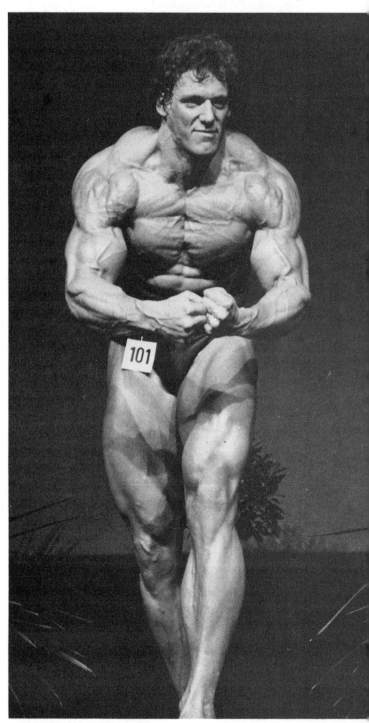

WHERE TO FIND FIBER

Vegetables	Fiber Content (percent)	Recommended Serving	Calories per Serving
Asparagus	1.7	½ cup	15
Bean sprouts	1.8	½ cup	17
Beans			
Brown	9.7	½ cup	95
Kidney	4.8	½ cup	94
Lima	3.7	½ cup	126
Pinto	10.0	½ cup	98
String	3.4	½ cup	12
Broccoli	4.1	½ cup	15
Brussels sprouts	2.9	½ cup	24
Cabbage	2.8	½ cup	11
Carrots	3.7	½ cup	19
Cauliflower	1.8	½ cup	12
Celery	2.9	½ cup	5
Corn	4.7	⅓ cup	41
Cucumber	1.5	½ cup	7
Eggplant	1.5	½ cup	17
Kale greens	3.7	½ cup	3
Onions	2.1	½ cup	25
Parsnips	4.9	⅔ cup	72
Peas	8.0	½ cup	44
Potatoes			
White	3.5	1 small	80
Sweet	4.0	½ cup	72
Radish	2.2	½ cup	9
Zucchini	3.0	½ cup	9
Tomato	1.4	½ cup	27
Turnip	2.2	½ cup	13

Fruit			
Apple	3.4	1 small	55
Apricots	1.7	2 medium	39
Banana	1.8	1 small	120
Blackberries	5.0	½ cup	30
Cherries	1.2	10	44
Grapefruit	1.3	½ average	41
Grapes	.8	10	34
Orange	2.1	1 small	45
Peach	1.3	1 medium	33
Pear	2.4	1 small	45
Pineapple	1.0	½ cup	41

Fruit	Fiber Content (percent)	Recommended Serving	Calories per Serving
Plums	1.8	2 medium	58
Strawberries	2.1	¾ cup	36

Grain Products

	Fiber Content (percent)	Recommended Serving	Calories per Serving
Bread			
Corn	3.4	1 square	151
Rye	10.8	1 slice	54
White	2.7	1 slice	74
Whole wheat	9.5	1 slice	63
Cereal			
Bran (100%)	33.1	½ cup	66
Corn flakes	11.0	¾ cup	64
Shreaded wheat	12.2	1 biscuit	84
Wheat flakes	13.1	¾ cup	75
Brown rice	5.5	½ cup	83
Noodles (egg)	3.0	½ cup	98
Oats (whole)	9.0	½ cup	61
Rye crackers	11.7	3	64

John Hnatyschak and Graeme Lancefield.   FACING PAGE: *Roy Callender, Barbados.*

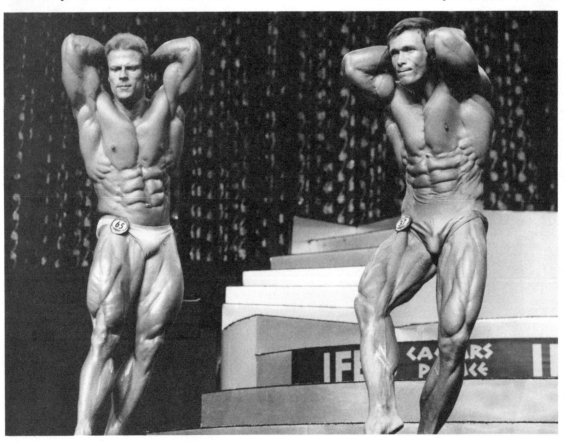

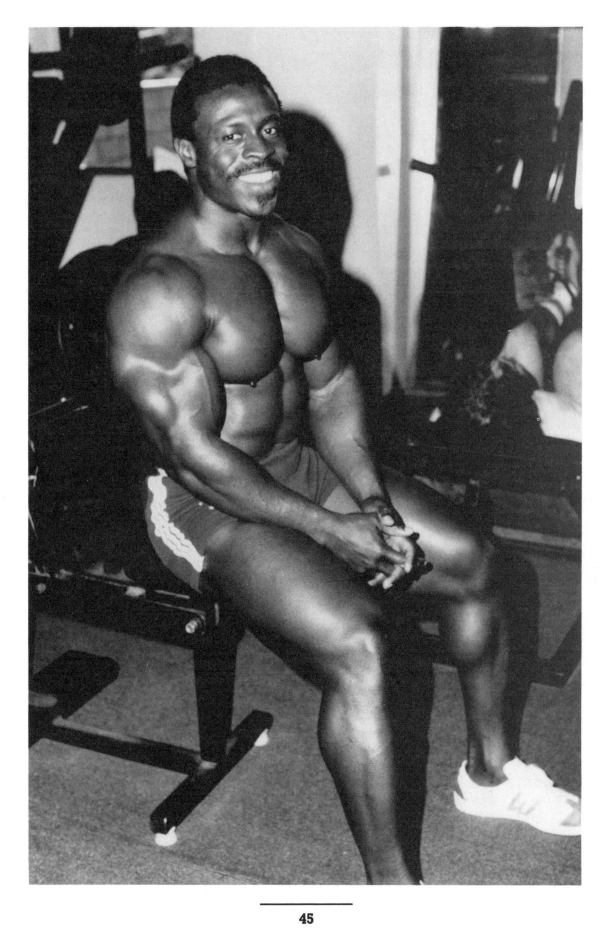

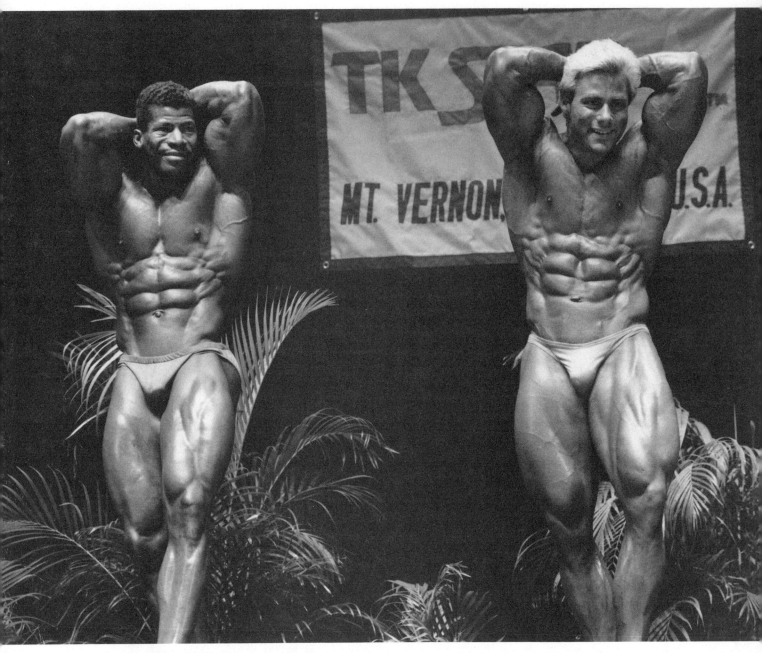

Ron Love and Dave Hawk.

Increasing your fiber intake is a simple task, and it will not add more than a few cents a day to take this step toward maintaining robust health. Half a cup of whole-bran cereal will go a long way to normalizing your fiber requirements in your daily diet. However, you may not be aware of all the various high-fiber foods, so I have compiled a list for easy reference. It is a good idea to draw on *all* food sources for your fiber, fruits and vegetables as well as wheat and bran. Bran alone, although almost 50 percent fiber, is inadequate as a sole supplier of fiber.

Remember now, as a bodybuilder you need optimum health and optimum nutrition. Substantial amounts of roughage will help you achieve success. Think fiber!

What's the nearest thing to nutritional magic? What one item do we absolutely, beyond any shadow of a doubt, require daily? Water. It is the most abundant macronutrient found in the body. Nothing survives without water. None of our body functions work without water. Our bodies need it to transport nutrients, to build tissues, and to maintain temperature. We require water for digestion, circulation, absorption, and excretion. Our hearts need it to beat, and our minds need it to think. We need water as much as we need air.

Many a person has fasted for days, weeks, and months on end without damaging the system. But try and go more than a few days without water and life will leave your body.

Of the six major nutrients we need to survive—water, carbohydrates, fat, protein, vitamins, and minerals—water constitutes the largest part of body weight. Muscle itself is about seventy percent water. So is your brain. Blood plasma is about 92 percent water and even your bones are 22 percent water.

Yes, pure water is our "lifeblood," almost literally. But there is an unhappy situation existing in our world. The dreaded modern-day evil, pollution, has reared its ugly head to spoil our most precious commodity.

According to Mike Synar (Democratic Congressman from Oklahoma), who chaired a committee formed to investigate water conditions in North America, "We are sitting on a time bomb, not only in my district, but in every congressional district and every locality in this country."

Ground water tables are becoming depleted. In addition, Synar's committee reported that over 3,000 wells in twenty-nine states have been contaminated in the past few years, while "almost daily" dozens of new wells are found unusable because of poisons leaching into the ground water.

Without going into the details of water contamination, which could fill the rest of this book, let it be known that few people's water supply is free of carcinogens. This sad state of affairs is

Rachel McLish.

9
THE DRINK OF CHAMPIONS
You Need It

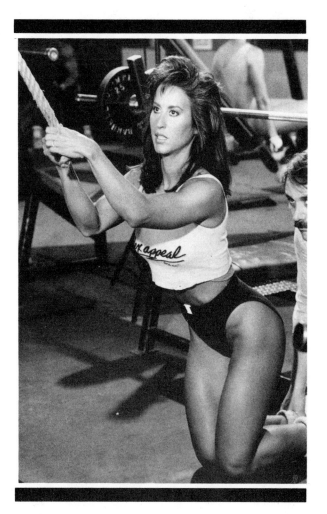

47

caused by several factors. One is pesticide use by farmers. Pesticides sink into the ground and accumulate to contaminate our natural underground waters. Another is hazardous waste dumps. Untold numbers of cancers have been caused by industrial poisons. There is general industry laxness in disposing of unwanted wastes. And then there is the ironic use of chemicals by government agencies to cleanse our water from all the man-made toxins previously mentioned; these chemicals, too, are potentially harmful to health. Mankind boasts of its "advanced ability" in producing over 10,000 new chemicals since World War II while forgetting to either fully control them or deal with their adverse biological effects on humanity, let alone the poor animals with whom we share our planet. What craziness! What stupidity!

We have inside our bodies a mechanism for regulating the water content of our systems. More water is required by athletes (about 1 milliliter per calorie expended); even more is needed if heavy sweating is induced, as is often the case with bodybuilders. Up to two quarts an hour can be lost by the system under certain conditions—for example, running a marathon in hot weather. It is up to us alone to replace what we use constantly. It is a good idea to drink six to eight glasses of fresh water daily. The rest of what we require can come from the foods we eat (all contain some water, and many contain a lot). It is far better to drink more water than you need, rather than too little. Do not, however, make a habit of drinking ice cold water. The cold temperature makes it difficult to break down fats, and it can lead to digestive disorders and discomforts. Drink your water cool by all means, but not freezing cold. No ice cubes, please.

If you have any doubts about the quality of water in your area, you can have it tested by an expert. You may feel safer to drink bottled water. Each brand of bottled water has its own particular flavor, but always pick those with low sodium levels. Spring waters are crisp, clear, and fresh. Sparkling waters have a tingling effervescence. And imported waters from France, Germany, or Italy can be an added, if somewhat expensive, touch to your diet.

The question of whether to drink plain old tap water or not is difficult to answer. Certainly it *is*

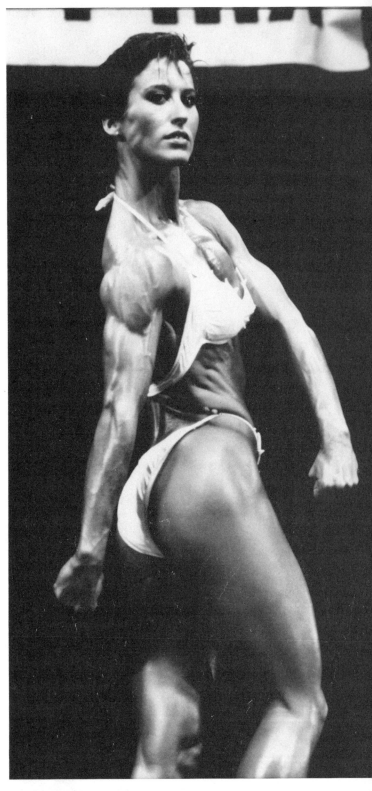

Rachel McLish, Ms. Olympia, advocates six to eight glasses of water per day.

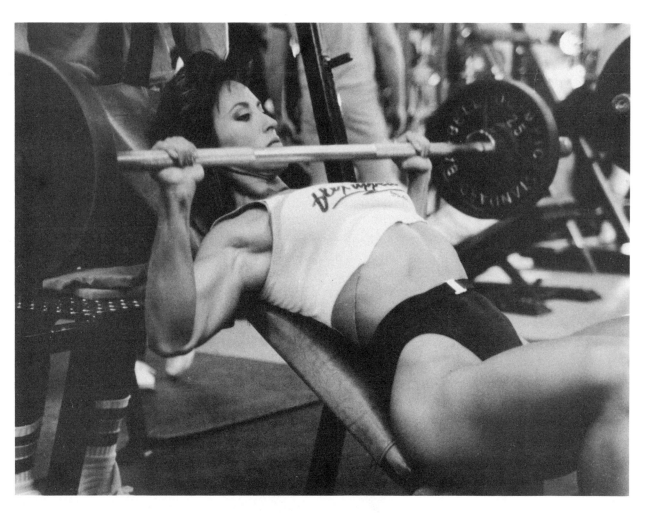

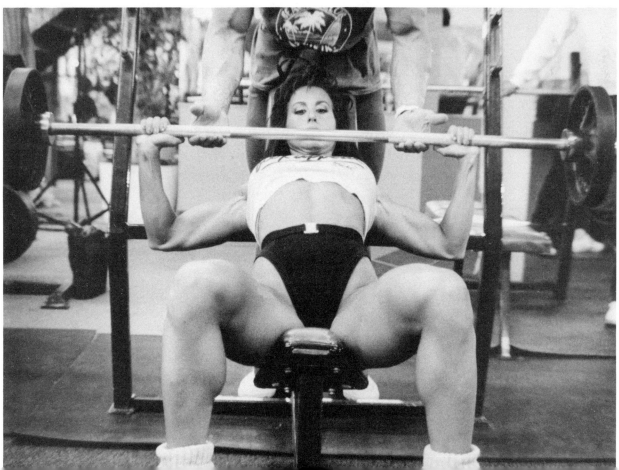

cheaper. If your city water tastes good and there has been no bad publicity in the local newspapers, then take the cheap way out and drink it. On the other hand, some tap water is so infused with chemicals that its taste is horrible. If this is the case, run off a few quarts from your tap and let it sit overnight, then boil for ten minutes. When it is cooled you can drink it safely. The negative side of this procedure, besides the added time needed to boil and cool your water, is the fact that boiled water definitely lacks sparkle and taste. It's flat and uninteresting.

Water plays an important part in your workouts. You cannot give your best if you are dehydrated. Make sure you not only drink water regularly during the day, but that you also drink during your training if the weather is excessively warm or you are shedding a great deal of sweat. Listen to superstar Rachel McLish: "Drinking six to eight glasses of water daily keeps my system like clockwork, which in turn keeps my system clean and pure. It's also great for the complexion. The hard trainer who really sweats out a workout must take in more water than sedentary individuals."

Years ago bodybuilders would totally dehydrate their bodies prior to competition. This is not done nowadays. Because most of our muscle size is made up of water, it just does not make sense to dehydrate by using water pills (diuretics) or by drastically limiting fluid intake. As a competition draws near, the bodybuilder's job is to take the water from underneath the skin and to put it into the muscle. Thus we end up with full, "loaded-up" muscles that pop out sensationally because they are covered by a very thin layer of skin. How is this done? I explain it all in the chapter on carbing up. It really works!

I often get asked whether it is better to take vitamins and minerals as a supplement or through normal food. My answer is, "Take them both ways." But ideally, of course, the ultimate and natural way to obtain these ingredients—and no doubt Mother Nature's way—is to get your vitamins from regular everyday food. This is fine for normal people, but the athlete, especially the physical culturist, is not a normal person. A bodybuilder's task in life is first to build larger muscles than average (abnormally large) and then, as a contest approaches, to cut calories (overall food intake) so that the skin becomes excessively thin and the muscles show up to maximum advantage.

During the off-season one can eat normally of a variety of foods, but when one is endeavoring to lose weight (fat) to "cut up" for a contest, there is a very strong case for supplementation. You simply cannot obtain all the vitamins and minerals needed when the calorie intake is greatly limited. At such time you have no other choice than to supplement your diet with vitamins and minerals. In this way you obtain these micronutrients without adding calories.

Both vitamins and minerals have known and unknown properties without which we cannot maintain healthy body function. To deprive ourselves of them leads to illness and, if enough time elapses, death.

If you have any doubt about your vitamin-mineral status, then by all means arrange to have blood, urine, hair, or tissue tests done. But even these may not show the complete picture, because *nutrients are only valid if they get to the areas of the body that need them.* Blood urine levels could show normal, and a deficiency could still exist in one or more tissues.

Note from the following synopsis of vitamins and minerals that your most important "vital-health" foods are organ meats, whole grains, fish, legumes, brewer's yeast, wheat germ, leafy green vegetables, seeds, nuts, eggs, and fruit. They crop up again and again as rich sources for essential nutrients.

Laura Beadry, Ms. USA.

10
VITAMIN AND MINERAL UPDATE
What Does What?

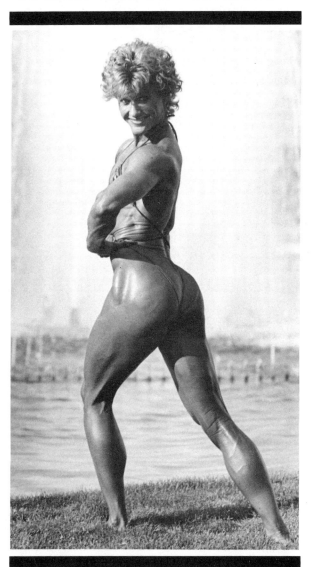

VITAMINS

Vitamin A

Have you ever experienced difficulty seeing in a darkened room or street? True, some people's eyes adjust to low-light situations faster than others, but vitamin A deficiency is a definite cause of night blindness.

Bodybuilders who experience difficulty seeing at night should consider that they may need more foods containing vitamin A. Usually, before the sight problem is noticed, a degree of anemia has already set in. And that can definitely hold back your progress.

Not only does vitamin A help the eyes, it also helps to keep the skin (and mucous membranes) healthy. And there is a positive need for vitamin A in the development of healthy teeth and bones. Stress is also combatted by this vitamin.

A Florida doctor randomly tested a hundred people and found twenty-six whose night vision was deficient. All of these night-blind people were given 25,000 units of vitamin A daily. Within ten days 90 percent of them "responded favorably."

Another negative result from insufficient vitamin A is increased susceptibility to infection. You cannot give your best to your workouts if your head aches, if your nose runs, or if your lungs ache from coughing.

The usual RDA (recommended daily dietary allowance) for vitamin A is 5,000 I.U. (international units) for men and 4,000 I.U. for women. Can we get too much vitamin A? Yes, as with vitamin D, you can overload on vitamin A and make yourself sick. This occurs because vitamin A is stored rather than excreted and toxic levels can be reached, although the safety margin is quite large. To produce toxic symptoms in rats, for instance, the rodents must be given 1,000 times more than the usual nutritional need. In humans several million units are required before symptoms of toxicity show up. However, children can be poisoned with a single dose of about 350,000 I.U.

Although vitamin A is a fat-soluble vitamin, that doesn't necessarily mean you must eat a lot of fatty foods to obtain it. You can find vitamin A in liver, egg yolks, and dairy produce. Tomatoes, yellow and green leafy vegetables, and fish liver oils can all supply your needs abundantly.

Thiamine (B₁)

Thiamine happens to be one of the coenzymes that help keep our energy levels high.

Whereas the classic syndrome of thiamine deficiency is beriberi, there are other signs that you may identify with more readily as a bodybuilder. Without thiamine, protein synthesis is depressed. The body's neurotransmitters fail to function properly. The first symptom of thiamine deficiency is nervous exhaustion. Often appetite, memory concentration, and initiative are dulled. You may become depressed. Pains in the abdomen and chest may follow, and as the deficiency worsens you will develop "pins and needles" in the feet and toes. This is a sign that the nerve pathways are degenerating. The next to go are the muscles.

The body's need for thiamine is dependent on two factors: the caloric content of the diet and the amount of energy expended. The baseline RDA is 1 milligram; active bodybuilders need more.

The richest natural sources of thiamine are organ meats such as liver, kidney, and heart. You will also find good sources in lean meats, yeast, eggs, leafy green vegetables, whole-grain products, berries, nuts, and legumes. Cooking in water, incidentally, contributes to thiamine loss. In case you are worried about overdosing on thiamine, this is quite unlikely. Thiamine is nontoxic and even allergic intolerance is rare. Doses as high as 500 milligrams per day have been administered for up to a month with no signs of toxicity.

Riboflavin (B$_2$)

Riboflavin, one of the B vitamins, is essential for cellular respiration. Your muscles need it to breathe; without it they suffocate. Growth failure, weight loss, eye problems, adrenal gland malfunction, and impairment of the nerves, skin, and mucous membranes have all been attributed to riboflavin deficiency.

Many bodybuilders have found that riboflavin deficiency has profound effects on the metabolism of carbohydrates, fats, and proteins. All three of these basic food elements require riboflavin if they are to be properly utilized by the body.

We all know that protein is needed to build muscle size and strength. However, few know that when riboflavin is undersupplied, protein utilization also drops off; more protein is excreted in the urine. This begins a vicious cycle of events, because as more protein is excreted the increased urinary output eliminates even more riboflavin from the body. (Any factor that increases urination also increases loss of water-soluble vitamins. The passing of feces and sweat has the same effect.)

According to medical authorities, riboflavin may have a beneficial effect on the muscles' ability to perform under stress. Experiments have shown that giving bodybuilders a moderate riboflavin supplement has increased their resistance to fatigue by 11 percent.

The recommended daily allowance (RDA) for riboflavin varies according to weight and metabolic rate. On average, male adults require 1.7 milligrams and female adults need 1.2 milligrams.

Riboflavin deficiency can be quite common among both men and women. One study showed that of women who had been on "the pill" for three or more years, 82 percent were riboflavin deficient.

You can find riboflavin in abundance in organ meats, fish, dairy products, eggs, leafy green vegetables, wheat germ, whole grains, and legumes. Too much exposure to light can destroy riboflavin, as can soaking foods or cooking them in water for long periods of time. Heat by itself does *not* destroy this vitamin.

Riboflavin is not toxic, so supplements in a wide variety of dosages are available (from less than 1 milligram to hundreds of milligrams). Taking riboflavin with food increases the absorption of the vitamin.

Niacin (B$_3$)

Without doubt niacin is one of the most important vitamins for assisting in cellular respiration and in the cells' utilization of all major nutrients.

As many bodybuilders know, niacin is a mild vasodilator, which means that it widens the diameter of the blood vessels and increases the blood flow. High doses of niacin lower high blood cholesterol and cause the well-known "niacin flush," in which the skin temperature increases, skin over the entire body and face reddens, and blood pressure temporarily drops. I have known bodybuilders who have taken high dosages of niacin just before a contest to pass out (some freaked out) from the effects. Several reported dizziness and mental confusion, nausea, and itching. In spite of this, the nutritional authorities insist that the niacin flush is not harmful, although it may be unsettling. It comes on within ten minutes and lasts about half an hour.

Why do bodybuilders take niacin before going on stage? It increases vascularity and adds color (redness) to the skin. Some claim that they get a better pump. Although every bodybuilder should have a diet including adequate niacin levels, I do not feel that a niacin flush is essential for looking your best on stage.

Rich, natural sources of niacin include organ meats, yeast, whole grains, dried peas and beans, fish, and nuts. Cooking foods by boiling can cause substantial loss of this vitamin.

Interestingly enough there are two forms of niacin: niacinamide and nicotinic acid (usually called simply niacin). Niacin comes from plants and niacinamide from animals. In the human body niacin is quickly converted to niacinamide. (Incidentally, if you are after a "flush" take niacin. Niacinamide doesn't do the job, although it is beneficial in every other way.) Both variations are

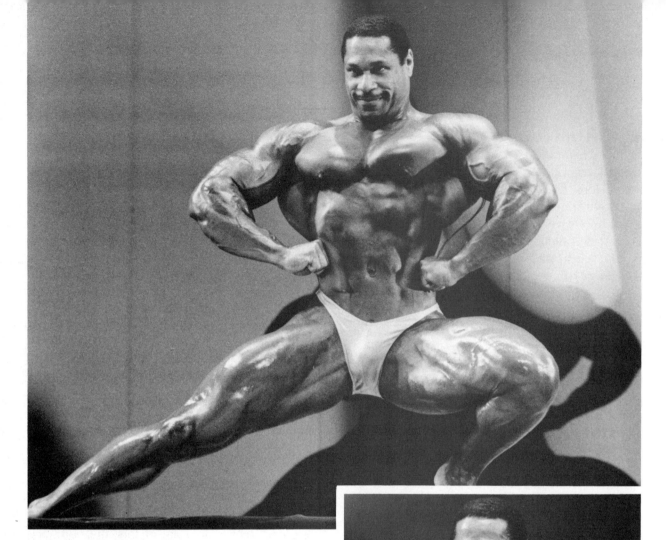

Power-plus. Mike Christian has it all.

available in a wide range of supplemental doses, from a few milligrams to 1,000 milligrams.

The RDA for niacin varies from 13 milligrams for adult women and 18 milligrams for men. High dosages should never be given to people with high blood pressure, peptic ulcers, diabetes, gout, or liver disease.

Pyridoxine (B$_6$)

This vitamin is an essential coenzyme for many, if not all the biochemical reactions involving amino acids, which make up cell-building protein. Pyridoxine also plays a vital role for the bodybuilder through its essential part in the body's metabolism of fats and carbohydrates.

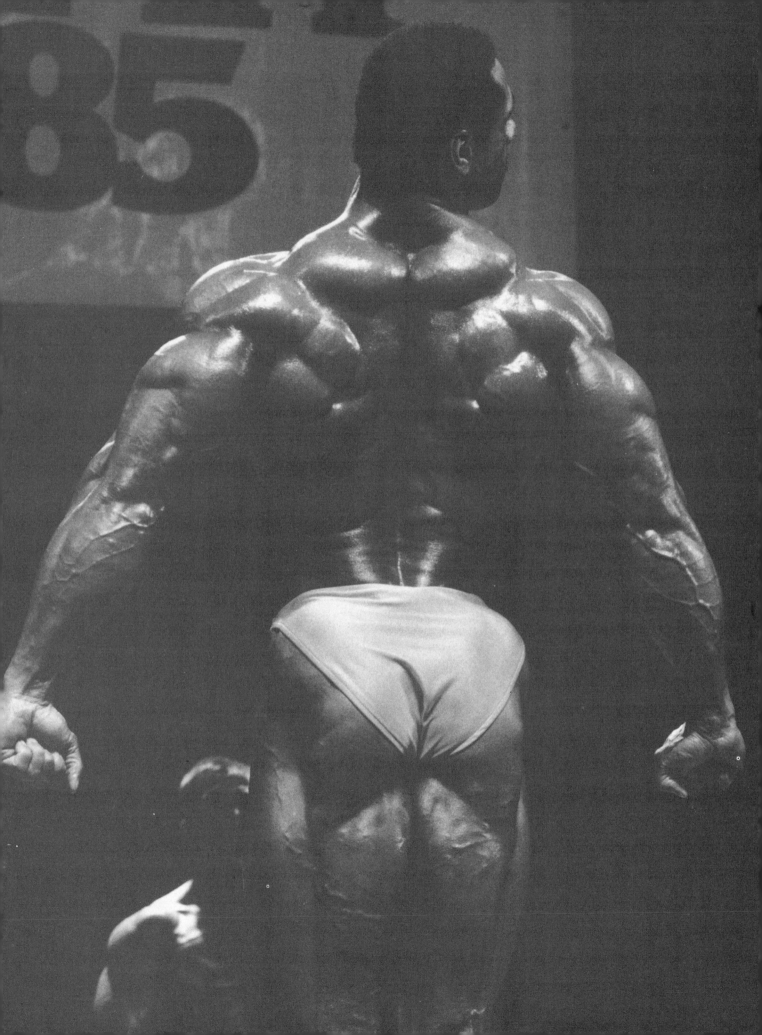

Without this vitamin, energy cannot be produced for body cells.

Because amino acids are the building blocks of all living tissue, and because they are needed by all, especially those who regularly use progressive resistance exercise to build their bodies, a deficiency of pyridoxine can do widespread damage. In fact, if you are getting less than is required, then your entire body development, including your brain, can suffer.

The RDA for pyridoxine is set at 2.2 milligrams for adult males and 2 milligrams for adult females.

Pyridoxine is not considered especially toxic, but megadoses should not be taken without a doctor's recommendation. The richest sources of this vitamin are liver and other organ meats, whole-grain cereals, wheat germ, soybeans, corn, yeast, blackstrap molasses, peanuts, cabbage, bananas, potatoes, peas, and green peppers. Pyridoxine is water-soluble and light-sensitive, so many canning, cooking, and processing procedures destroy substantial amounts of it. For maximum benefit, vegetable sources of the vitamin should be eaten raw.

Pyridoxine is available in supplements in a wide range of doses, from 5 milligrams to over 500 milligrams.

Folate

Also known as folic acid, folate is not currently fully understood. Certainly it has an important role in the maintenance of normal metabolism. We do know that it is necessary for the synthesis of the essential nucleic acids DNA and RNA. These protein substances are required for cell reproduction and division, so it isn't hard to imagine how devastating a deficiency of this vitamin could be for the bodybuilder. For one thing, you will suffer chronic anemia and a debilitating effect on the nervous system.

The classic symptoms of folate deficiency include weakness, inflamed and sore tongue, numbness or tingling in the hands and feet, indigestion, diarrhea, depression, drowsiness, and a slow, weakened pulse.

The RDA for folate for adults is .4 milligram.

Folate is relatively nontoxic, but if you are epileptic or suffering some serious illness, you should not take folate indiscriminately without first consulting your doctor, since folate stimulates RNA and DNA.

Rich, natural sources of folic acid include dark green leafy vegetables, organ meats, asparagus, yeast, lima beans, whole grains, wheat germ, lentils, and oranges. Cooking, canning, storage, and processing can cause folate destruction, since the vitamin is sensitive to heat, sunlight, and acids.

Cobalamin (B$_{12}$)

Also known as cyanocobalamin and vitamin B$_{12}$, cobalamin has the largest molecule of all vitamins. It is the only vitamin to contain the metal cobalt. Like folic acid, a deficiency of cobalamin impairs the formation of red blood cells and negatively affects the nervous system. Pernicious anemia can follow…and prove ultimately fatal—hardly a good situation for the aspiring bodybuilder.

Symptoms of cobalamin deficiency include weakness, inflamed tongue, weak pulse, stiffness, drowsiness, depression, diarrhea, and numbness and tingling in the hands and feet.

The adult RDA is .3 microgram. Medical professionals frequently point out that vegetarians often suffer from cobalamin deficiency because the primary sources of the vitamin are animal products.

Cobalamin is not toxic. The best sources are organ meats, muscle meats, fish, and milk. There are some vegetable sources (seaweeds such as wakame and kombu, and fermented soybeans, tempeh).

Cobalamin is not normally destroyed in cooking unless drastically overheated. It is available in supplemental form ranging from a few micrograms up to a milligram (1,000 micrograms).

Biotin

The thyroid and adrenal glands are dependent on biotin for perfect function, as are the reproductive tract, the nervous system, and the skin. Severe dermatitis results when insufficient amounts of biotin are ingested, and there is an adverse effect on the heart and reproductive system. A deficiency also takes away your ability to withstand stress. Biotin is essential for the synthesis of proteins and fatty acids in the body, and to the metabolism of carbohydrates—heavy-duty information for the physical culturist.

Those who take *raw* eggs frequently may find their levels of biotin drastically reduced, due to the phenomenon called "egg white injury." A substance in raw egg white, *avidin*, binds with the B vitamin biotin and renders it unavailable to the body. Cooked egg whites do not have this effect.

The RDA for biotin is 300 micrograms (.3 milligram) per day for adults.

Biotin is not toxic. No human (or animal) experiments have demonstrated a toxic reaction to excessive dosages of biotin.

You can find biotin in abundance in liver and other organ meats, egg yolk, peanuts, mushrooms, cauliflower, whole grains, and rice (unprocessed). You can obtain available supplementation of biotin in health food stores, ranging from doses of a few micrograms to several hundred micrograms.

Pantothenate
(Pantothenic Acid)

Pantothenate is the essential part of coenzyme A, which is required for cellular metabolism. As an aspiring bodybuilder, you will readily accept its importance since *every* cell in the body depends on pantothenate for its working vitality.

The effects of pantothenic acid on humans were revealed in a classic experiment on four healthy young men fed a diet free of pantothenate. Within weeks their blood pressure dropped, causing dizziness when standing up. Their pulses would race after simple exertion and they became excessively tired. By the fourth week, the men suffered from constipation and they grew irritable and aggressive. Their balance, coordination, and reflexes diminished, and soon they began getting respiratory infections one after the other. One man got pneumonia. In fact, the symptoms were becoming so severe that the experiment was brought to an abrupt halt.

The RDA for pantothenate ranges from 5 milligrams to 10 milligrams for adults. It is relatively nontoxic. No researcher has ever succeeded in producing toxic symptoms in humans. (In animals, however, doses of over 2 to 3 grams per kilogram of body weight have proved lethal.)

The richest sources of pantothenate include organ meats, egg yolk, peanuts, cauliflower, cabbage, whole grains, bran, and broccoli. Fair sources include milk, meat, and fruits, but the all-time richest source so far discovered is *royal jelly*, the substance worker bees feed to the queen bee.

Although pantothenate is not normally destroyed by cooking, processing, canning, and freezing can result in considerable losses. Pantothenate supplements are available in a wide range of doses from a few milligrams to several hundred milligrams.

Choline

Choline is an important vitamin (although some say that it isn't a vitamin at all, since it can be synthesized in the body from the amino acid methionine).

Choline is needed to maintain a sharp memory. In fact, college students have shown better memory performance after supplementing with choline, as have sufferers of Alzheimer's disease. Choline is also used to combat certain heart diseases (but there is more to maintaining a healthy heart than the taking of a choline pill).

Bodybuilders have taken choline (with inositol) to help them cut up (lose fat) for a contest or a photo session. There have been no scientific tests to support choline's value in this regard. However, the trial-and-error brigade of bodybuilding generally conclude that choline supplementation (with inositol) does help define the body *slightly*. "It works best," says Larry Scott, two-time Mr. Olympia, "when used in conjunction with a low-calorie diet and a combination of aerobic and high intensity training."

No RDA for choline has been set, although average diets have been found to contain 250 milligrams to 600 milligrams. The richest source of choline is lecithin. Good sources of choline include whole grains, fish, yeast, eggs, legumes, and organ meats (liver).

Choline is relatively nontoxic, and supplements can be purchased ranging from doses of a few milligrams to several hundred milligrams.

Inositol

Like choline, inositol is another B complex factor with a nebulous status: Is it or is it not a true vitamin? In any case, research has indicated that inositol is necessary for good motor nerve conduction. It is also needed to maintain resistance to illness and has even been shown to lower cholesterol levels in humans.

Inositol has been used by bodybuilders in conjunction with choline (in supplement form) to reduce body fat percentages prior to bodybuilding competition. Both substances are lipotrophic agents (fat emulsifiers). They work to help your body utilize fats, particularly cholesterol. Their use appears to improve appearance by reducing body fat percentage *slightly*. The results are more evident when the bodybuilder is following a precontest diet. To take choline and inositol without lowering overall calorie levels would not serve much use. You would not notice any significant lowering of body fat.

No RDA for inositol has been set. An average diet supplies about 1 gram daily. Good sources of inositol include lecithin, yeast, organ meats, fruits, vegetables, nuts, and whole grains.

Inositol supplements are available in a wide range of doses, from less than 100 milligrams up to several hundred. There are no reports of inositol being toxic.

PABA
(Para-aminobenzoic Acid)

This ingredient is only tentatively accepted as a vitamin—that is to say, its absolute "essentiality" has not been established by the government. There is, however, evidence that its removal from the diet can produce gray hair.

The most common use of PABA is as a *sunscreen*. In solution (usually with alcohol), it is applied to the skin to effectively screen out harmful portions of ultraviolet light, rays that cause sunburn and cancer. In experiments with animals, PABA has been shown to protect the skin completely from cancer-causing rays. Skin cancer is the most common form of cancer. Over 300,000 cases develop yearly, 5,000 of which are eventually fatal.

Sunburn also contributes to aging, and many doctors advise staying out of the sun as much as possible. If you must sunbathe—and many bodybuilders like to tan in the sun rather than use artificial colorings—then use PABA to protect your skin.

No RDA has yet been set for PABA. The best natural sources are liver and yeast and other B vitamin sources. PABA can be obtained in supplemental form from dosages ranging from a few milligrams to several hundred milligrams. It is considered nontoxic.

Vitamin C
(Ascorbic Acid)

"You can't overestimate the importance of vitamin C to the bodybuilder," says *Muscle and Fitness* editor Bill Reynolds. Actually, vitamin C is vital to everyone, since it has many important functions within the body. It has a role in the metabolism of amino acids, but its most essential role is its part in the formation of collagen and other fibrous tissue. Collagen is the main supportive protein of skin, tendon, teeth, bone, cartilage, and connective tissue. Capillary walls depend on vitamin C for their strength. Vitamin C is used by bodybuilders to repair broken down tissue and to help speed up postworkout recuperation. Virtually all tissue in the body depends on vitamin C for proper maintenance, growth, and development. There is some evidence to show that large amounts of vitamin C can speed up the healing process of broken down tissue.

If you don't get enough of this vitamin in your diet, you will find that you first start to bruise easily. Then there is a swelling of the gums, loosening of teeth, swollen joints, anemia, weakness, aching joints, and weight loss. Scurvy results from prolonged vitamin C deficiency.

Also, evidence has been mounting for decades that vitamin C plays a key role in heart disease. It helps protect against cardiovascular disease by means of its role in the clotting of blood. Some researchers have indicated vitamin C's role in helping to withstand the stress of heat and cold, and preventing cancer, diabetes, bone disease, arthritis, and mental ill-health. No wonder it has been referred to as the miracle vitamin.

Smoking depletes blood levels of vitamin C. This depletion could be one factor in the high death rate among smokers as a result of heart disease and cancer. The RDA for vitamin C is 60 milligrams for adults.

Vitamin C is nontoxic. The richest sources are citrus fruits, strawberries, cantaloupes, rose hips, raw vegetables (especially peppers, parsley, broccoli, kale, brussels sprouts, cauliflower, cabbage, tomatoes, potatoes, and bean sprouts). Since this vitamin is water-soluble, prolonged cooking in water, steaming, washing, soaking, and canning can result in a high rate of vitamin C loss.

Because of its popularity (and genuine value), vitamin C is available in supplement form in a wide range of doses, from a few milligrams to over 1 gram (1,000 milligrams).

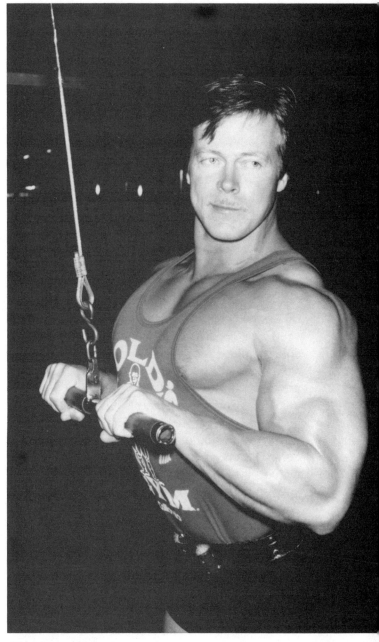

Olev Annus, Finland.

Vitamin D

Often referred to as the sunshine vitamin, vitamin D is unique for two reasons: It's synthesized by the body when the skin is exposed to sufficient sunlight; and since it is involved in regulating the function of specific organs, it is also a hormone.

Vitamin D plays a role little understood as yet in the proper mineralization of bones. It is also important to the structure and function of the thyroid and pituitary glands. Its main function is to enhance intestinal absorption of calcium and phosphorus.

A deficiency in vitamin D can cause rickets (malformed bones) and a "pigeon-chest" deformity of the rib cage. Prolonged deficiencies can lead to hyperirritability, spasms of the extremities (wrists and feet), general spasticity, and convulsive seizures.

When vitamin D deficiency occurs in adults, the bones lose vital minerals, causing them to soften and bow (bend out). Osteoporosis (brittle bones) is also a symptom of too little calcium and vitamin D.

The RDA for Vitamin D is 200 international units (I.U.) daily.

Yes, vitamin D is toxic. Too much can cause loss of appetite, thirst, urgency of urination, vomiting, headache, and diarrhea. Some adults observe signs of toxicity when only 50,000 units per day are taken in for a few weeks, whereas others can tolerate ten times that dosage for a year with no ill effects. Curiously, an excess of sunshine does *not* lead to vitamin D toxicity. Apparently our bodies regulate the amounts that are synthesized, stored, and used.

Natural sources of vitamin D are scarce, unless you include sunshine. Fish, especially fish with heavy amounts of oil in the flesh (sardines, herring, salmon), are good sources. Other sources include liver, egg yolk, and summer milk. Ironically, most current dietary sources of vitamin D are actually foods to which synthetic vitamin D is added. Vitamin D supplements are available in doses ranging from a few units to several hundred units.

Vitamin E

Not so long ago vitamin E was publicized as the "sex vitamin." Everybody started taking it to improve performance, virility, stamina, you name it.

Vitamin E hit the headlines as a sex pill because of an experiment with rodents. When rats were maintained on a diet free of vitamin E, no physical symptoms appeared, unlike in most other deficiency tests. They appeared bright-eyed, sleek, and active and maintained good size. However, it was observed that practically all of the test animals became sterile. The researchers

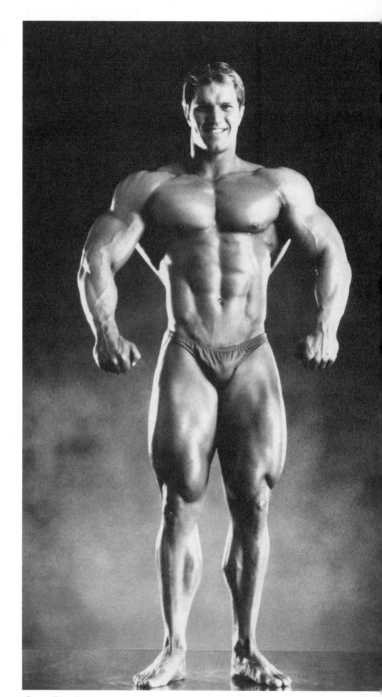

Gary Strydom.

concluded that the missing substance (found in fresh lettuce leaves, whole wheat, oats, wheat germ, and meat) was responsible for enabling the rats to bear young. They took the Greek words *tocos* and *phero,* meaning *childbirth* and *to bring forth,* and named the substance tocopherol. Vitamin E, the "sex vitamin," was born.

Deficiency of vitamin E can impair your reproductive system and promote the degeneration of sex glands. There is also a degeneration and dystrophy of the skeletal, striated, and cardiac muscles. The most widely recognized deficiency symptom of vitamin E is a decreased survival time for red blood cells.

Does vitamin E really enhance sex life? No tests have proven conclusive as yet. However, it does seem reasonable that a vitamin whose deficiency adversely affects a person's sex life will in turn enhance it if quantities are provided to offset any possible deficiency.

Vitamin E also appears to help in stressful situations. It aids the immune system and the healing process. And vitamin E is still used extensively by some doctors in treatment of heart disease because of its role in decreasing blood clotting. (Canadian physicians Evan and Wilfrid Shute have been using vitamin E treatment for various cardiovascular disorders for over thirty-five years.) There are also several research studies showing that vitamin E can partially offset the effects of air pollution and exposure to some of the toxic chemicals found in the environment we inhabit.

The RDA for vitamin E was changed in 1974 from a *maximum* of 30 I.U. to 15 I.U. Today it's even lower, standing at 10 I.U. for men and 8 I.U. for women. Why the change? Dietitians and doctors were finding that it is difficult to actually obtain 30 I.U. of vitamin E daily. When patients asked for a "well-balanced" diet the doctors were at a loss as to what to do—not surprising when we realize that the refining of flour removes just about *all* of the vitamin E!

Although vitamin E is a fat-soluble vitamin and stored in the body, it does not appear to be toxic. However, one study showed that high doses of vitamin E can lower basal metabolism rate.

Whereas storing foods can cause vitamin E loss, as can deep frying, it is not generally destroyed in the cooking process. Vitamin E supplements are available in doses ranging from a few I.U. to over 1,000 I.U. The richest natural sources are found in wheat germ oil, soybean oil, cottonseed oil, sunflower seed oil, and corn oil. Smaller quantities are found in nuts, eggs, fish, and organ meats.

Vitamin K

This vitamin is needed for proper bone mineralization and for the correct clotting of blood. Vitamin K is synthesized by intestinal bacteria. Accordingly, there is no set RDA for vitamin K, since authorities feel that a deficiency is not possible under normal conditions. This seems somewhat of a cop-out because deficiencies, however rare, *do* occur. In one hospital researchers reported vitamin K deficiency in one out of every 2,000 patients admitted to their hospital for whatever reason. In patients admitted for bleeding disorders, 2.3 percent had vitamin K deficiency.

The richest natural sources of vitamin K are leafy green vegetables such as cabbage, cauliflower, and spinach. Liver and soybeans are also good sources. Cooking does not destroy vitamin K.

Although there has been no reported case of toxicity with natural vitamin K in adults, the vitamin is available in supplemental form only through a doctor's prescription.

MINERALS

Calcium

Calcium makes up about two and a half to three pounds of our weight (mostly in the bones and teeth). It is the main structural mineral in the body. All bodybuilders need an adequate supply of calcium, since our muscles are supported by our bones. Men tend to start losing bone mass between the ages of forty-five and fifty-five; women start the same process ten years earlier. Actually, calcium is replaced at the rate of about 20 percent yearly, so it's easy to see why a constant supply is needed.

Good sources include milk and milk products, egg yolk, soybeans, leafy green vegetables, broccoli, kale, roots, tubers, seeds, turnips, and stews and soups made with bones.

The adult RDA for calcium is 800 milligrams. There are many people who suffer from calcium deficiency.

Chromium

Chromium deficiency can lead to high incidence of plaque buildup on the aorta (the main artery from the heart). A restricted growth rate and even a shortened life-span can result from too little chromium in the diet.

Best sources include brewer's yeast, whole grains (except rye), blackstrap molasses, black pepper, liver, cheese, seafood, meats, and nuts.

Chromium is nontoxic, since the body eliminates excess amounts.

Copper

A deficiency of copper, which is rare, causes abnormal skin and hair pigmentation and defects in blood vessels, which can lead to rupture. Anemia, faulty bone and nerve development, and loss of a sense of taste are other results of deficiency.

Best sources of copper include nuts, organ meats, seafood, mushrooms, and legumes. Most fresh foods contain some copper.

Fluorine

This mineral is the most controversial of all. To many people fluorine is the best thing to come along (through our water pipes) since antibiotics. It is prized for its preventive effects with regard to tooth decay. On the other hand, there's no evidence to show that fluorine is essential to the diet, and there is a sizable body of evidence that fluorine, or fluoride, increases the risk of cancer, heart disease, and genetic mutations. Most fluoridated water supplies contain about 1 ppm (part per million) fluoride. Several countries have outlawed fluoridation, including France, Denmark, Italy, and Norway. In Britain, Canada, and the United States, the controversy continues.

Iodine

Iodine's role in health and well-being is in the formation of thyroxin, the thyroid hormone. This regulates the body's basic metabolic rate (BMR). The presence of iodine affects the amount of hormone secreted. An iodine deficiency causes goiter, an enlarging of the thyroid gland, but the same thing can happen if too much iodine is ingested.

The best sources of iodine are seafood of all kinds, kelp, and onions.

The RDA for iodine is 150 micrograms (.15 milligram). Two grams of iodized salt supplies at least this amount. Iodine is an essential mineral, but the best way to make sure you are getting adequate supplies is to eat seafood regularly without increasing your salt intake.

Iron

Iron is essential to the production of red blood corpuscles (hemoglobin), red pigment in the blood (myoglobin), and certain enzymes. Iron (along with calcium) is frequently deficient in the diets of North American and British women. Often those deficient in iron suffer from tiredness and cannot gain from bodybuilding exercise. Among other things, the capacity to train diminishes. Resistance to disease can also be lowered.

Good natural sources of iron are heart and liver, raw clams, red meat, peaches, oysters, dried beans, egg yolk, whole grains, and nuts.

The RDA for iron is 18 milligrams for adults. Excesses of iron are excreted from the body, so toxicity is not usual, but it has been known. Do not indulge in excesses.

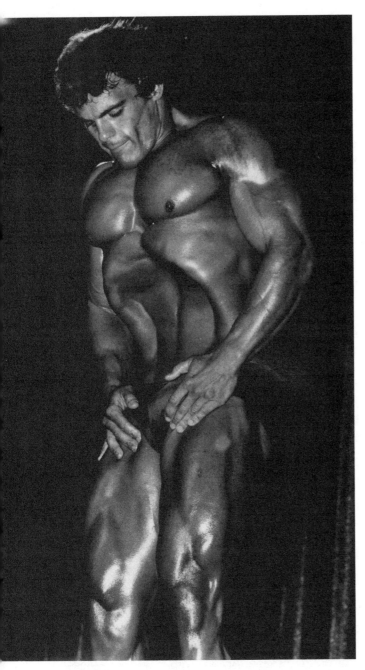

Gary Leonard demonstrates the vacuum.

Magnesium

Almost all chemical reactions via the cell depend on magnesium. This mineral is vital for regulating cell metabolism. Your muscles must have a correct balance of magnesium (and calcium) to function properly. Without proper amounts of magnesium a wide variety of symptoms can occur, including muscular weakness, lethargy, knotting of muscles, and a variety of seizures and jerks—and mental problems.

The RDA of this mineral is 350 milligrams for men and 300 milligrams for women. Researchers have found that males are particularly susceptible to magnesium deficiencies. Excess magnesium taken orally has a laxative effect.

The best natural sources include legumes, nuts, whole grains, and shellfish.

Supplements of this mineral are available in doses ranging from 50 to 500 milligrams.

Manganese

Manganese is essential for healthy, strong connective tissues. A deficiency of manganese causes skeletal deformities, impairment of growth and loss of muscular coordination among other things.

Manganese is one of the most common elements in the earth's crust, and all animal and plant tissues contain it. Good natural sources of manganese are nuts, whole grains, seeds, wheat germ, bran, peas, tea, ginger, and sage.

As yet no RDA has been determined for this mineral, but manganese is sometimes included in multimineral supplements.

Molybdenum

Although rare, molybdenum appears to be essential to our well-being. It shows up in all plant and animal life. Major sources of this mineral are legumes, organ meats, and milk.

There are few if any reports of molybdenum

deficiency in humans, and accordingly no RDA exists. Molybdenum is toxic in excessive amounts, but few supplements exist, so risk of overdosing is limited.

Phosphorus

There is more concern over getting too much of this mineral than too little. It is very common, and very important, too! Phosphorus teams with calcium to give bones (and teeth) their strength. *Every* metabolic process in the body requires phosphorus, including muscle energy production. Carbohydrate, fat, and protein metabolism rely on phosphorus.

The problems surrounding phosphorus concern its potential toxicity. The RDA is 800 milligrams for adults, but amounts in excess of this are easily obtained from processed foods, since additives often include phosphates.

Natural sources of phosphorus include meat, fish, poultry, eggs, nuts, legumes, milk, and cheese.

Potassium

Potassium is one of the most abundant minerals in the human body; a 150-pound person has about nine ounces (250 grams). It is known to most competitive bodybuilders because it is used in the final stages of preparing for the day of competition (see chapter 25 on contest preparation and carbing up).

Many cellular enzyme systems depend on potassium, and muscular contraction itself depends on it. A deficiency can cause muscular weakness, nervous irritability, mental disorientation, and cardiac irregularities. If levels of potassium get low enough, the heartbeat can falter, vibrate rather than pump, causing sudden death. Excess can cause the same symptoms as deficiency—cardiac arrhythmia, weakness, anxiety, low blood pressure, confusion, etc.

Potassium has no established RDA, but authorities recommend an intake equal to that of sodium (about 2.6 grams per day).

Probably the most useful thing about potassium is that it can counteract the blood pressure–raising effects of sodium. Potassium may not—and should not be expected to—protect you completely from the harmful effects of excess salt consumption, but it may help significantly.

Bodybuilders in particular should be aware of potassium, since strenuous exercise and the sweat it causes can lead to potassium depletion. In addition, the taking of diuretics (which some bodybuilders do in order to lose weight for a contest) can also deplete potassium reserves. One bodybuilder, Hans Salmeyer of Austria, died during a bodybuilding event in Europe, probably as a result of diuretic use and subsequent potassium depletion.

The best sources of potassium are bananas, lettuce, broccoli, fresh fruit, potatoes, peanuts (unsalted), wheat germ, and oranges.

Potassium is available in supplementary form in a wide range of doses, but observe caution when taking supplements. Acute toxicity can occur with daily doses of as little as 25 grams of potassium chloride per day.

Selenium

In the early days of bodybuilding selenium was considered a poison. Today it is considered to play a very important role in fighting two of the most ominous threats to modern health: cancer and heart disease. Among other things, selenium has an essential role in maintaining the integrity of muscle cells and red blood cells.

The adult RDA for selenium is 50 micrograms (.05 milligram). Like most other trace minerals, selenium can be toxic in excessive amounts.

The richest natural sources of selenium are organ meats, seafood, whole grains, and brewer's yeast.

Silicon

All living tissue contains silicon—at least, traces of it. It is present in rocks, dust, clay, water, and sand. Human blood contains the same concentrations of silicon as seawater (1 to 5 parts per million).

Deficiencies of silicon can cause depressed growth and brittle bones. Some scientists tie silicon deficiency in with aging, although hard evidence of that is not yet available.

No RDA for silicon has been determined, but it seems clear that most diets provide adequate amounts to meet general needs. Silicon has not been found to be toxic, so there is little concern about possible overdose.

Whole grains are a good source of silicon and so, ironically, is beer. Although muscle and organ meats contain only small amounts, the connective tissues, bones, and skin of animals we eat rate as good sources.

Sodium

Yes, sodium is important, but it can also be dangerous. Taken in as sodium chloride (salt), it is added to almost everything, and enough is enough. You won't find many processed or manufactured foods that have not had loads of sodium added. Avoid excessive sodium intake by refusing to use table salt and by saying no to processed foods.

The primary purpose of sodium is to help push nutrients in and out of cells through the cell membranes. Sodium is vital; a deficiency can cause muscle cramps, headaches, weakness, and even collapse of blood vessels. But most sodium-related problems in our civilized world are caused by sodium overload rather than the opposite. Too much raises blood pressure to dangerous highs. (There is, as mentioned earlier, evidence to show that dietary potassium can offer *some* protection against the blood pressure—raising effect of salt.)

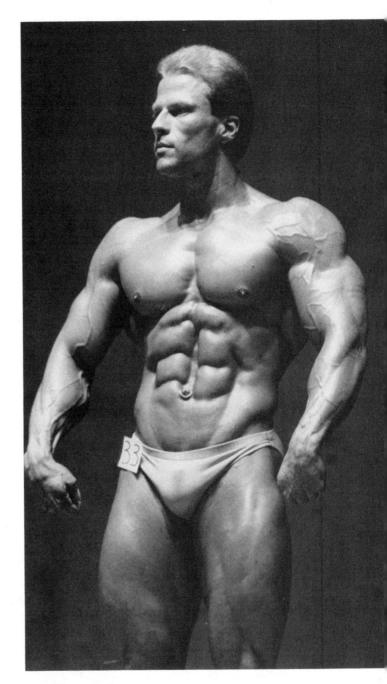

John Hnatyschak.

Zinc

Nature's complexity is apparent when we consider that scientists have already isolated zinc as a cofactor in at least forty-five different enzyme systems. That is too many to mention, but one is of paramount importance to the bodybuilder: zinc's vital role in protein synthesis. And we all know that, aside from its water content, muscle is built primarily of protein.

You are certainly not going to build to your fullest potential if your ingestion of zinc is inadequate. Because zinc is necessary for cell growth and rapid cell proliferation, your intake must always stay above the 15-milligram RDA for adults. Research has shown that many Americans and Canadians may be marginally deficient in zinc. Even hospital meals have been found to contain less than the RDA for adults. A point of interest to bodybuilders: Evidence suggests that high-protein diets may increase zinc requirements.

Zinc is relatively nontoxic; no side effects have been reported from studies in which varying doses of zinc supplements were administered.

The best natural sources of zinc include seafoods (especially herring), liver, meats, milk, nuts, eggs, legumes, and brewer's yeast. It is also avail-

Diana Dennis, California.

FACING PAGE: *Dr. Lynn Pirie.*

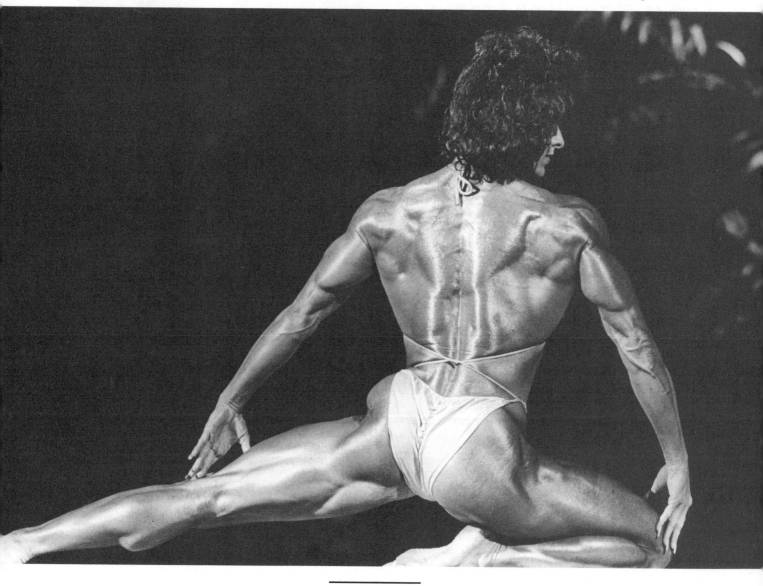

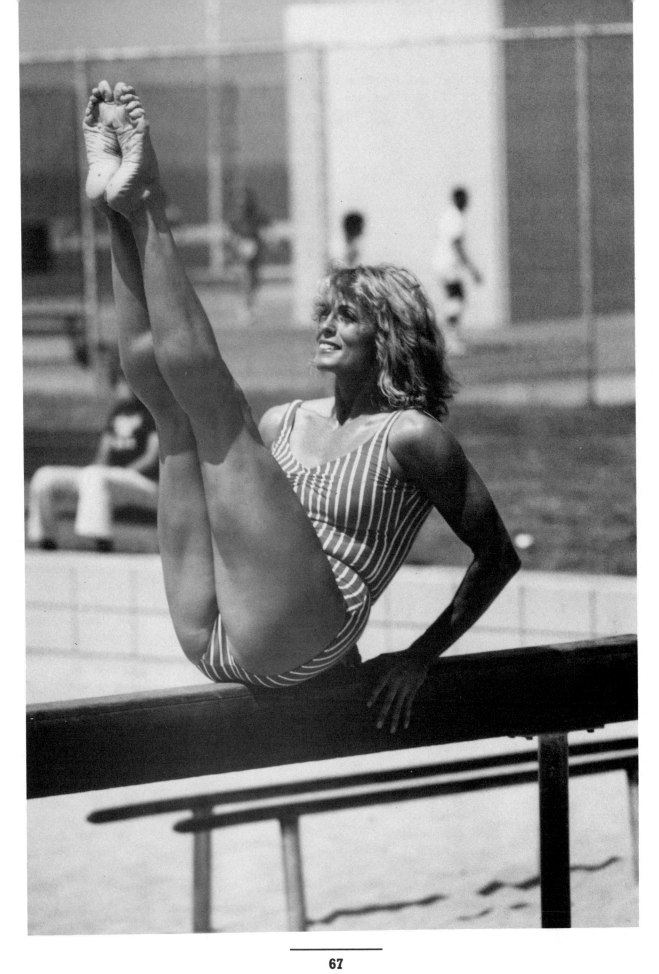

able as a supplement in various doses. Regrettably, much of the soil in the United States has been found deficient in zinc.

Other Minerals

More! Well yes, but who knows how many? Besides the fifteen minerals I have briefly discussed, there are numerous others, but deficiencies in these are uncommon in humans. Sulfur and chlorine, for example, are used by the body, yet no scientist has shown anyone deficient in them. There are probably other mineral nutrients out there that we have not yet discovered. Are they vital to health? Must we have them for optimum strength, energy, and development? I think it's safe to say that the minerals that we have not mentioned, plus others we have not yet isolated and named, are required in such small quantities that our diets almost certainly supply adequate trace amounts. As one scientist put it, "There may be micronutrients that we have never heard of, so small that they could ride in on the smallest speck of dust."

BIOFLAVONOIDS

Bioflavonoids are found in the leaves, fruits, flowers, stems, and roots of most plants. They are neither vitamins nor minerals, but they do contribute to optimum health. Their essentiality has yet to be proven. When bioflavonoids were first discovered, they were named vitamin P, but this term was discarded later and the name *bioflavonoids* (or flavonoids) was adopted.

The principal role of flavonoids is to keep capillaries strong and healthy. This is pretty important stuff you'll agree, yet flavonoids are still considered only "semi-essential."

Another role attributed to bioflavonoids is that of decreasing the tendency of blood cells to clump together or aggregate. Blood cell clumping can impede the blood's passage through the microscopic capillaries and increases the possibility of dangerous blood clots.

Bioflavonoids also have antiviral properties. Daily treatment with bioflavonoids (1,000 milligrams) and vitamin C (1,000 milligrams) has been effective in promoting the healing of herpes sores on the lips.

Bioflavonoids are being used in the treatment of cardiovascular disease under the rationale that they may be able to increase the strength of the blood vessels while decreasing the tendency for the blood to clot. There is no hard evidence to support this relatively new theory as yet.

You will find the white rind of oranges, lemons, and other citrus fruits to be rich sources of bioflavonoids. Supplements are available as *rutin* or *bioflavonoids* in doses up to 1,000 milligrams. They are nontoxic.

11
SUPPLEMENTS
The Added Ingredients

Supplementation for bodybuilders used to be a matter of yea or nay. In fact, the titanic Arnold Schwarzenegger has pronounced more than a few times that he won the IFBB Mr. Olympia contest both while he was supplementing his diet heavily and when he was taking no supplements at all. (Of course, steroid intake was never denied in either case. For more on that subject, see chapter 13.)

Food supplementation for bodybuilders probably arrived through the food faddists writing in the latter part of the last century. But its real sophistication seems to have started with Rheo H. Blair in the 1950s. He was the bodybuilder's savior at that time, when he introduced his original milk and egg protein mixture. It was taken by Larry Scott, Don Howarth, Dave Draper, and Arnold Schwarzenegger, all successful bodybuilders. Scott actually went so far as to claim that a large percentage of his incredible size was due to mixing Blair's protein with half milk and half cream. Blair had a great following in the fifties, sixties, and seventies, and even though he is now dead (he died in 1983), he is still regarded by bodybuilders in the U.S. as the guru of supplementation.

Looking back at bodybuilding since I've been involved in it over the last thirty years—as a competitor (no great shakes), a writer (no bestsellers), and a magazine publisher (no great distribution)—I will admit that in the early days there were bodybuilders who just relied solely on their spouse's cooking. They took no supplements. There were, at the height of the steroid era (the 1970s), numerous bodybuilders who achieved success while taking drugs but no supplements. Today I know of no top class or even state, province, or county-level bodybuilder who does not see the necessity of using supplements. Many claim that their training time is wasted unless they combine it with food supplementation.

Because competition is so intense today, we cannot neglect supplementation. No matter what our condition, age, ambitions, or genetic poten-

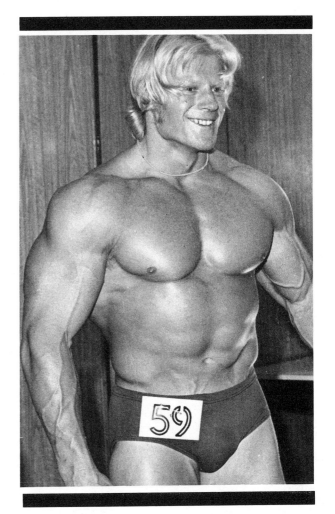

Dave Draper, Mr. World.

tial, we all train to improve. If we fail to use modern scientific supplementation to help us along the way, we are forfeiting at least half our chances for bodybuilding success.

The following is a list of recommended types of supplements to give bodybuilders ultimate nutrition.

- Vitamins A and D—should be obtained from fish liver, such as cod or halibut liver oil.
- Vitamin E—check label to be sure that the source is natural not synthetic.
- Vitamin B complex—the brand should contain all the B vitamins.
- Vitamin C—look for the bioflavonoids type, preferably time-released.
- Minerals—look for amino acid chelates.
- Proteins—milk, glandular, or egg protein powders are best. Check the label to make sure that sodium caseinate is used in any milk products, not calcium caseinate.

Supplements, with the exception of amino acids, should be taken with meals and spread out throughout the day rather than taken all at once. If you take supplements, especially in pill form, on an empty stomach and with no other food, they simply do not excite the digestive system and are not utilized properly. Amino acids are different. Their effect is neutralized by food, and they should be taken on an empty stomach.

VITAMINS

The most efficient way to take your vitamins is by investing in a multipack product. These provide insurance against nutritional deficiencies that will adversely affect your progress. North America is the most well-fed continent on planet Earth, yet at least one-third of the population is malnourished. You are a hard-training bodybuilder, expending more energy, burning more calories than most, and requiring extra nutrients to build up your muscles and strength. Chances are you are undernourished, too.

A multipack product is your answer to any possible vitamin deficiency. Check the labels carefully. Make sure the minerals in the multipack are *chelated*. Chelation is a process by which protein molecules are bonded chemically to inorganic minerals (making them far more usable by the body). The most trusted names in multipacks include the Weider Good Life Mega Packs, the Hardcore Line, Super Spectrum, Beverly International, and Natural Source products.

Never doubt for one second the importance of vitamins in your training. They are absolutely essential, not just for gains but for basic health and life itself. Scurvy is caused by a vitamin C deficiency, pellagra is caused by a niacinamide deficiency, beriberi is caused by a vitamin B deficiency, and rickets is caused by a vitamin D deficiency. All these diseases are particularly gruesome and in their worst stages can cause death. But they are only some of the illnesses that can be caused by vitamin deficiency.

Here is the point that I would like to write in mile-high letters across the sky: To sustain good health, robust energy, and the constitution to benefit from bodybuilding training, you must have the chemicals your cells need to perform the task of tissue repair and muscle growth. If any one chemical is not made available, your body will suffer accordingly. For example, insufficient vitamin A can cause night blindness (or total blindness). Even moderate deficiencies of many other vitamins can leave you vulnerable to infection, increased likelihood of injury, mental slowness, depression, and many other conditions, all of which, as you can readily see, would impede your making ultimate bodybuilding progress.

Many people are confused about both the number of vitamins and the designations of letters, names, and numbers that they are given. For example we have vitamin A by itself and then a confusing array of B vitamins—B_1, B_2, B_6, B_{12}. And then there's the vitamin niacinamide, which has no letter or number designation. It's confusing isn't it?

Well, the reason that it is such a jumble is that ever since Polish biochemist Casimir Funk first discovered vitamins and their role (in 1911), there has been a flurry of activity in the field, with input coming from all corners of the globe.

Discoveries came so quickly, especially in the 1930s and 1940s, that even the scientists got confused. The B vitamins are particularly mixed up. B_1, B_2, B_6, B_{12}, for example, are all *different* vitamins. The fact that they have been designated with the letter B is simply an accident of history. Biochemists agree that if they were naming them today they would give them all separate chemical names. I suspect this will happen in due course.

There are more vitamins than you think—far more than the alphabet has letters to accommodate. At the last count (and depending on whom you talk to) there were forty-one kinds of vitamins. But it doesn't end there. There are unquestionably ingredients in food vital to our health but not as yet identified.

What is a vitamin anyway? A vitamin is a chemical present in extremely small amounts in our food with these characteristics:

- It is an *organic* compound, rather than inorganic. (Minerals are inorganic.)
- It is *essential* for normal health.
- A specific *disease* or *malfunction* will occur if it is absent.
- It *cannot be completely manufactured* by the body processes alone (unlike hormones, which the body can make).

PROTEIN

Your main protein, like your vitamins, should come from natural foods. However, if you are impatient to pack on weight, it is a good idea to try a powdered protein product.

The best type of protein supplement is one formulated solely from milk and eggs, although desiccated liver tabs (and other glandulars) can be useful. Desiccated glandulars are usually in pill form and constitute 38 percent protein. Milk and egg protein is more often than not in powdered form, always superior to pills in that no binder (glue) is used to hold the grains together.

Nutritionists have established a protein efficiency ratio (P.E.R.) so that the usefulness (assimilability) of a product can be evaluated. The P.E.R. is based on egg albumin (egg white), the most assimilable source of protein available for human consumption. The protein in *milk* is second, and *fish* and *meat* follow closely in biological value. Nutritional science has recorded that egg white (albumin) is about 80 percent usable by humans. It is very expensive and you'll find that most so-called milk and egg proteins actually include very little egg. Most of the product is made up of calcium caseinate (about 95 percent protein), although sodium caseinate is superior. Those proteins containing considerable amounts of yeast or soya-based proteins are inferior to pure milk and egg products. Yeast and soya proteins are cheap ingredients and are often included to hold down the initial cost of the product to the manufacturing company. The savings may or may not be passed on to you, the consumer.

Shop with care when buying a protein product. Avoid purchasing simply by percent, which may seem impressive on the label. For example, a manufacturer could package a 100 percent protein product made of cellulose. However, as you cannot digest cellulose, the protein is totally unusable. A protein should be purchased according to its ingredients or P.E.R.

At one time the York Barbell Company promoted a "Protein from the Sea" product that undoubtedly would have been a useful supplement had it not had the most vile odor this side of rancid catfood. They dropped the line several years ago, but I understand their sales to bodybuilding enthusiasts were quite significant. It has been said more than once that bodybuilders would eat horse dung if they knew for certain it would pack on muscle size quickly. I have yet to hear a top bodybuilder dispute this statement, incidentally.

MINERALS

Like vitamins, minerals are chemicals needed by the body for ultimate health and performance. Unlike vitamins, which we still do not fully understand, minerals are relatively simple chemicals. They are dead substances that can be dug out of a rock. Vitamins are organic, found in living things. But you will still suffer poor health if you don't get adequate minerals regularly.

If you are eating a wide variety of fresh fruits and vegetables, it is most unlikely that you are getting insufficient minerals. However, those who live on overprocessed foods should change their eating habits now, and meanwhile take a mineral supplement to get them back on track nutritionally.

Unlike vitamins, minerals are cheap, but even so, read the labels carefully before supplementing. The following is a simple chart of the essential minerals and recommended dosages:

Mineral	Dosage	Symptoms of Deficiency
Calcium	800 mg.	Bone weakness and disease
Phosphorus	800 mg.	Muscular convulsions
Magnesium	325 mg.	Growth retardation
Iodine	120 mg.	Goiter
Iron	14 mg.	Anemia

AMINO ACIDS

Amino acids are a buzz-phrase today. They are the building blocks of your body, derived from the protein you eat. In other words, meat, fish, eggs, beans, and milk all contain protein, which is made up of combinations of different amino acids. After ingestion these amino acid building blocks are utilized in a complex manner to build your hair, fingernails, bones, and—more relevant to this book—your muscle tissues and cells. In all there are twenty-two different amino acids that your body requires. There are two kinds: "nonessential" (those that can be synthesized by the body) and "essential" (those that cannot be synthesized by the body). You must get the essential amino acids from what you put in your mouth, or else your body will not work properly. Here's a list of both types:

Essential	Nonessential
Histidine	Alanine
Isoleucine	Arginine
Leucine	Asparagine
Lysine	Aspartate
Methionine	Cysteine
Ornithine	Cystine
Phenylalanine	Glutamate
Threonine	Glutamine
Tryptophan	Glycine
Valine	Proline
	Serine
	Tyrosine

Not long ago there was a trend—no, it was more than that, it was a thundering onslaught of craziness—surrounding the use of L-arginine and L-ornithine to build muscle size to the same degree as with anabolic steroids. The combination of these two amino acids was purported to trigger the natural growth hormone within the body to produce conditions whereby additional muscle growth resulted.

I recall Arnold Schwarzenegger taking amino acid tablets way back in 1968. Vince Gironda and Frank Zane were taking them, too (they were Blair's product). Few other bodybuilders even knew about amino acids. They were just getting into soy protein tablets.

I have talked to scores of bodybuilders about their use of amino acids. When working on *Super Pump* (Sterling Publishing), a book on

FACING PAGE:

Corinna Everson, Carla Dunlap, and Mary Roberts.

Corinna and Mary share a moment while the judges decide a winner.

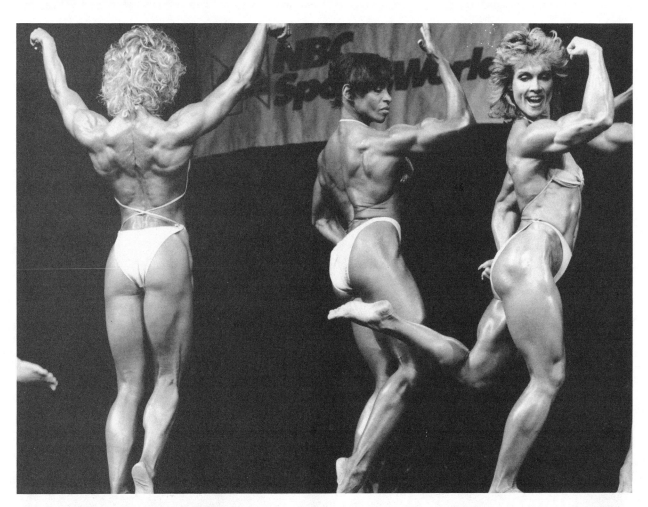

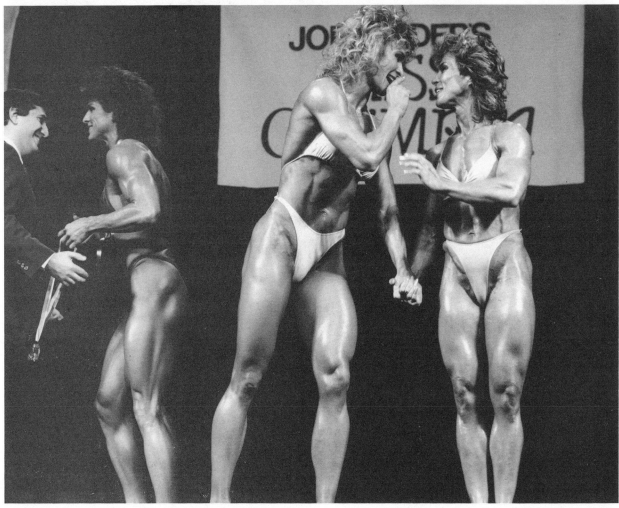

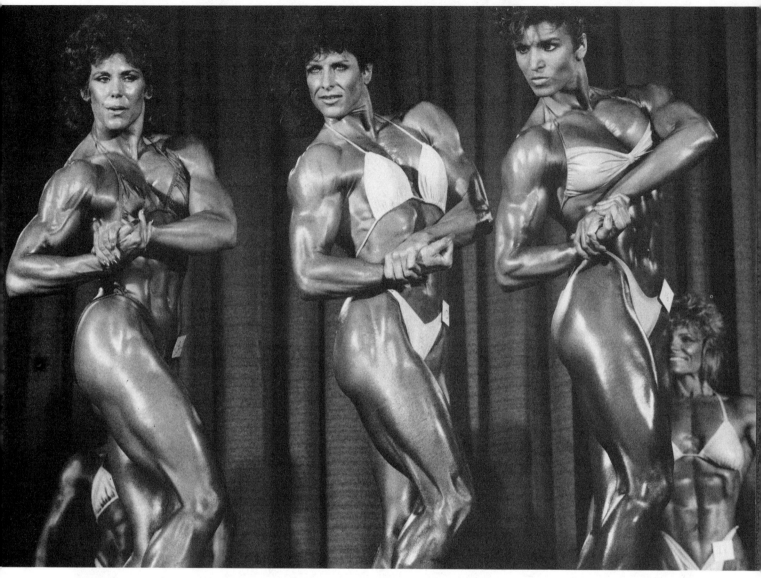

Sue Ann McKean, Diana Dennis, and Marjo Selin compare side chest poses.

advanced women's bodybuilding that I wrote with Ben Weider, 95 percent of the top professional women I interviewed told me that they took amino acids in their training for the coveted Ms. Olympia crown. At least 80 percent of male champions I've talked to admit to taking amino acids, especially when a contest is looming up. The brand name most mentioned was Tyson, reportedly good because its formulations were "pharmaceutical strength."

As publisher and editor of *MuscleMag International,* I have talked and corresponded with literally thousands of "lesser lights"—the bodybuilding neophytes, the intermediates, and be-

ginning contestants. Although a few openly declared that they had seen *no* gains at all from trying amino acid supplementation, most did notice that they (1) hardened up, (2) gained strength, (3) gained some muscle size, (4) lost fat. I should caution you that none of these advantages were hugely dramatic. The results were not comparable to heavy anabolic steroid intake. Let's face it, mix steroids with plenty of food and hard training and you'll blow up like a balloon. I've seen it too many times to doubt it. Trouble is, like the overfilled balloon, the person who takes large amounts of steroids will one day burst. And don't you ever doubt that either.

Personally, I am very much against steroid use; although I have never taken any myself, I have seen the results firsthand. In many cases they lead the bodybuilder up a dead end street. They increase your size, weight, and strength so dramatically that you don't want to let go. And unfortunately, more and more are needed to get the same effect. This ultimately puts you on a pathway to self-destruction. You have to take more to stay the same, and more is bad for you. Steroids also cause bodybuilders to be super aggressive, and this in itself can lead to trouble. Additionally, I am convinced (though I have no concrete or scientific evidence to support my thoughts) that heavy steroid takers somehow run the risk of throwing their minds out of balance and can be susceptible to sociability problems and even mental illnesses such as schizophrenia, depression, and anxiety.

But I am against steroid abuse for other reasons, too. Assuming even that they aren't harmful, I do not see them as enhancing the body when they are taken in huge quantities. They make everything grow, and I mean *everything!* Not only your shoulders, legs, arms, and chest, but also your intestines. So what results? The intestines push out the waistline and it hangs out all over the stage. Scores of times I have seen nice looking balanced physiques ruined by steroid abuse.

Think of your thickest waisted bodybuilders, men and women. Chances are they are among the heaviest steroid users in the field. They look better when they get off the stuff—1,000 percent. I am happy that steroid testing is with us.

Britain's comeback bodybuilder Frank Richards tells of his supplement intake. "I take liquid amino acids, free form amino acids, and liquid liver. Also, each day I take three mega B complex capsules, three grams of vitamin C, 1,200

Frank Richards of England, the "Comeback Man."

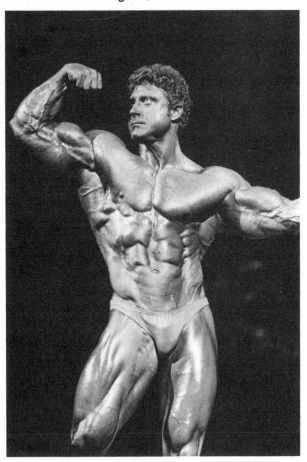

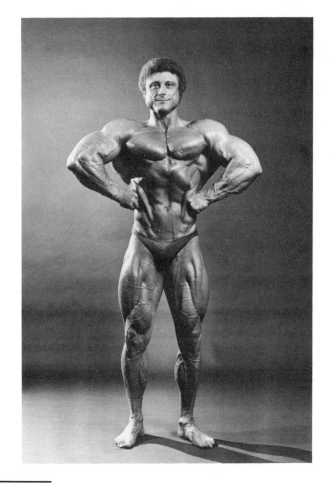

I.U. of vitamin E, three iron tablets, three mega-mineral tablets, three zinc, three potassium, and about thirty brewer's yeast tablets."

Lydia Cheng, a star of the film *Pumping Iron II, The Women,* takes the following supplements with her breakfast: amino acids (ornithine, gly-cine, tryptophan), desiccated liver capsules, multi-vitamin/mineral tablet, vitamin C, enzyme pill.

Super physique woman Mary Roberts always takes a daily vitamin multi-pack at breakfast and dinner, and she takes four amino acid tablets after every meal except her midafternoon snack.

Durk Pearson and Sandy Shaw, the renowned authors of *Life Extension: A Practical Scientific Approach* (Warner Books), really opened a few eyes with their chapters on improving athletic performance. In *Life Extension,* they talk about growth hormone: "It is released by the pituitary gland in the brain in response to exercise, fasting, hypoglycemia, sleep, trauma, dopaminergic stimulants, and other factors. Growth hormone (GH) has many functions, including maintaining the immune system, *stimulating muscle growth* [my emphasis], and burning fat. Exercise in which there is a briefly sustained muscular *peak* output releases growth hormone; exercise at less than peak effort, even when prolonged, releases little or no GH."

This statement set the athletic world, especially the bodybuilding fraternity, wild with excitement. Why? Because in the very next paragraph in their book Pearson and Shaw wrote: "There are several nutrients and prescription drugs which cause GH release." So now we were all ears. This sounded like a bodybuilder's dream. The next sentence didn't disappoint; we got the information we wanted: "These include the amino acids arginine and ornithine and the prescription drugs L-Dopa (another amino acid) bromocriptine (Parlodel® by Sandoz) and vasopressin (Diapid®, Sandoz nasal spray). In one study ½ gram per day of L-Dopa increased the growth hormone output of men in their sixties (who were not suffering from Parkinson's disease) back up to near young adult levels.

As a result of *Life Extension*'s revelation that certain amino acids could trigger the body's mechanism to release more growth hormone, the craze for combining amino acids hit the Western world like a ton of bricks. Bodybuilders *had* to have arginine and ornithine. Subsequent tests on Pearson's and Shaw's findings were carried out and it was reported as conclusive that very large amounts (10 grams or more) of arginine and ornithine injected into human beings *will* trigger the release of human growth hormone (HGH).

Gladys Portugues, New York.

12
GROWTH HORMONE
Metabolic Effects of Amino Acids

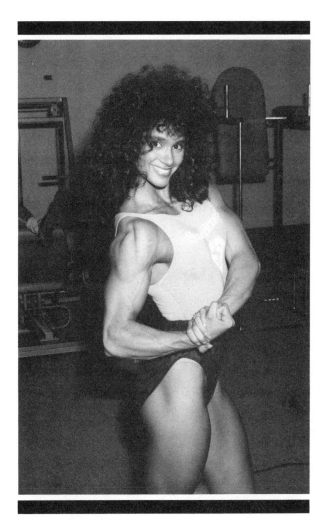

Unfortunately, the vast majority of amino acid products that surfaced to feed muscle-hungry bodybuilders (especially those loath to resort to taking potentially dangerous anabolic steroids) contained insufficient amounts of the amino acids to stimulate extraordinary growth hormone release.

Frank Zane, writing in *Zane Nutrition* (Simon and Schuster), says, "When you consider that all animal proteins come packaged in fat, it makes sense to use amino acids in free form, and eat smaller amounts of animal proteins if you want to keep calories to a minimum."

I remember that Vince Gironda was taking amino acid supplements already back in 1962, and he had such an advanced physique for his era that many considered him too muscular! The next time I heard of bodybuilders taking amino acids was in 1968, when I visited California. After a workout with Arnold Schwarzenegger, then a fast-rising star of the day, I went to his small apartment (which he was sharing with Frank Zane), and he told me that as well as taking plenty of milk and egg protein, he was also taking the "new" (and very expensive) amino acids—supplied free, incidentally, by Rheo H. Blair, who was making a small fortune selling amino acid pills for $1.50 each to bodybuilders throughout North America.

I never heard Arnold make much of a claim for their usefulness—perhaps he was keeping quiet because he thought they gave him a competitive edge—but Zane and his wife, Christine, openly admitted that free form amino acids gave them an improved feeling of well-being, more energy, alertness, and stamina, plus increased fat loss, faster recuperation, better sex drive, improved muscle tone...and more muscle growth!

In 1986 I made a concerted effort to interview many of the world's greatest women bodybuilders for a book project I was involved with in conjunction with IFBB President Ben Weider. These women included Juliette Bergman, Erika Mes, Dinah Anderson, Tina Plakinger, Cory Everson, Clare Furr, Carolyn Cheshire, Gladys Portugues, and many others. I was surprised to find that almost all of these women religiously supplemented their diets with free form amino acids.

My own observations and conclusions about the use of amino acids, especially combining arginine and ornithine to stimulate growth hormone release, are limited to answers I have obtained from hundreds of unbiased users. The general consensus is this: *Using free amino acids does cause loss of body fat, increased muscle hardness, and some noticeable gain in size and strength.* This use must be over a period of six weeks. This is not a scientific conclusion, merely my report of others' observations.

It is generally acknowledged that free form amino acids do *not* compare in effect to anabolic steroids, which accelerate muscle growth and strength enormously. But then again, steroids come with risk factors (side effects) that to me are totally unacceptable. Every prescription drug has some form of side effect (the contraindications).

There is no doubt that when taken in conjunction with a high-protein diet and rigorous progressive resistance exercise, steroids do help build muscle mass and density at an almost unbelievable rate. The side effects, however, read like a horror story: liver damage, hair loss, acne, testicular shrinkage, predisposition to early heart attacks, cancer, hardening of the arteries, etc. It is obvious that steroids should not be part of any athlete's supplement program. (See the next chapter for a more complete discussion of steroid use.)

Free form amino acids come in many varieties. All are on the expensive side. Frank Zane has his own "Super Body Formula," which consists of the following 16 free form amino acids in capsule form:

L-lysine	L-tyrosine
L-tryptophan	L-aspartic acid
L-arginine	L-vatine
L-isoleucine	L-glutamic acid
L-histidine	L-phenylalanine
L-cystine	L-glycine
L-methionine	L-serine
L-glutamine	L-cysteine

"When my wife and I are in hard training for a contest or exhibition," says Zane, "we take one to ten capsules half an hour before meals. This

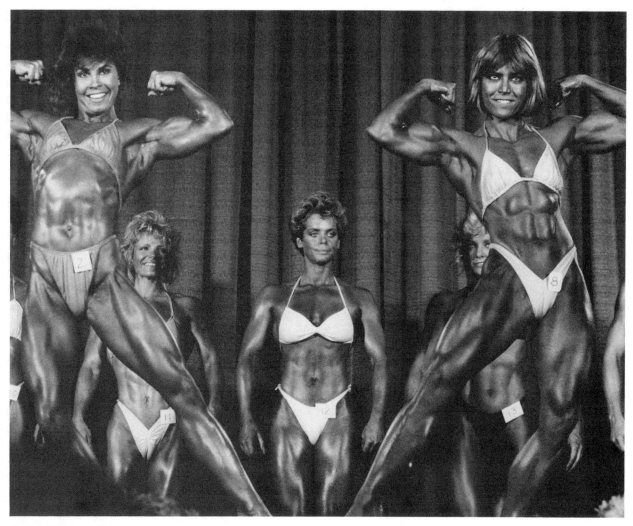

Janice Ragain (USA) and Juliette Bergman (Holland).

gives the amino acids plenty of time to be absorbed into the tissues of the body."

It is important to start out with low dosages of amino acids, gradually increasing them until optional dosage is achieved. Amino acid supplementation should be accompanied by a B-complex vitamin supplement (especially B_6). A multivitamin (A, D, E, and C) should also be taken, plus a mineral complex pill. The majority of bodybuilders can benefit from amino acid supplementation. However, it is always a good practice first to review your health situation with a clinical nutritionist or a medical doctor known for his or her study of diet (and in sympathy with the value of optimum nutrition). A few people have congenital amino acid metabolism disorders.

Taking amino acids with milk is not a good idea. Milk coats the stomach lining and hinders absorption of these nutrients into the body. It also forms complexes with many of the amino acids. Take your amino acid capsules with vegetable juice or water.

Human growth hormone (also called somatotropic hormone, or STH) itself can be obtained through a doctor's prescription. Actually, the accepted medical use of this drug is to help growth hormone—deficient children reach normal height. It is a rare commodity and, needless to say, every time a bodybuilder uses it a needy child goes short. (Dr. Robert Kerr claimed in the June 1983 issue of *Flex* to have supervised the use of growth hormone in 150 bodybuilders.)

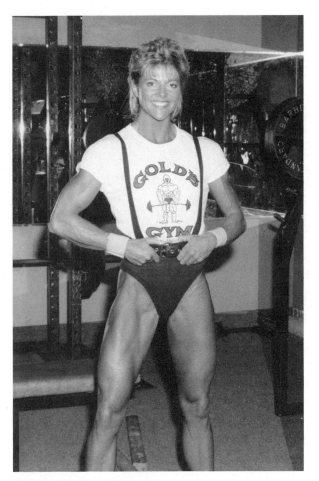

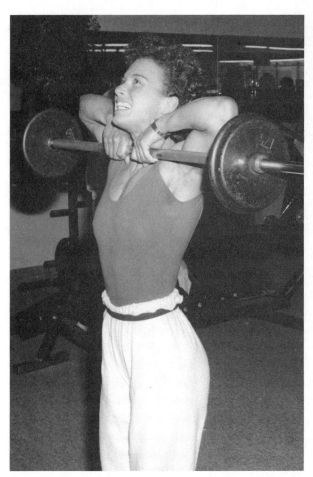

Carolyn Cheshire, England.

Erika Mes, Holland.

The supply is finite since it is obtained only from human pituitary glands. Dr. Louis E. Underwood, Professor of Pediatrics at the University of North Carolina at Chapel Hill, says, "Worldwide only a fraction of the children who need STH treatment have access to this precious material. Every unit of growth hormone used by bodybuilders denies a short, growth hormone—deficient child the chance to achieve normal growth and acceptable adult height."

Incidentally STH does not increase height in adults, who by the age of twenty or so will have reached their normal height (and closed their epiphyses, the growth portion of the bone length). Nothing will elongate the bones of adults further.

There is little evidence that STH actually builds muscle dramatically, although there appears to be some evidence that it hardens muscle and chases away fat. Certainly there is evidence that STH thickens bones (widens jaws, deepens fore-

heads) as can be evidenced in some top male and female bodybuilders whose jaws have grown so dramatically outward that the gap between their front teeth has widened significantly.

Human growth hormone is a potent metabolic agent that has diverse effects on the body. Prolonged use can cause diabetes, cardiac disease, selective overgrowth of bone, and neurological disability. There are doubtless other, unknown risks.

Further, apparently much of what is sold to bodybuilders as STH is not really STH. It is either hormone taken from animals or, worse, it is an agent that is dangerously contaminated. One person known to me tried out what he was told was growth hormone only to suffer illness with symptoms similar to AIDS (constant diarrhea,

FACING PAGE: *Dinah Anderson.*

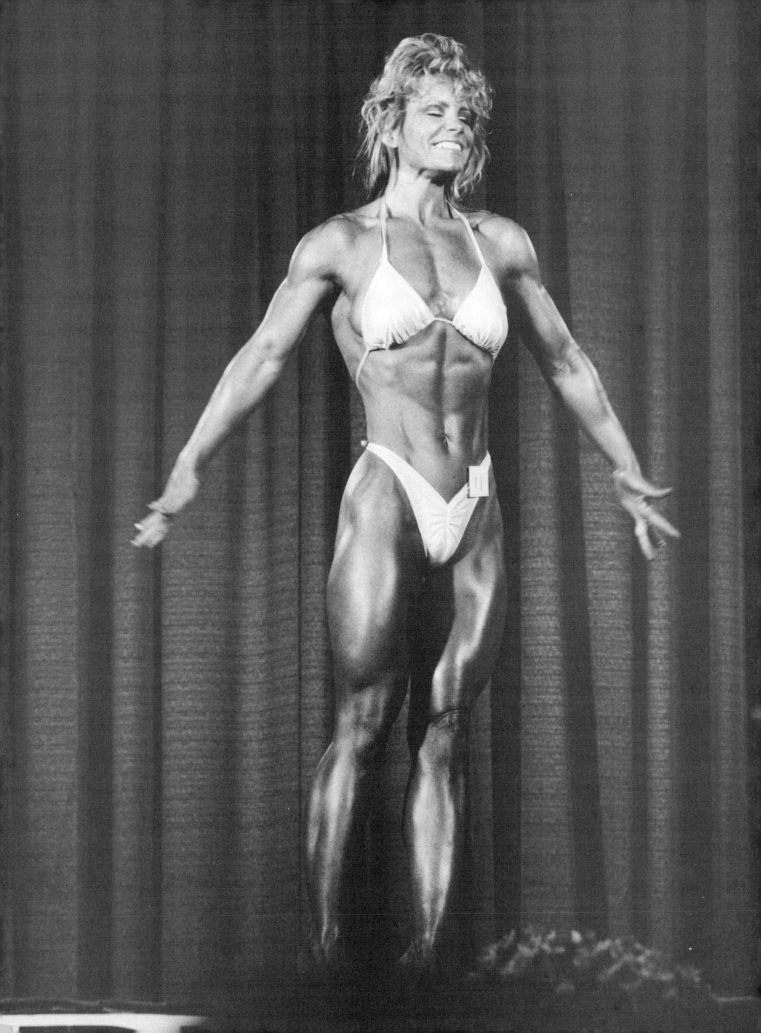

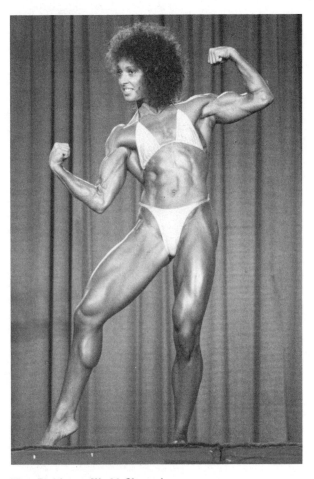

Tina Plakinger, World Champion.

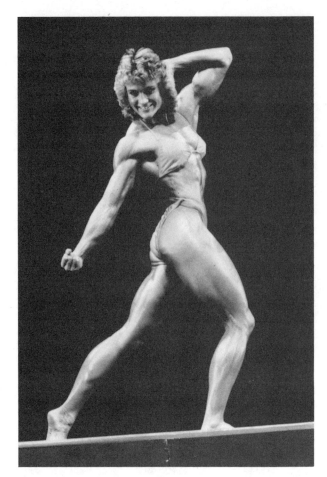

Cory Everson, Ms. Olympia.

nervous attacks, etc.). His doctors neither knew what his problem was, nor how to treat it. As of this writing he has still not recovered.

In these days of drug testing at the Olympic games and at bodybuilding shows, STH is a popular agent because, at this writing, there are no tests to identify those who are taking it. I desperately hope this situation changes.

An interesting fact about growth hormone is its relationship to exercise. The *European Journal of Applied Physiology* reported that Canadian researchers Vanhelder, Radomski, Goode, and Casey recently conducted an experiment which compared three different types of exercise in relation to their effect on the production of human growth hormone. The exercises were: seven sets of squats, with ten repetitions per set; continuous cycling at the rate of 50 revolutions per minute; and intermittent cycling at the rate of 70 revolutions per minute. Each exercise session lasted twenty minutes.

Continuous cycling (an aerobic exercise) led to the lowest levels of growth hormone output. Intermittent cycling was responsible for more growth hormone release than continuous cycling, but heavy ten-rep free weight squats were responsible for the *greatest* growth hormone release. Interesting stuff.

Besides mood-altering drugs such as marijuana, LSD, speed, cocaine, crack—you name it—there is a series of drugs called hormonoids. These substances are synthetic reproductions of chemicals the body produces in varying amounts for normal body functioning. Bodybuilders and other athletes have been using these drugs to enhance their appearance and performance for years. To his credit perhaps, Arnold Schwarzenegger was the first top bodybuilder to admit publicly, and on national television no less, that he did take steroids when preparing for a contest. He did it during a Barbara Walters interview ...no sweat.

Roy Rose, an Australian IFBB-NPC judge and longtime bodybuilder, sees it this way. "With the IFBB already instituting major steps in contest drug testing at top level, future competitors may well be looking very seriously at the art of fine tuning their supplementation in order to gain that extra contest edge." Anabolic steroids have been the answer to many a skinny person's dream. They have enabled both men and women to cheat their way to muscle gains and blatantly rob competitors who did not take steroids of their winners' trophies.

However, steroids are not a supplement. They are drugs, legally available only through a doctor's prescription and based on synthetic male hormones. When taken in conjunction with progressive resistance exercise, they measurably improve muscle size, strength, workout stamina, and even recovery ability. Like any drug they have side effects. Writer Bill Reynolds, who has experimented with steroid programs, lists these in his book *The Gold's Gym Book of Bodybuilding* (Contemporary Books) as follows:

- Liver and kidney dysfunction and damage
- Possible liver, kidney, and prostate cancer
- Testicular atrophy and increased or decreased libido (in men)
- Masculinization and clitoral enlargement (in women), largely irreversible.

Rich Gaspari.

13
HORMONOIDS
Chemical Bodybuilding

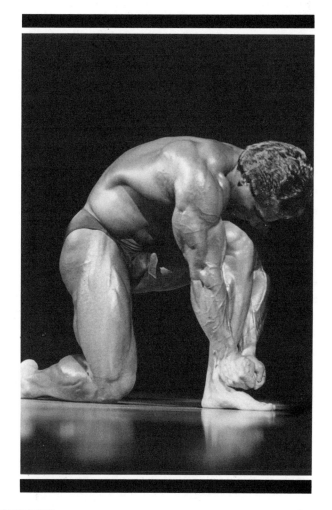

- Masculinization of a fetus (not too pleasant if the fetus is female)
- Premature closure of bone growth plates in pubescent individuals (could stunt height)
- Water retention and consequent high blood pressure
- Acne
- Hair loss
- Osteoporosis (weakening of bones due to depletion of bone calcium)
- Increased aggression
- Death

CORTICOID HORMONES AND ACTH

These chemicals help to overcome extreme exhaustion. They also help to reduce swelling and pain in a specific area. I remember that in an early Mr. Olympia contest Arnold Schwarzenegger strained his shoulder muscle while twisting and flexing during the posing routine. Arnold knew that he had to pose off against Sergio Oliva at the evening show later that day, so he had a cortisone shot to relieve the pain. (Incidentally, cortisone can smooth out the physique in a hurry.) That night he posed like he'd never posed before. Without the shot I doubt he could have done anything. As it was, he beat the great Sergio Oliva.

Pain, of course, is an indicator of trouble. It's the body's way of warning against further activity. Coaches who give their players a quick cortisone shot and send them back out to compete are taking a chance. The player's pain is suppressed, but the muscle tear or other damage could be made far worse by continuing to be active. When used judiciously in a moment of true need, these hormones are acceptable.

THYROXIN

This drug has a stimulating effect on the metabolism. It speeds up the metabolism, which results in increased combustion of glycogen, fat, and other metabolites and a corresponding increase in the body's oxygen requirement and an increase in heat production.

Thyroxin is taken by some bodybuilders because it burns fat, but this drug is harmful. Heavyweight pro boxer Muhammad Ali admitted to having taken thyroxin to lose weight for one of his fights. The result? He ran out of steam early on and lost the match. He had shed weight, all right, but in doing so *artificially*, he had lost his normal high stamina.

Losing pounds to make a certain body weight should be done by natural means, such as reducing calories and increasing aerobic activity. I know several pro bodybuilders who took thyroxin for more than the usual three weeks prior to a bodybuilding show and actually shut down their own thyroid production permanently. Each now has to take a daily thyroxin pill for the rest of his or her life.

Rich Gaspari, one of the most ripped men in bodybuilding, says, "I never use cut-up drugs like thyroxin. They just rev up the metabolism and wear you down. I cut up by training extra hard while reducing calories."

INSULIN AND ADRENALINE

Both these drugs are taken to speed up the normal metabolic rate. This helps the body to lose fat, but as with thyroxin, taking them is potentially lethal.

Insulin and adrenaline are related drugs. Insulin enhances the uptake of glucose and potassium by the tissues, while adrenaline stimulates glucose metabolism in the cells. There are legitimate medical uses for these drugs, but healthy iron pumpers using them to lose weight risk disturbing their own metabolic functioning.

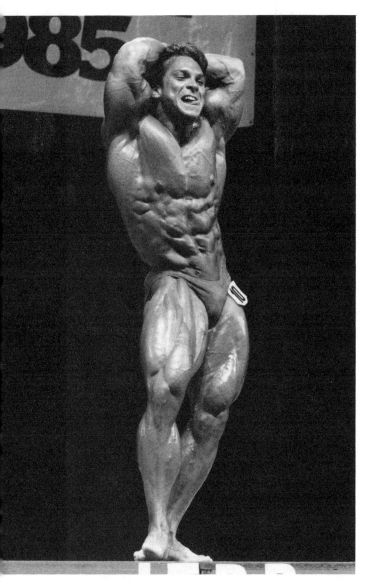
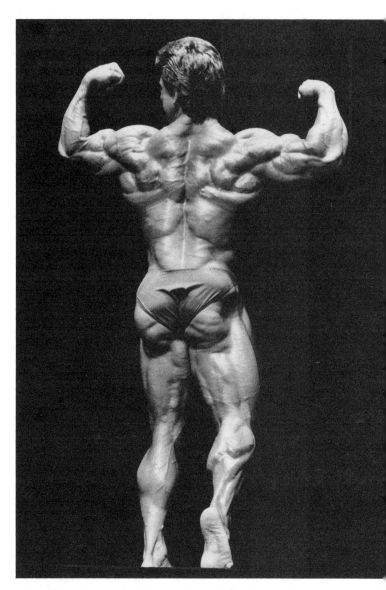

Rich Gaspari: "I never use cut-up drugs like thyroxin. . . . I cut up by training extra hard while reducing calories."

ANABOLIC STEROIDS

It has been said that 80 percent of competitive shot putters, javeline throwers, weight lifters, discus throwers, and bodybuilders use these substances, which improve protein assimilation and increase muscle mass and strength. They also enhance the formation of large glycogen stores.

Dr. John Ziegler was the man who pioneered steroids use in America. He had noticed that the Soviet weight lifting team had suddenly increased their "totals" by substantial amounts as a result of using hormones. Ziegler then worked in co-operation with CIBA Pharmaceutical Company to develop anabolic steroids in the United States. They were administered to the U.S. weight lifting team (York Barbell Club) to help team members compete on an even ground with the Soviets. It wasn't long before every athlete who required additional strength was talking about the new

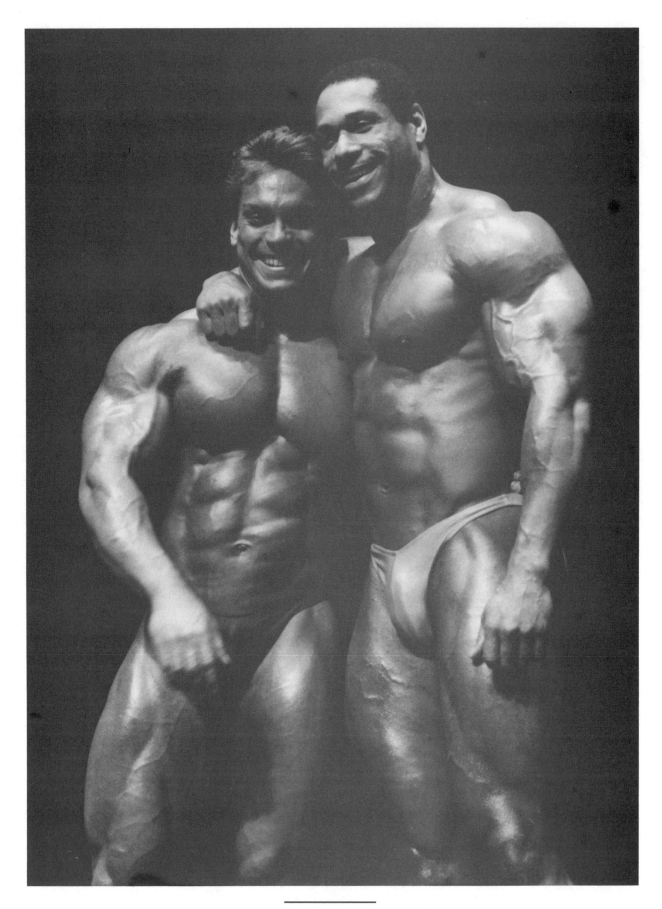

wonder drugs. Football players took them, basketball players, bodybuilders…A survey of thirty-eight track and field athletes and weight lifters at UCLA discovered that fully half of them had taken or were taking anabolic steroids. In many cases the amounts consumed were up to four times the prescribed therapeutic doses. (The normal recommended daily dose is 2 to 10 milligrams.)

I recall reading in *Sports Illustrated* years ago that all the strength athletes were taking steroids. The magazine reported that most of the top men in track and field had either publicly or privately admitted to having used these drugs. According to *Sports Illustrated,* this list included Randy Matson, the 1968 Olympic champion and world record holder in the shotput; Dallas Long, the 1964 Olympic shotput champion; and Hal Connolly, the 1956 Olympic champion in the hammer throw. So we can see that athletes were using steroids way back in the fifties.

Several old-time bodybuilders have told me that they took testosterone and other synthesized hormone supplements way back in the late forties and early fifties. Among them are several Mr. America, Mr. Universe, and Mr. U.S.A. title winners. (They did not give me permission to divulge their names so I will respect the confidentiality of their statements.)

Today steroid use by athletes of all types is rampant. Sadly, the use of steroids is not limited to professionals and college athletes but has spread to the high school athlete.

The athlete himself is not always to blame. Coaches, friends, and drug pushers have ways of persuading…The main selling point, of course, is the promise of winning as opposed to the misery of losing. I have personally known scores of bodybuilders who did not want to take steroids but were nagged into taking them by coaches and friends. Numerous women have been talked into "just trying a little" by boyfriends who wanted them to harden up via the shortcut of synthesized male hormones.

Do steroids work for the bodybuilder? Yes, when used in conjunction with a relatively high-protein diet and a high-intensity progressive training routine. The gains steroids give you are far more than the much touted 10 percent figure. Steroids give you size that you would never get from normal training. They add strength, chase fat away, and give you a vastly improved recuperative ability. They add vascularity and even allow you to train longer with less fatigue.

It is generally accepted today that the androgenic formulations (containing testosterone) are more risky than anabolic steroids that have had most of the androgenic properties removed. Testosterone was available in injectable water-based form already in the early part of this century. It was the first anabolic (tissue-building) drug. It is still used by bodybuilders today—but should not be, because the side effects are potentially devastating. Dr. Fred Hatfield ("Dr. Squat"), an expert on steroids and related drugs, states, "Testosterone is to be avoided. True, it adds some size and strength, but this is temporary and potentially dangerous because of the high androgenic quality. Far better the aspiring bodybuilding champ who wants to build dense, long-lasting muscle cells use good nutrition and quality training patterns. There is considerable empirical evidence that low-androgenic/high-anabolic drugs increase myofibrils most efficiently, particularly when applied with a planned, long-term approach to bodybuilding drug use."

Among oral anabolics, Anavar is considered one of the least androgenic. Where injectables are concerned, the least androgenic are Deca-Durobolin, Winstrol, Primobolin, and a veterinarian drug called Equipoise, developed for use with horses.

Bodybuilders who *continually* take steroids run the risk of shutting down their own body's natural hormone supply and delivery systems. It is far less dangerous to take a four- to six-week program under a qualified doctor's supervision—the doctor can test to see if you are a genetically suitable candidate for a steroid program, and then he can monitor your condition with regular blood tests.

Yes, steroids work for the bodybuilder. Don't let anyone tell you it's just a placebo effect. They could legitimately be described as miracle drugs—

Platform buddies: Rich Gaspari and Mike Christian.

if they didn't have the reputation for side effects such as those already mentioned. Steroids can also aggravate and stimulate the growth of any preexisting cancers or hormone-sensitive tumors. Gynecomastia (breast development) is another likelihood. In women the effects lean toward overall masculinization, much of it irreversible.

At a top contest for men that I recently observed, seven out of eighteen competitors showed evidence of gynecomastia, commonly known among bodybuilders as "bitch tits."

Today the IFBB under the auspicies of President Ben Weider is testing for drugs in most of the important contests. This was first initiated by the IFBB in 1985, at that year's Ms. Olympia contest, a brave step in view of the fact that the athletes may well have chosen to leave IFBB ranks to compete in contests run by other orga-

nizations who do not impose drug testing on their athletes. Fortunately, because the IFBB is well organized and has built up a good reputation, this did not happen. The best men and women bodybuilders are still to be found in IFBB organizations.

The only problem with drug testing is that it is not quite foolproof. The tests today can only go back so far. Those who take drugs and stop a couple of months before being tested can often "beat" the tests. There are also so-called "blockers," which can mask a steroid that would otherwise be picked up by traditional tests. I have personally heard athletes boasting after a contest about beating the test. It made me sick, because a competitor who did not take steroids was robbed of a trophy as a result of a cheat's deviousness.

IFBB president Ben Weider looks on as Rich consoles his training buddy.

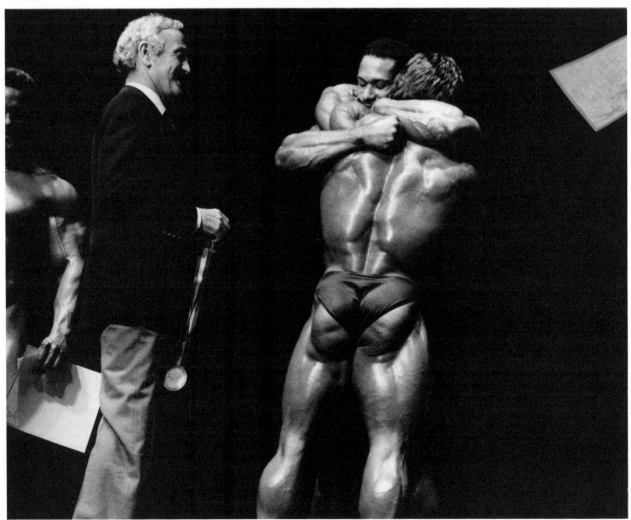

A heck of a lot of people seem to do very well on a vegetarian diet, yet curiously few bodybuilders are vegetarians. Bill Pearl, Roy Hilligen, Chuck Sipes, and Andreas Cahling come to mind. Most bodybuilders eat meat, the more the better, sometimes up to six times daily, ingesting as much as 300 to 400 grams of high-quality protein each day. "Way too much," says Bill Pearl. "A growing bodybuilder just doesn't need that much protein, and he or she can do very well without any meat whatsoever."

Actually, vegetarianism comes and goes. One decade it's popular. The next it's passé. Right now, as we close off the century, it is enjoying renewed growth. Today most people don't have the willpower to live an entirely meatless life, even if they wanted to. But a growing number of *semi*vegetarians—people who eat less meat and more vegetables—are becoming a decisive force in shaping the nation's taste in food. And it's possible that their way of eating may be the healthiest of all.

There are three categories of vegetarians. *Vegans* are those who eat *only* vegetables and fruits—no animals, animal products, or animal by-products whatsoever. *Lacto-vegetarians* include milk and milk products in with their vegetables. *Lacto-ovo-vegetarians* go one step further and include eggs with their milk and vegetables.

All four top bodybuilders just mentioned—Pearl, Hilligen, Cahling, and Sipes—take milk and milk products in their diets, so they are not true vegans. They do ingest animal products and by-products. None of these men is lacking in muscle size. The fact that they do not eat meat cannot be seen by studying their bodies. Bill Pearl says that veteran bodybuilder Steve Reeves is almost a vegetarian. "I never saw him eat much meat. Whenever I ate with him he seemed to prefer eating salads, avocados, fresh fruits, vegetables, plus some occasional milk products." Reeves himself has reported that during his competitive days he ate *lots of protein-high gelatin,* which he obtained from health food stores.

Roy Hilligen at fifty-eight years of age.

14
VEGETARIANISM
It's Your Choice

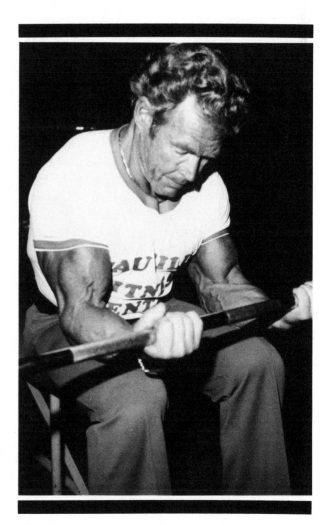

Dr. Peter J. Van Soest, from the division of Nutritional Sciences at Cornell University, says, "We were most likely meant to dine mainly on food derived from plants." This is probably true, but there also appears to be some benefit, especially to the hard-training bodybuilder, in including some meat in the diet. Even Bill Pearl admits that when he wants to get into his best contest shape he will make a conscious decision to include some meat in his diet for a few weeks in order to maximize development. Pearl, incidentally, became a vegetarian while conditioning astronauts for NASA. "One day—just as a lark—the doctor checked my cholesterol level. It was 307, an unbelievably high level, so my blood was running almost as thick as soup. The doctor told me that I could just as easily keel over at fifty from high cholesterol as anyone else, even though I was in great shape physically. He got me thinking. I trained and won the 1967 Mr. Universe contest and then decided to change my eating habits. I thought that I would lose a lot of muscle size by not eating meat, but this didn't happen at all. I became *lacto-vegetarian,* felt much better, almost immediately. My cholesterol levels went down to normal (198) and my blood pressure was markedly lowered. I'm in better shape now approaching sixty than I was in my twenties."

Roy Hilligen enjoys life almost more than any other bodybuilder I know. He has been Mr. America, Mr. South Africa, and Mr. Canada...Amazing, isn't it? He also won Mr. World, which, considering his traveling habits, seems quite appropriate! Roy lived just up the road from me for several years, and I occasionally spent time with him while he was training...or eating. He loved fruits and vegetables and would take his share of milk and milk products, but he never consumed meat. His training output at fifty-eight years of age was stunning. When he went to the squat racks and loaded up, the entire gym held its breath. Everyone had to watch, perhaps to convince themselves that what they were seeing was real. Roy would end up squatting a dozen reps with nearly 500 pounds—awesome, especially for a man who declines to eat meat.

It is generally considered that any type of strength athlete should eat other animals to be truly strong. Current evidence does not seem to

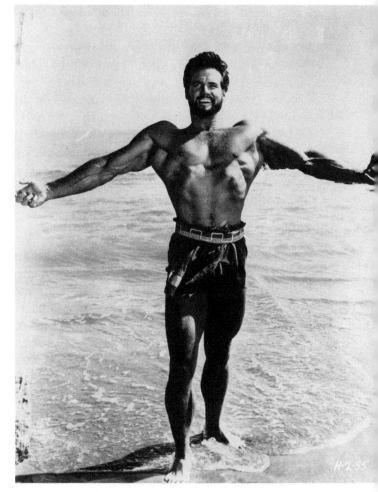

Bodybuilder and star of the silver screen Steve Reeves.

support this theory, however. What does seem likely is that a bodybuilder may not be able to make it to the very top on a pure vegetarian (vegan) diet. Most who do turn toward vegetarianism are lacto-ovo-vegetarians—they include eggs, milk, and milk products in their diet.

At age fifty-five, after several years as a lacto-vegetarian, Bill Pearl, who won the Mr. America contest and four Mr. Universe contests, said, "Today my energy levels are incredible, and I feel like a million dollars all the time. There's nobody I've trained with whom I couldn't stay up with in a hard workout. My energy is greater than ever, and they don't need to knock off fifteen cows a year to keep me fed!"

Ron J. Goodman, writing in *Iron Man* magazine, debates the concept of whether a competitive bodybuilder can be a vegetarian. "One unsupported opinion often expressed by vegetarians is that, yes, an individual with potential to achieve a championship physique will achieve it just as readily on a vegetarian diet as on the more normal high-protein diet. Oh yeah? Really? Let's see the evidence for the opinion. Show me one such champion!"

Actually, Goodman goes on to challenge readers to produce *any* champion in *any* sport that's not pure endurance who is also a true vegetarian. "They're all lacto-ovo-vegetarians; and eggs and milk are known to have higher quality protein than even meat, so what's the big deal?"

The record shows that those athletes who have tried true vegetarianism, eating nothing that doesn't grow in or from the ground, fall miserably short in their overall performance lev-

Andreas Cahling of Sweden, another champion lacto-vegetarian.

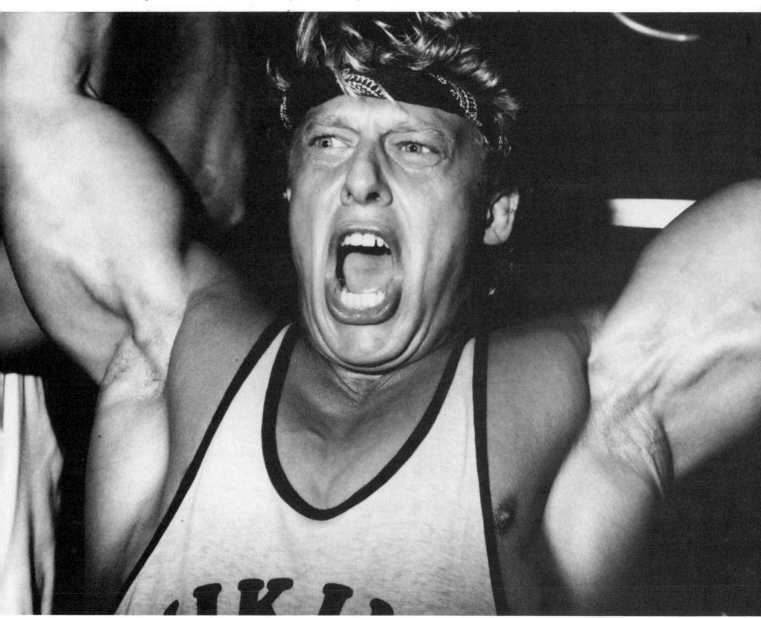

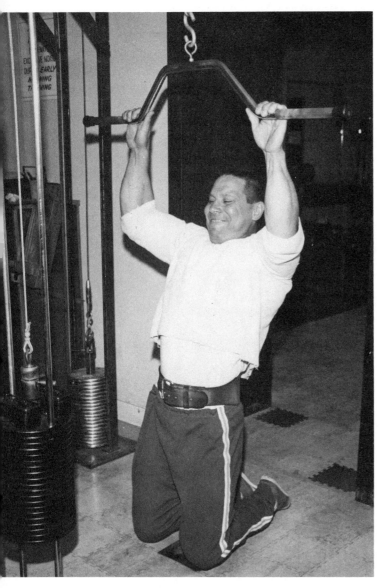

Bill Pearl, a champion lacto-vegetarian.

els. They are forced to dispense with their ideals and either return to meat or else to take a compensatory approach and adopt a "fleshless diet" that allows for the consumption of milk and eggs. A few allow themselves milk only.

Many vegetarians try to prove the value of vegetarianism by observing that horses and cows and gorillas are vegetarians, yet at the same time possess massive muscle development with enormous strength to boot! What they fail to comprehend is that the farm animals have more than one stomach and cannot even loosely be compared to human beings in any physical sense. As for gorillas, they are constantly eating worms, insects, rodents . . . anything they can catch, and all animal protein. They also steal eggs from bird nests whenever the opportunity arises. Ask any zoo keeper and he will tell you that gorillas will steal and eat whatever flesh food they can get when the opportunity presents itself.

Getting back to Ron Goodman, here is more of what he has to say: "Vegetarians always imply, and sometimes state, that you can get all the protein you need from a vegetable diet. Now, it's pretty generally agreed in bodybuilding circles that you need about one gram of protein per pound of body weight daily on which to build muscle. A 170-pound athlete can get 170 grams of protein by eating 2 pounds of beef chuck, lean and fat, weighed raw without the bone. Or . . . he can eat 12.88 pounds of raw, shelled chestnuts, 16.96 pounds of broccoli, 35.34 pounds of cauliflower, 55.70 pounds of celery, 15.60 pounds of green peas, 26.50 pounds of lettuce. Which would you prefer?"

Actually, you would have to eat more than the above amounts of vegetables to get the equivalent of meat because the vegetable proteins are of a poorer quality and have a protein efficiency ratio (P.E.R.) of well below 100 percent.

True vegetarians often state that the elements (micronutrients) not available in their vegetable-based diets can be manufactured or somehow transmuted from their food intake. Scientists have no hard evidence of this. Natural law dictates that changing one element into another by any chemical process is a flat impossibility. It just can't happen.

It seems to me that there is a movement toward eating less meat today. I agree in principle with the practice of eating fewer land animals. It may well be a healthy trend. On the other hand, judging from the evidence, the bodybuilder would be ill-advised to adopt a *true* vegetarian diet. You can be one of the growing millions who are eating less meat and more vegetables. You may even want to drop all flesh entirely. But it could be a mistake to try for pure vegetarianism. Only 3.7 percent of Americans consider themselves to be vegetarians, and of those only a fraction of 1 percent are purists. In the bodybuilding world of champions that percentage is currently . . . zero!

oday we see more confusion about the foods we eat than ever before. There are scores of books on the subject. Read them all and you will be even more confused. Almost everyone recommends a different approach to eating. And even if you are able to sort out the reasonable from the ridiculous, you still face the problem of adjusting your present eating habits so that you are not only eating what's good for you but at the same time avoiding what's bad for you.

This is particularly important for the bodybuilder, who cannot afford to eat foods that do not contribute to progress in a positive way.

15
TEN BEST, TEN WORST
Foods to Build On, Foods to Avoid

THE TEN BEST FOODS FOR BODYBUILDERS

Well, there's no time like the present. I have rounded up what I consider the ten best foods to maximize your health and to put you to your all-time peak of readiness so that your training will not be wasted. These foods actively promote health and well-being. They ready your constitution for the building of the ultimate body. Here's my list of the ten best foods:

The Orange

Plus-value: vitamin C, fruit fiber

Not to be confused with orange juice, which is most definitely *not* the same as eating an orange with all its fibrous qualities and added goodness. Orange juice is absorbed too quickly and has more concentrated sugar, so does not provide a sustained energy release. Oranges

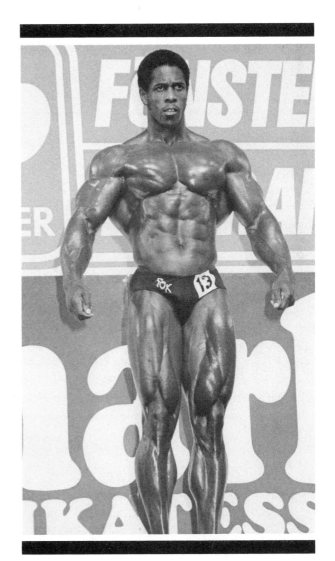

Bertil Fox, England.

also have the added bonuses of potassium and calcium, two very important nutrients for the bodybuilder.

Qualities per 5½-ounce orange

Protein	1.1	grams
Carbohydrates	13	grams
Fat	.16	gram
Vitamin A	270	I.U.
Vitamin B$_1$	.1	milligram
Vitamin C	67	milligrams
Calcium	52	milligrams
Potassium	235	milligrams
Magnesium	13	milligrams
Calories	58	

Whole-Wheat Bread

Plus-value: carbohydrates and fiber

Formerly known as the staff of life, good unadulterated bread is still one of our best foods. It was once considered fattening, but, made with whole-grain flours in natural unrefined form, it is an excellent source of carbohydrates, the chief source of fuel supplying energy for all physical functions—breathing, digestion, assimilation, walking, sitting, weight training, etc. Because of its natural fiber and bulkiness, whole-wheat bread takes a goodly amount of time to digest, which helps to promote balanced blood sugar levels, necessary for good health. It also results in sustained release of energy, vital to the bodybuilder who needs additional stamina for workouts.

Qualities per slice of whole-wheat bread

Protein	3	grams
Carbohydrates	15	grams
Fat	1	gram
Vitamin B$_1$	.06	gram
Vitamin B$_2$	.1	milligram
Niacin, a B vitamin	1	gram
Calcium	15	milligrams
Phosphorus	60	milligrams
Iron	0.7	gram
Calories	72	

The Potato

Plus-value: complex carbohydrates

For a long time potatoes have had a "bad guy" image. This is because traditionally they have been fried in fat or eaten with either sour cream or butter, all of which catapulted their calorie rating through the sky. Today almost everyone believes that potatoes will make you fat, when in reality they are an excellent food with only moderate calories (a 4-ounce potato has only 82 calories).

In addition to being a wonderful source of bodybuilding carbohydrate, potatoes supply loads of minerals. Maximum advantage is gained if you eat your potatoes baked in their (fiber) skins. Don't fry or roast them in fat.

Qualities per 4-ounce potato

Protein	2.12	grams
Carbohydrates	17.4	grams
Fat	.2	gram
Niacin, a B vitamin	1.5	milligrams
Vitamin C	16.5	milligrams
Magnesium	40	milligrams
Potassium	417	milligrams
Phosphorus	53	milligrams
Calories	82	

Turkey

Plus-value: low in fat, high in protein

Turkey, chicken, and other poultry meats generally contain substantial levels of tryptophan, an essential amino acid and a precursor to the brain neurotransmitter serotonin. Serotonin can actually control (stimulate or inhibit) nerve impulses in the brain, invariably acting to calm overactivity. Studies have shown that serotonin can also improve concentration, memory, judgment, and overall thinking ability. Frank Zane supplements his diet with tryptophan, which he calls his tranquility formula. It helps him relax and sleep better at night, relieving him of nervous tension.

Four ounces of white meat poultry delivers about 27 grams of high-class protein (amino acids), which is about as much as the body can assimilate at any one feeding.

Needless to say, a naturally raised turkey that

Samir Bannout and Frank Zane compare biceps at the IFBB Mr. Olympia contest.

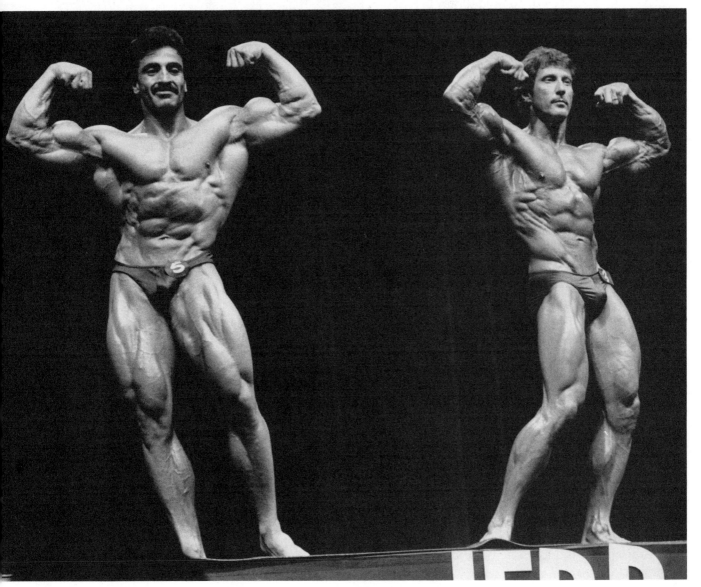

scratches around in the earth for its food (or at least is fed natural grains) is far superior to a closely caged bird that never sees the earth, feels the wind, or experiences natural light. The drugs and chemicals pumped and fed into the poor creatures raised in batteries of cages hardly make them suitable consumption for health-minded humans.

Turkey and other poultry are ideal both as meals and snacks for the bodybuilder. They are very low in fat, especially when the skin is taken off before cooking. The white meat (breast) has less fat and calories than the dark meat (legs and wings).

Qualities per 3 ounces of cooked turkey breast

Protein	20	grams
Carbohydrates		trace
Fat (unsaturated)	.30	gram
(saturated)	.69	gram
Vitamin B_6	.49	milligram
Vitamin B_{12}	.34	microgram
Niacin, a B vitamin	9.33	milligrams
Iron	.65	milligram
Potassium	210	milligrams
Phosphorus	164	milligrams
Calories	102	

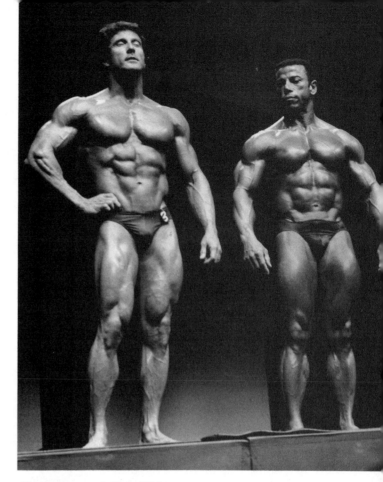

Frank Zane and Chris Dickerson.

Broccoli

Plus-value: vitamin A, low in calories

Yes, broccoli is a sensational source of vitamin A. One cup provides almost 80 percent of the suggested daily adult requirement. Vitamin A keeps the liver in good condition, helps maintain perfect eye function, and supplies the body's immune system with essential nutrients. Broccoli also contains vitamin C, essential for proper tissue repair and maintenance and, in tandem with vitamin A, thought to help in cancer prevention.

Broccoli can be cooked and eaten with meat or fish, or it can be used raw in salads, as a side dish, or as a mixed salad main dish. Broccoli is extremely low in calories, so it becomes a popular item during the precontest countdown period, when you are doing your best to rip up those hard-earned muscles. Consume both the stems and the flower when eating broccoli.

Qualities per cup of broccoli (steamed)

Protein	4.7	grams
Carbohydrates	7	grams
Fat	.5	gram
Vitamin A	3,800	I.U.
Niacin, a B vitamin	1.2	milligrams
Vitamin C	140	milligrams
Calcium	136	milligrams
Potassium	414	milligrams
Iron	1.2	milligrams
Calories	40	

Sole

Plus-value: high in protein, unsaturated fat

Health research indicates that sole and similar flat fish (flounder, plaice) contain high amounts of eicosapentanoic acid (EPA), a fatty acid that helps improve general health by enhancing the state of the cardiovascular system and helping to control levels of blood fats.

Flat fish provide lower levels of potentially dangerous saturated fats and higher levels of the better unsaturated fats than red meats or even chicken and turkey. It is an excellent source of bodybuilding protein, so necessary for tissue repair after strenuous training. Five ounces supply a full 25 grams of protein.

Qualities per 4 ounces of steamed fillet

Protein	20	grams
Carbohydrates	0	
Fat (unsaturated)	.63	gram
(saturated)	.31	gram
Vitamin B_{12}	1.3	micrograms
Niacin, a B vitamin	1.9	milligrams
Pantothenic acid, a B vitamin	.96	milligram
Phosphorus	220	milligrams
Iron	.9	milligram
Potassium	385	milligrams
Calories	92	

Milk

Plus-value: high in calcium and phosphorus

Calcium is vital for perfectly functioning muscles, and phosphorus is needed for nearly all metabolic processes including muscle contractions. Everyone needs calcium to maintain bone mass. This is especially true of women over forty and athletes of all ages. Bodybuilders in particular need strong bones. What adults do not require is the high fat content found in whole milk. Fat-free milk (99 percent fat-free) is usually ideal. There is still enough fat for nutrient absorption (especially of the fat-soluble vitamins A and D) and also high levels of the carbohydrates and protein needed for muscular growth.

Qualities per 8-ounce glass

Protein	8.3	grams
Carbohydrates	11.7	grams
Fat	1	gram
Vitamin A	500	I.U.
Vitamin B_2	.4	milligram
Vitamin D	100	I.U.
Calcium	295	milligrams
Magnesium	33	milligrams
Phosphorus	232	milligrams
Calories	104	

The Bran Muffin

Plus-value: fiber and energy

Probably Mike Mentzer is most responsible for "bringing back" the bran muffin. Wheat bran boasts a healthy amount of cellulose, the natural fiber so important for intestinal fitness. Serum cholesterol levels can also be kept at their proper levels by regularly eating bran muffins. They can be eaten at any time of the day—breakfast, lunch, or dinner, or as an in-between snack.

Muffins made with white flour and loaded with sugar are not an acceptable substitute for whole-wheat, natural grain muffins, especially if the latter include raisins, nuts, or seeds, all of which add different types of fiber. It may be a good idea to bake your own. (Muffin recipes are included in this book.)

Qualities per 3-ounce muffin

Protein	6.2	grams
Carbohydrates	34.4	grams
Fat	7.7	grams
Vitamin A	185	I.U.
Vitamin B$_2$	.2	milligram
Niacin, a B vitamin	3.1	milligrams
Calcium	114	milligrams
Potassium	345	milligrams
Iron	3	milligrams
Calories	200	

The Banana

Plus-value: potassium

Bananas can be eaten raw by themselves or mixed in with fresh fruit salads to make a perfect snack and dessert. They are ideal in that they are high in natural carbohydrates and extremely rich in potassium, one of the body's most important elements, found in each and every cell. Potassium provides a counterbalancing action with sodium and is directly connected to proper fluid balance and overall muscle tone. Potassium is used extensively by the world's top bodybuilders during their last week prior to competition.

A banana a day, whether sliced in a bowl of whole-grain cereal, added to a protein drink, or merely peeled and eaten whole, is a super idea for all enthusiastic bodybuilders. It's great for you.

Qualities per 6-ounce banana (weighed with skin)

Protein	1.18	grams
Carbohydrates	26.7	grams
Fat	.54	gram
Vitamin B$_6$	.64	gram
Biotin, a B vitamin	6	micrograms
Vitamin C	10	milligrams

Iron	.35	milligram
Potassium	451	milligrams
Magnesium	33	milligrams
Calories	100	

The Mushroom

Plus-value: low-calorie nutrition

Although a few people are allergic to the mushroom family, it is rich in essential food components and a plus for most bodybuilders. But eat mushrooms with caution if you are sensitive to yeasted foods in general.

Like carrots and celery, mushrooms are wonderful to munch on as snacks or to include in a big (or small) salad bowl. They make fine additions to clear soups or steamed vegetarian dishes, although they do not take as long to cook as other vegetables.

Most people find that mushrooms (the most common is the white mushroom) provide pleasant-tasting nourishment for the body, but their real value is for the calorie-restricted dieter who wants high nutrition together with low calories. Like the banana, mushrooms are relatively high in potassium.

Qualities per cup of mushrooms (uncooked)

Protein	1.9	grams
Carbohydrate	3.1	grams
Fat		trace
Niacin, a B vitamin	2.9	milligrams
Biotin, a B vitamin	11.2	milligrams
Vitamin C	2	milligram
Copper	1.97	milligrams
Potassium	290	milligrams
Zinc	.91	milligram
Calories	21	

Sue Ann McKean.

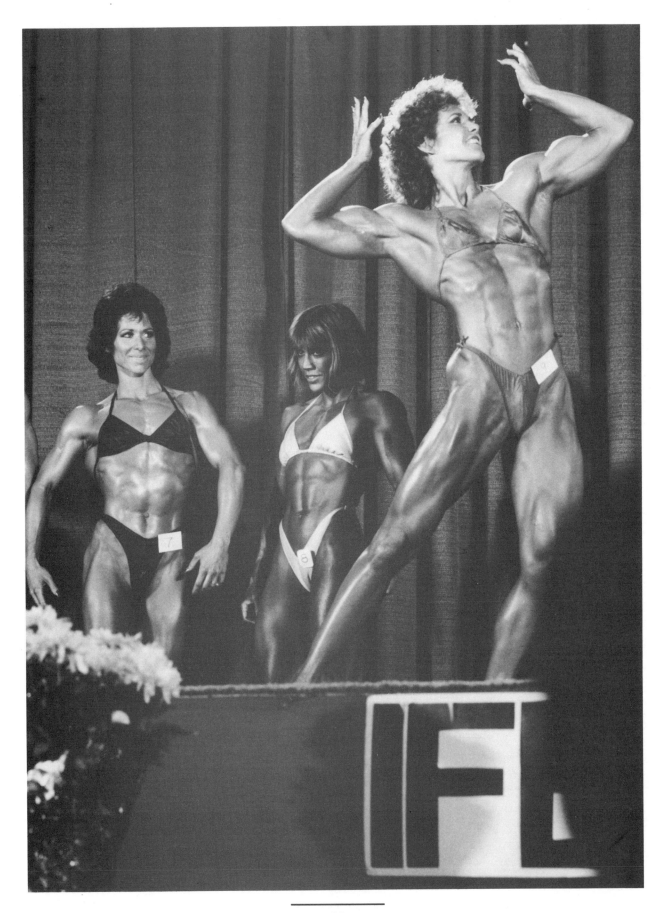

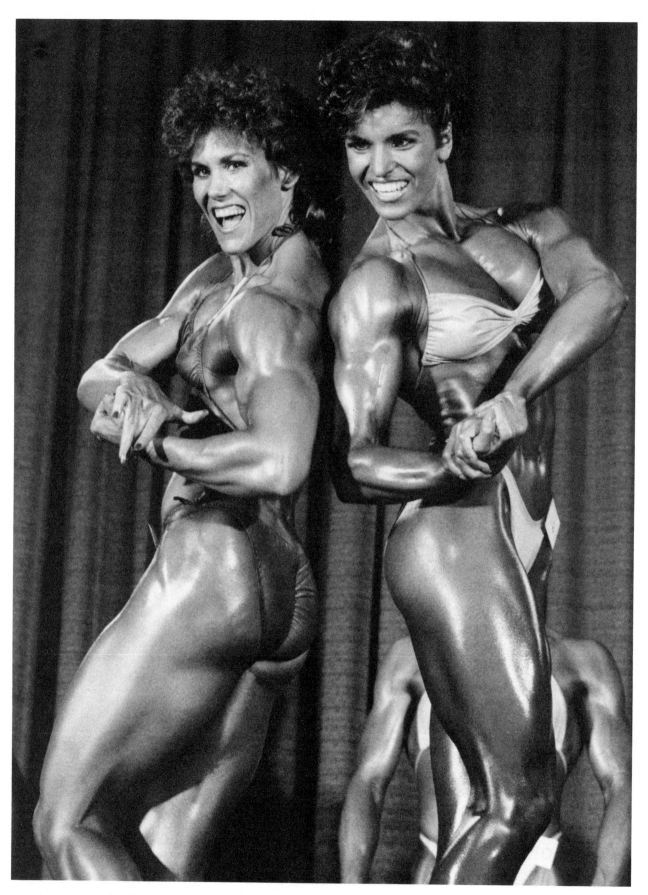

Sue Ann poses off against Marjo Selin at the 1986 Women's World Championships.

Did you expect "miracle foods" among my top ten? Disappointed that every item I listed was entirely known to you? Well, believe it or not, I would love to have listed special unknown, exciting, hard-to-find foods for you; it would have made this chapter the talk of the town—"Kennedy's secret list of rare foods that will make you a champion overnight." But somewhere along the line I would be challenged. That's why I gave you the honest truth. Ordinary as they may seem, these foods really are the superstars of the nutrition arena.

It all reminds me of the Swedish bodybuilder who journeyed to California to watch Bertil Fox train. He was breathless with anticipation as he climbed the stairs of World's Gym on Ocean Boulevard in Venice. When Fox came to the gym floor to commence his workout, our enthusiastic friend's heart almost stopped. But as the British giant went through his workout, the Swedish man's mouth dropped open not with astonished awe but with uncontrolled disappointment. Fox's training consisted of squats, bench presses, curls, presses behind neck, dips, and bent over rowing. "He just trains with ordinary basic exercise," said the Swede. "I thought he would have some special secret exercises that he uses to get so big!"

THE TEN WORST FOODS

Who hasn't succumbed to the temptation of a chocolate bar, piece of fudge, or candy at a checkout counter in a convenience store and bought it, knowing full well that it would do nothing positive for your health, fitness, or appearance? You know it's not good for you, but you do it all the same. Paradoxically, your "just this once" excuse has been used scores of times previously. You act in spite of yourself.

I could have included rich desserts and synthetic pastries, imitation meats, and thousand-calorie-dense foods in this "bad news" category, but the limit is ten, and they didn't (couldn't) make it! The so-called foods that did make the list have in common a high degree of processing that obliterates almost all nutritional value that may have been present in the original ingredients. Also included in most of the items listed here are high amounts of preservatives, "fresheners," refined sugars, salts, fats, and artificial coloring agents. All bad news, folks!

The Food and Drug Administration (FDA) does monitor food ingredients used in our nutrients and approves virtually all ingredients currently being used. However, questions remain. Tests have shown that some ingredients being used today may be unsafe for human consumption. Saccharin, for example, was to have been banned way back in 1977, but that ban has been indefinitely postponed due to pressure brought about by powerful food industry groups. Nitrites, too, were to have been phased out of bacon, sausage, ham, and other cured meats in the late 1970s. Again, because of food industry pressure the phase-out was put on hold. It seems the food industry doesn't mind slowly poisoning us as long as they make the big bucks. I wonder if their company directors eat their own junk? I wouldn't think they make a habit of it, would you?

If you are concerned with health and maximum performance, avoid the following foods as much as possible. Not all are devastatingly unhealthy, but they aren't going to *promote* ultimate health, vitality, and peak performance, that's for sure. And in the long run, especially if you are one of those who are genetically unable to cope with the additives and changes in composition brought about by overprocessing, it could spell the end of the road to the Olympia.

The Doughnut

Minus-value: additives, including artificial color and chemical preservatives

There's virtually nothing but bad news when you read the label of almost any commercially packaged doughnut. Doughnuts are usually kept

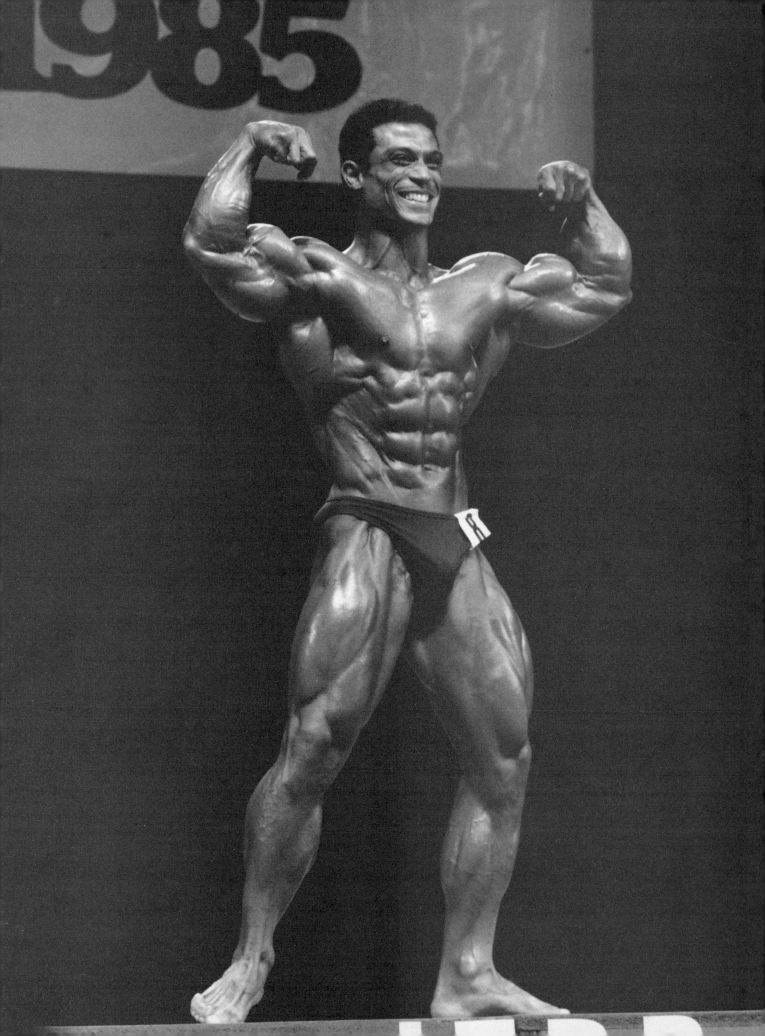

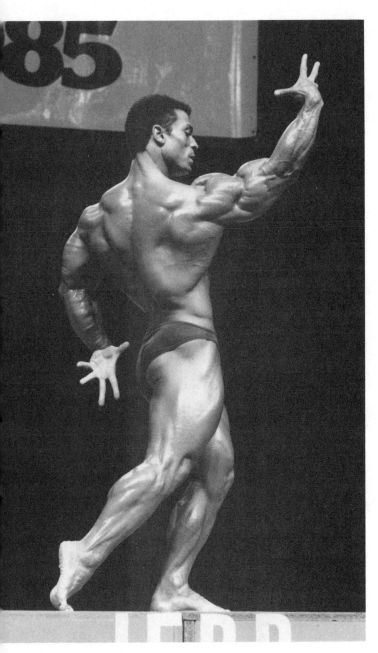

Canada's fabulous Mohamed Makkawy.

tumor formation and cellular membrane damage. These findings were reported by the Environmental Health Perspective, and similar conclusions were drawn by the Oak Ridge National Laboratory; Loyola University concluded that there is a possibility of neurological effects resulting in altered behavior patterns. England and Japan have already banned BHT, but it is still considered safe in the United States.

Alternative: whole-grain muffin or raisin bran

Bacon

Minus-value: nitrites, sugar, fat

Many people never have breakfast without bacon. It's the accepted starter for most North Americans who bother to take more than coffee for their first meal of the day. After all, bacon is about 38 percent protein. But there's more. Fat is a main source of bacon's calories, and that brings cholesterol into the picture: 16 milligrams in the average three-strip serving. Then there's the curing process, involving salt-and-sugar processing (also used with corned beef and frankfurters), which is of increasing concern among nutritionists. Cancer research warns us daily of the dangers of eating salt-cured, salt-packed, smoked, high-fat foods like bacon.

Alternative: slice of lean fresh ham or beef

Sodas

Minus-value: sweeteners and other additives

Soda manufacturers are in a race to produce a noncaffeine formula that is both tasty and thirst quenching as well as 100 percent safe from potentially harmful ingredients. They may be fighting a losing battle. The artificial sweetener aspartame is gradually replacing saccharin,

"fresh" by the use of chemical agents designed to keep them spongy and soft. These include mono- and diglycerides, propylene glycol mono- and diesters, and vegetable gums. Coloring agents include FD&C yellow number 5, long suspected of causing allergy reactions, and preservatives such as BHT and BHA. Even though both of these are considered safe, in one 1983 test on animals BHT, for example, was found to cause

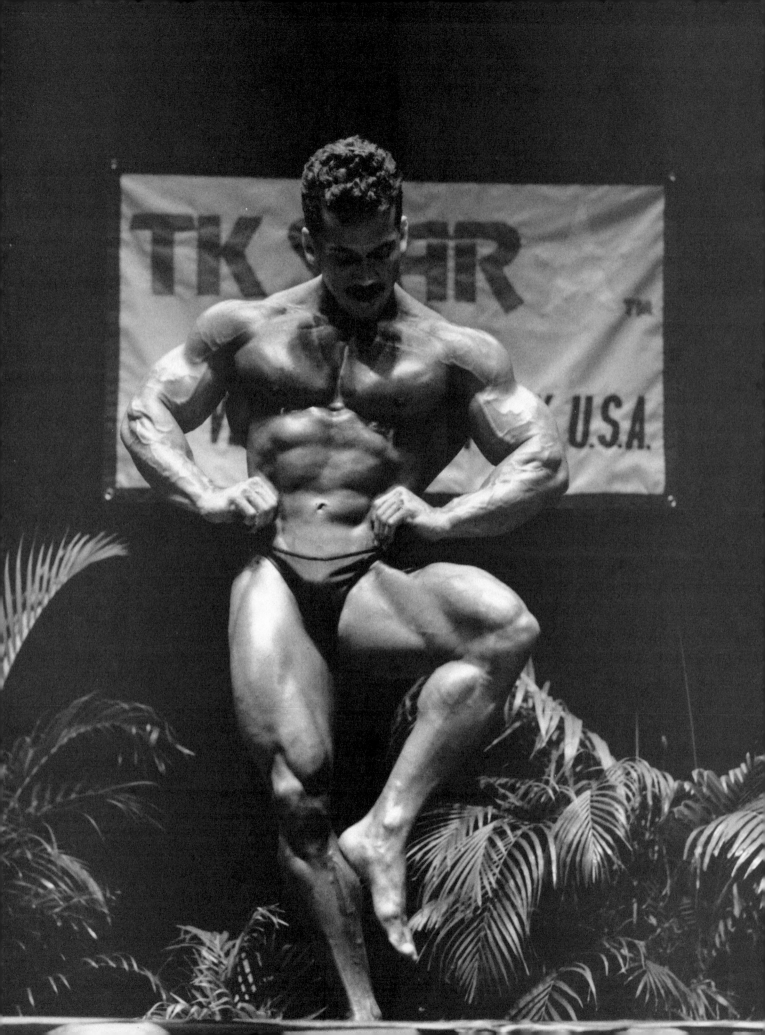

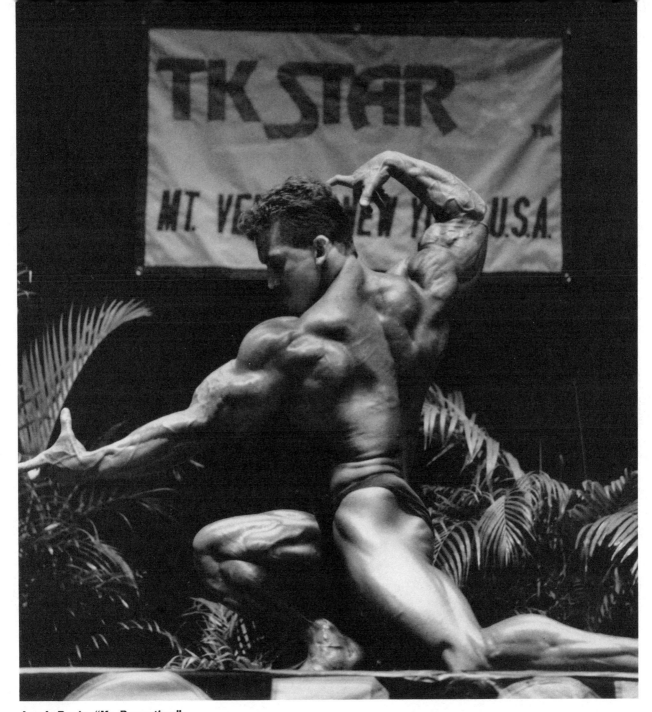

Lee LaBrada, "Mr. Proportion."

which can cause cancer under certain laboratory conditions. However, aspartame itself is now under study. Unfortunately, all sodas contain preservatives and other chemicals. In many cases the cans themselves could be the cause of unhealthy trace ingredients entering the body. Non-diet sodas usually contain an abundance of sugar and artificial flavors, and coloring agents are common in most varieties.

Alternative: plain mineral water with a twist of lime or lemon

Granola Bars

Minus-value: preservatives, sugars

Granola bars are usually high in oats, which sounds positively healthy. But invariably granola bars are high in sugars and fats as well, and they almost always contain preservatives that could be damaging to your health and well-being. Do

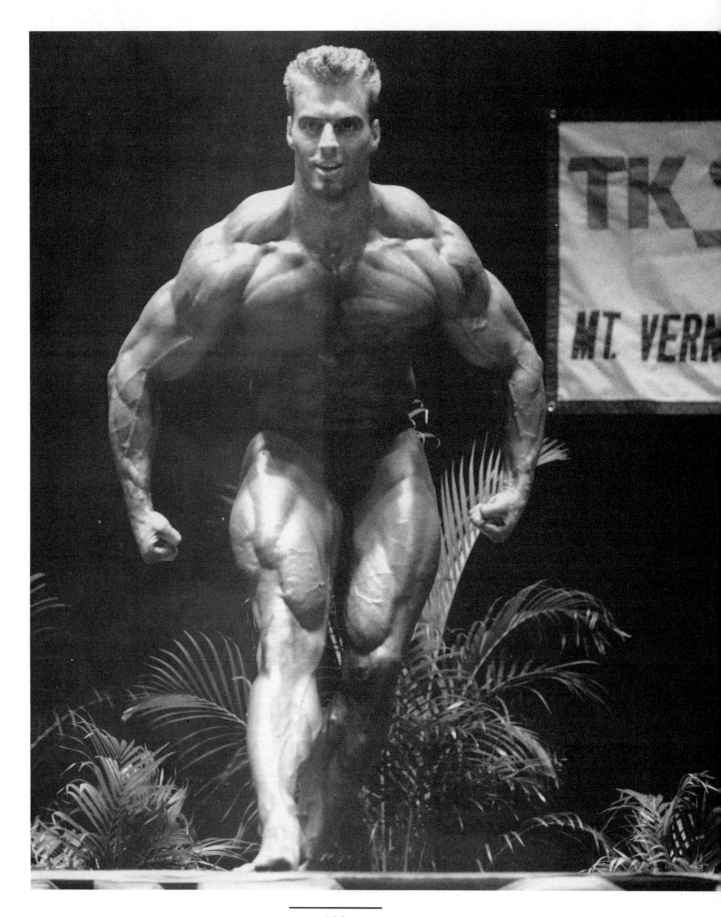

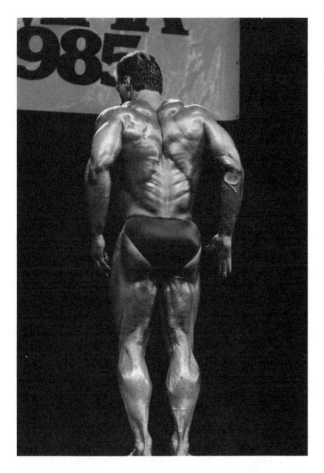

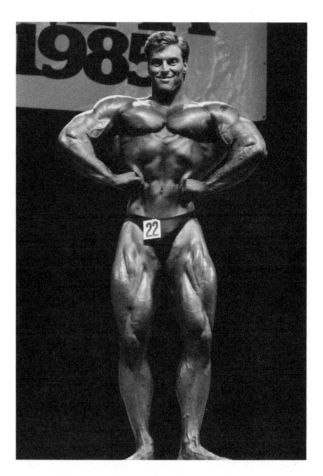

Awesome is the only apt description for Holland's Berry Demey.

not confuse granola bars with granola, a dry mixture of cereals, nuts, dried fruits, etc., that is often eaten with milk for breakfast.

Granola bars commonly contain sugar, corn syrup, corn-syrup solids, invert sugar, sorbitol, and the preservative BHA, suspected of causing allergic reactions.

Alternative: carrot muffin

bacterial contamination that could lead to food poisoning, have been linked to cancer. They combine with natural stomach juices to create carcinogenic nitrosamines. The American Institute of Cancer Research has identified the curing process as a health hazard. Furthermore, corned beef is usually full of chemicals, including monosodium glutamate, which can cause severe allergic reactions in some people.

Alternative: fresh roast beef

Corned Beef

Minus-value: sodium, nitrites, sugars, and additives

Corned beef, which is high in fat to start with, is also subjected to numerous chemicals in the curing process. Sodium nitrites, used to prevent

The Frankfurter

Minus-value: nitrites, sodium, sugars, and additives

If you thought the corned beef assessment was bad, add to the disadvantages listed for that product the frankfurter's flavor enhancers, including potentially unhealthy hydrolyzed vegetable protein. Cheap frankfurters add fillers to take the place of meat. Those dreaded nitrites are right here, too. Serious health problems could result over the long haul from any diet regularly incorporating frankfurters.

Alternative: whole-wheat turkey sandwich

Breakfast Cereals

Minus-value: added sugars, chemical preservatives

The billion-dollar breakfast cereal industry has probably spoiled more kids' teeth than almost anything else. Ironically, most people add sugar to the popular breakfast cereals, many of which are 50 percent sugar already! The only good thing about this devitalized junk is the milk that is taken with it. Don't be fooled by any added vitamins used to "enrich" the product. You still get sugar-loaded junk of very poor nutritional value, even if the advertising appears to suggest differently.

Alternative: whole-grain unsweetened cereal or homemade granola

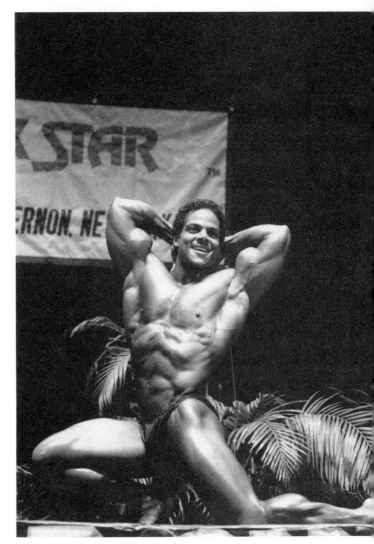

Sean Jenkins.

Artificial Fruit Drinks

Minus-value: sugars and artificial coloring and flavoring

Many of these drinks contain no real fruit, only chemicals that imitate the taste of fruit. The rest is sugar-loaded water or, in the case of diet drinks, chemical sweeteners. No protein is offered and the "simple" carbohydrate content is useless as a source of energy, which your body properly gets from natural complex carbohydrate sources. Artificial coloring agents are almost always used in these drinks.

Alternative: mixed fruits pureed in a blender, with water added to dilute to taste

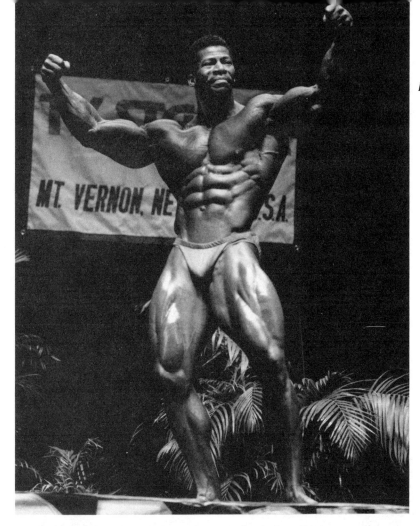

Ron Love.

Appi Steenbeek, Lary Leonard,
Berry DeMey, and Bob Birdsong.

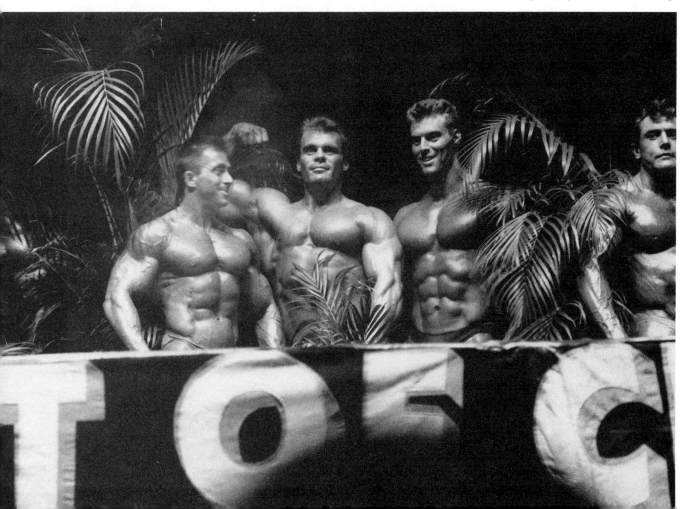

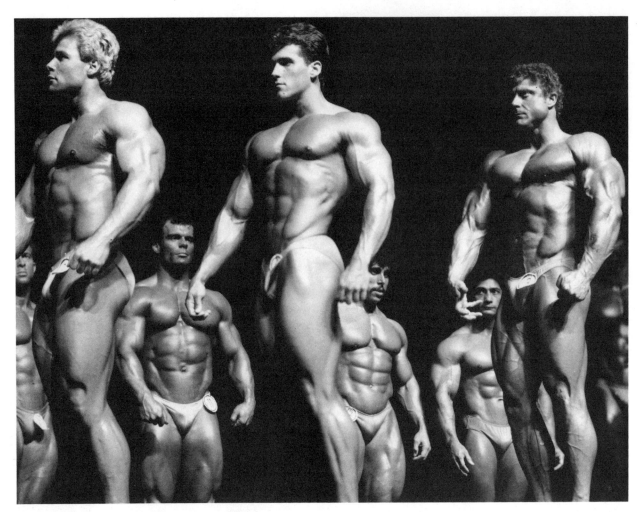

Dave Hawk, Bob Paris, and Frank Richards.

Potato Chips

Minus-value: sodium, fats

Far too high sodium content makes this snack food almost lethal, especially if you are predisposed to high blood pressure. One popular brand contains 680 milligrams of salt, compared to the 4 milligrams of sodium one finds in an average baked potato. In addition, most of the nutrition is burned out of this product. The bulk of the calories come from the refined oil used in the cooking process. Flavor additives are also widely used to enhance taste, since this is a very competitive product.

Alternative: plain unbuttered, unsalted popcorn

Cotton Candy/Candy Floss

Minus-value: dyes, sugar, chemicals

Another disgusting variety of calorie-dense, sugar-loaded foodless food, treacherously stacked with wild artificial colors to attract the buyer. Worse than marshmallows and candy (which are bad enough), this product should be avoided. The artificial flavors and colors used in it push it beyond the limits of food acceptability. Cotton candy is sold most commonly at fairs and tourist resorts, so chances to review a label listing its ingredients are rare.

Alternative: Nothing so disgusting as an alternative. Eat an apple instead.

16

BREAKFAST
The Nutritional Head Start

Answer this question honestly. Do you currently have a substantial well-balanced breakfast every day of the week? Probably not, if you're like most people. Yet nutritionists, physiologists, coaches, and dietitians unanimously stress the importance of breakfast. Scientific studies have shown that a good breakfast is mandatory for maximum mental and physical efficiency, and overall health is benefited as well. People who do not eat breakfast put themselves at a greater risk of illness than those who start the day with a comprehensive meal.

I'm constantly amazed when consulted by bodybuilders regarding their desire for better results to find that 80 percent of them miss having a decent breakfast. Not only is breakfast essential for those who want to gain mass; it is equally important for those wishing to lose weight. Missing meals, especially after a ten- to twelve-hour period with no food, forces your body to reduce its basic metabolic rate. Toronto nutritionist Rose Schwartz confirms: "Not eating slows your metabolic rate." People with already slow metabolisms wind up burning off calories even less quickly, which can lead to obesity.

Bodybuilders I have talked to miss breakfast for one of two reasons. They are either in such a hurry to get to work that they "just don't have the time," or they claim that eating first thing in the morning makes them feel sick—they either feel nauseated or have no appetite for food.

Being in a hurry to the extent you have to miss breakfast is bad planning. For the bodybuilder hoping for a career in the sport it's suicide.

I am firmly in favor of bodybuilders sleeping an extra thirty to sixty minutes on nights following heavy, vigorous workouts. I feel that our bodies tell us they want a little more sleep for recuperation, so whereas some people can exist happily with six or seven hours' sleep, most hard-training men and women I know are happier with seven and a half to eight hours each night. But still this should be no excuse for missing breakfast.

Juliette Bergman.

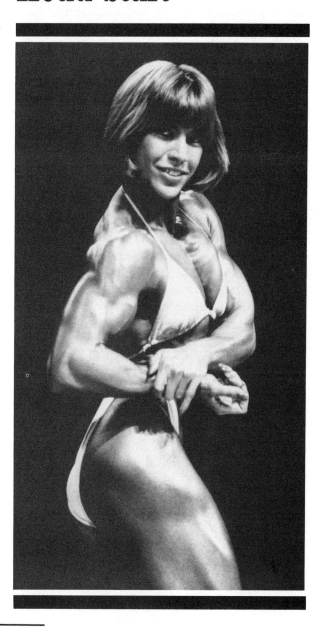

Often the "no time to eat" brigade chase off to school or work knowing that they will be able to grab coffee and a doughnut shortly after they arrive. My reaction, of course, is that coffee and a doughnut are *not* breakfast but nutritional sacrilege! The only thing worse would be coffee and a cigarette...and, believe me, there are millions who start their day with that health-destroying combination.

If it seems you can't get up in time enough to have breakfast, go to bed half an hour earlier. Set your alarm to get up a half hour earlier—and get up. No, you don't have to have a four course meal. If you can't get interested in cooking oatmeal or an omelette, then have a piece of fruit, a glass of skim milk, and whole-wheat toast with peanut butter. That's a well-balanced breakfast and it's not time-consuming to prepare. Just make sure you don't spread the peanut butter with a trowel.

Are you one of those people who just can't face food in the morning? Does the thought of scrambled egg that early turn your stomach? Dr. Harvey Anderson, chairman of the Nutrition and Food Sciences department of the University of Toronto, says, "This is a common complaint, epecially with obese people." Actually feeling nauseated in the mornings is often a result of poor eating and living habits. Face it, you are not going to feel bright and perky at the dawn of a new day if you eat poorly, smoke excessively, get drunk regularly, or go to bed too late.

Also, feeing sick or nauseated in the morning is often as much a psychological as a physiological problem—a habit. But the habit can be broken. Breakfast can make you feel nauseated simply because you are not used to it. Once you get used to it, you overcome the nausea. Your body adapts itself to breakfast—if you make a point of eating it. Why not start with some dry toast and a glass of milk? Gradually you can add other goodies—grapefruit, bananas, oats, eggs ...you name it.

I've found that most of the no-breakfast types really don't wake up properly. They are not wide awake and full of energy, so they don't eat breakfast. This leaves them in a semidepleted, lethargic state. Coffee becomes the standard wake-up ingredient, a poor substitute for a nutritional breakfast. Then when they decide to

eat something around midmorning, it's usually doughnuts and more coffee.

It is important that your breakfast include both complex carbohydrates and proteins. The combination will set you right for the rest of the day. Your blood sugar levels will stay high; you won't experience sudden drops that cause shaking, total loss of energy, etc. Above all, avoid sugar-rich breakfasts—frosted cereals, sugar-loaded tea or coffee, fruity-chocolaty breakfast bars. A poor, sugar-rich breakfast overstimulates the pancreas. Very shortly after a "sugar high" energy kick, the blood sugar level drops dramatically...to the point where you run out of fuel and energy. Statistics show that a person who grabs a regular coffee and a doughnut in the mornings actually feels hungrier within two hours than the person who has no breakfast at all.

The energy you receive from complex carbohydrates and proteins lasts longer and doesn't cause your pancreas to overreact. Your blood sugar levels stabilize. Today complex carbohydrates are enjoying a new popularity. Those high in fiber are superior. A good breakfast could include bran cereal or oatmeal (porridge), skim milk, low-fat yogurt, and whole-wheat toast. Instead of butter, use peanut butter, which is high in protein. Eggs, of course, are an excellent source of protein, although people on a low-fat diet or who are predisposed to high cholesterol levels in the blood should eat eggs only infrequently. Or, to avoid the high fat content of eggs, do as some bodybuilders do: Make a three- or four-egg omelette using only one or two of the yolks. (Since the egg's cholesterol content is also concentrated in its yolk, this is a good technique for restricting cholesterol intake, too.)

Remember that skipping breakfast is neither a good way to lose weight nor a workable way to bodybuild. Breakfast energy is vital. It sets you right for the day. As the late Adelle Davis used to say, "Eat breakfast like a king, lunch like a prince, and dinner like a pauper."

Dr. Michael Walczak, medical adviser to many California bodybuilders, concurs. "Breakfast must be our best meal. This is essential for bodybuilders." Walczak slams the average high-sugar American breakfast of eggs, bacon, cereal, toast, jam, orange juice, and coffee. "The blood sugar goes up within fifteen minutes. We get a quick energy boost, but this is followed by a sudden drop. We become listless, tired, and grouchy. We think we need a coffee break, Coke that refreshes, a doughnut, a cigarette, alcohol. All of these merely serve to whip a tired horse. They make the condition worse." At the end of the day we have run a gauntlet of unsatisfying pick-me-ups. By dinnertime we are famished and exhausted. We tend to eat big, watch television, and drag ourselves off to bed, hoping for a better tomorrow.

But when we eat protein and complex carbohydrates for breakfast and avoid the midmorning sugar traps, insulin is secreted gradually. It steadily drips into the bloodstream rather than suddenly gushing out and then stopping abruptly.

A normal blood sugar level is thus maintained for hours; we have a steady flow of energy and a sustained sense of well-being.

Modern day champion bodybuilders know the importance of a good breakfast, but probably the biggest breakfast eater in the entire muscle field is veteran strongman Milo Steinborn. He's a magnificent ninety-five years of age and still going strong. And what's more, he eats a humongous breakfast; according to experts who have known him most of his life, he always has. He starts with an enormous bowl of rolled oats, and then it's eggs, ground beef...and a variety of other energizing, bodybuilding foods. I do not mean to imply that eating a massive breakfast is your key to the longevity and health enjoyed by Steinborn. Perhaps one can have too much of a good thing, although it certainly hasn't hurt him. I am convinced, along with the world's most respected nutritional experts, that a substantial well-balanced meal first thing in the morning is good policy.

Here's what British bodybuilder Frank Richards eats for breakfast when he's training to add muscle size: "First thing in the morning I have porridge [hot oatmeal], then I eat six eggs [scrambled or poached], a half pound of ham with some kind of beans...and I finish up with whole-grain pancakes. The entire meal is over 2,000 calories."

Fabulous physique woman Juliette Bergman from Holland has her own brand of breakfast. It consists of two *eierkoeken,* a light, nonfat bread made with eggs. Juliette adds unsweetened jam for taste. She then eats a mixture of müsli,* yogurt, and banana. That's a pretty substantial breakfast, you'll agree.

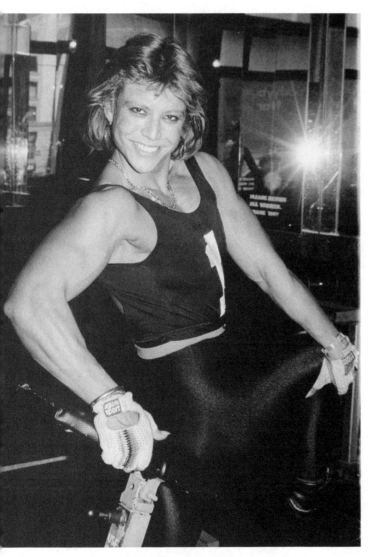

Holland's Juliette Bergman starts her day with a substantial breakfast.

---

*A mixture of raisins, prunes, apricots, grated apple, chopped nuts, lemon juice, and honey; mixed with rolled oats that have been soaked overnight in boiling water; served with milk or cream.

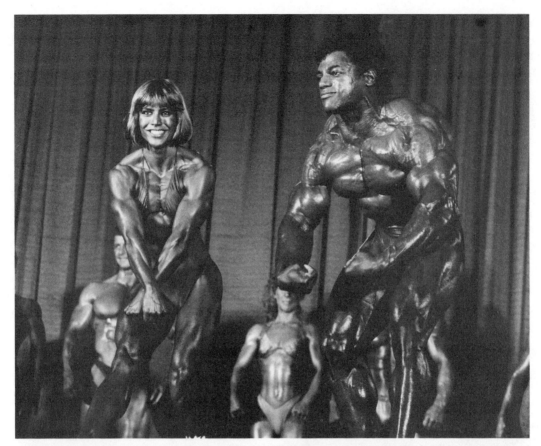

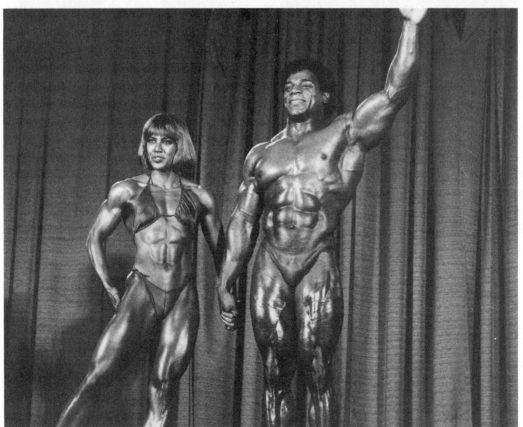

Mixed Pairs champions Juliette Bergman and Tony Pearson.

American superwoman Corinna Everson, two-time Ms. Olympia, also enjoys a hearty breakfast. She told me that after talking to Al Beckles she gave porridge a try...and discovered she loves it. Her breakfasts now consist of a bowl of hot oatmeal, six eggs (but only three yolks), and a protein drink made from skim milk and 100 percent egg whites. That's lots of protein and plenty of complex carbs, right? Right!

Ming Chew, New York City.

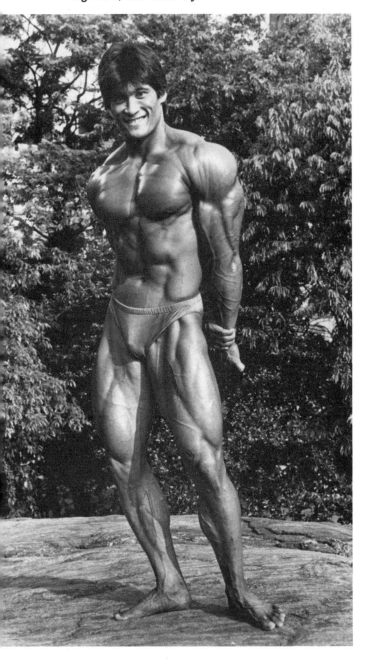

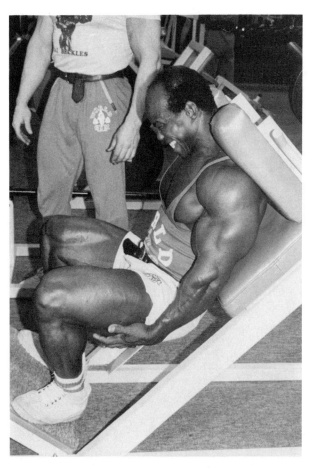

England's Al Beckles works at the hack machine to keep his legs looking great.

IFBB World Champion Lee LaBrada explains his breakfast: "I take in approximately 3,500 calories per day in the off season. My breakfast is a big meal. It consists of six egg whites [scrambled], one ounce of cheddar cheese, one slice of whole-grain toast, and a bowl of mixed fruit [for example, bananas and oranges], one glass of skim milk."

Chinese-American bodybuilder Ming Chew, who was born in New York and is currently making a name for himself in commercials for Coca-Cola, eats the following breakfast during the last ten weeks before a contest: a large bowl of oatmeal with skim milk and one sliced banana plus a large cup of decaffeinated coffee. He also takes a multivitamin/mineral tablet and 5 grams of amino acids at breakfast.

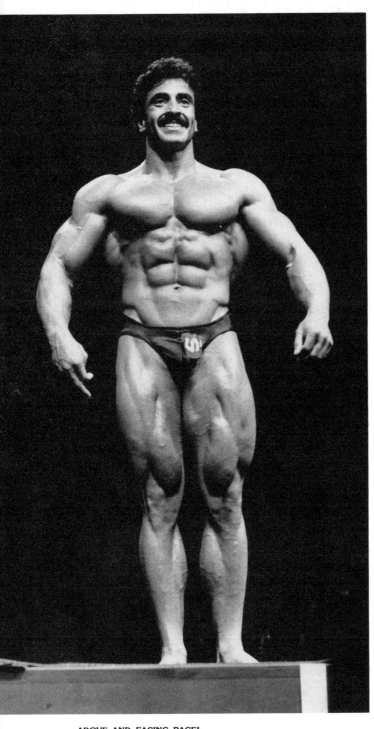

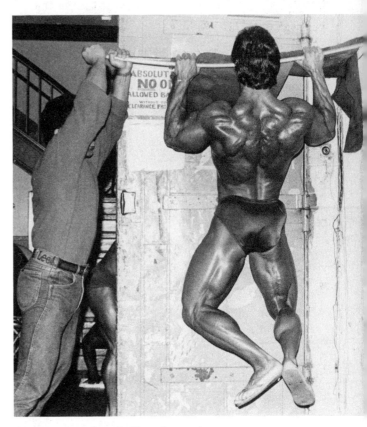

Samir assists Greg DeFerro in a unique way of pumping up backstage.

ABOVE AND FACING PAGE:
IFBB Mr. Olympia Samir Bannout.

"My off-season breakfast," says Mr. Olympia Samir Bannout, writing in *Muscle and Fitness,* "consists of high complex carbs to stoke my furnace for morning workouts. (I always eat complex carbs two hours before a workout.) I start with a cooked whole-grain cereal with just a little nonfat milk on it, and perhaps some cinnamon sprinkled over the cereal. I usually have two eggs or a small piece of low-fat meat. I then have a toasted bran muffin or a slice of whole-grain bread." Samir, like most top bodybuilders, eats at least four or five times a day.

For a selection of good bodybuilding breakfast foods, see the recipes section at the end of this book.

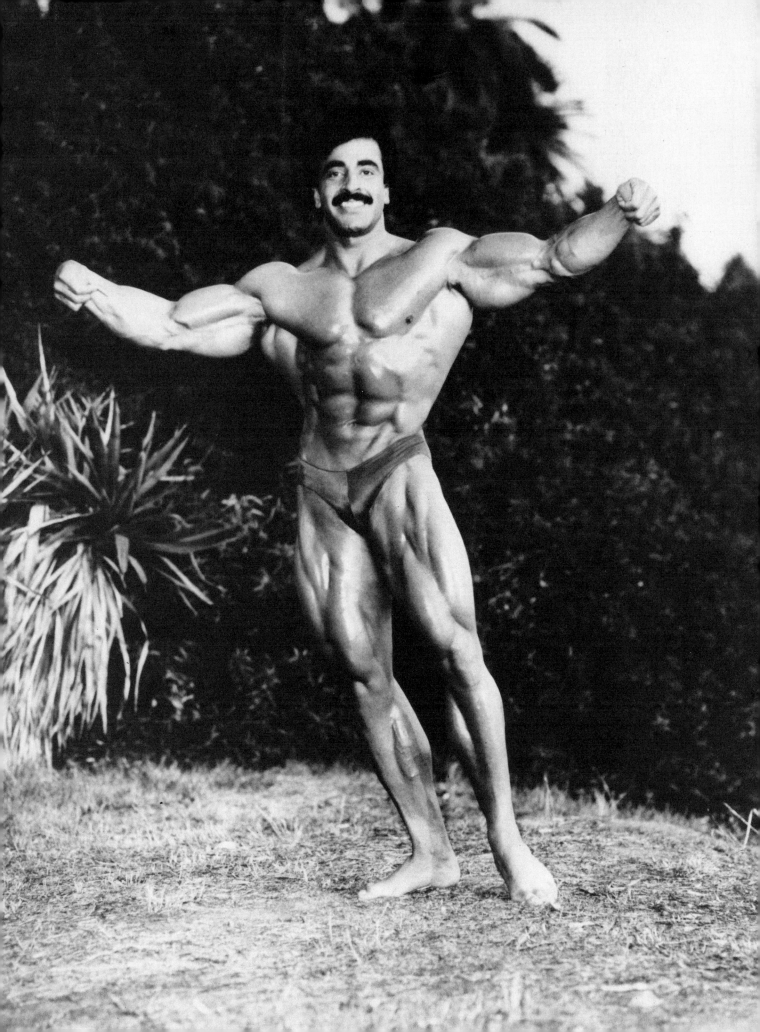

17
SNACKS
Upping the Nutrition

What is a snack? According to most dictionaries, it is a "small portion of food or drink (or a light meal) eaten between regular meals; anything that can be eaten quickly and without formality to appease the appetite, such as potato chips, crackers, or the like."

As a youngster, I was always taught by my parents that snacking was bad, yet at the same time they saw to it that I had a cookie and a glass of milk around midmorning and fruit or a sandwich at night, all in addition to the three main meals of the day!

There seems to be an implication when one talks of snacking that eating extra food is a more or less unscheduled response to some sudden hunger pang or near desperate need for sustenance. In fact, when snacks are regularly taken as supplement to usual mealtimes they can quickly become *necessary*. Many people, especially bodybuilders and other athletes, feel that they don't have any energy for their training if they don't have their customary snack. Some go so far as to say they feel faint without it.

There has been a renewed interest in snacking of late. MRCA Information Services, private research firm, surveyed 5,500 people about this national pastime. They concluded that most North Americans snack frequently and that snacking habits are changing slowly to eating more nutritious foods—from potato chips to yogurt, for example.

The question remains: Is snacking bad for us, an unhealthy aberration, or is it a reasonable way to get good nutrition? We can answer that with reference to one thing we know for sure: Enormous, stomach gorging, heavy meals are bad for us. They stretch the stomach and overload the digestive system. As a logical extension of this conclusion, we can see that snacking, or partaking of five or six smaller meals instead of three big meals, is a preferable way of satisfying our nutritional needs. It certainly works well for bodybuilders. And, curiously, it works well for those who want to progress quickly whether they want to *gain* or *lose* weight. (The modern

Tony Pearson.

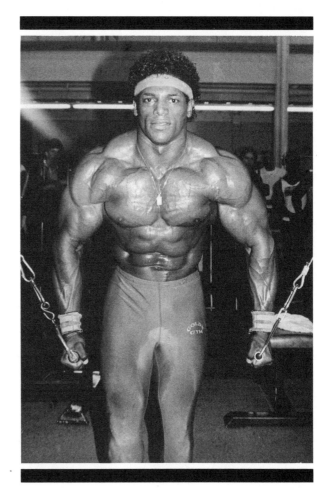

119

name for taking more frequent small meals is *grazing*.)

MRCA Information Services find that Southerners snack less than most. People in the Great Lakes area do it all the time. Northeasterners tend to snack on pizzas and popcorn, while Westerners prefer apples and oranges. The British like their biscuits and tea, while their continental cousins snack on a variety of pastries, bread, cheese, and wine.

For the bodybuilder snacking has to be different. It is either good or bad for us depending on the answers to two questions. First, do we need the added food we are putting into our mouths? And second, is the snack itself of high nutritional value? It goes almost without saying that a typical potato-chip-and-cola snack is pretty worthless, and yet it is a daily food combination for millions around the world, especially school-aged youngsters.

I should clarify that I believe it's best to observe the "three main meals a day" format, but with the proviso that those meals are never large to the extent of causing even mild discomfort. Snacking between these meals will help your bodybuilding progress—provided snack items are appropriate, high in nutrition. Naturally, an eye must be kept on the overall amount of calories consumed. This is as important for the person wanting to gain weight as it is for those of us who are endeavoring to lose weight.

Like your set meals, a scheduled snack or between-meal eating plan must be based on good nutrition. Don't waste your snacking with worthless, empty-calorie foods. Except in the most dire emergency, forget about snacking on hot dogs, potato chips, packaged cakes and cookies, chocolates, candies, etc.

It is very important to plan your snacks ahead of time. Whether you are a student, teacher, truck driver, laborer, or office worker, you cannot rely on getting a suitable snack simply on the off chance that it will be available when and where you want it. Snacking has to be thought out in advance. Prepare your snack at home. Not only will you be eating exactly the right food you need, you will also be eating the correct amount. And it will also be less expensive. "Coffee trucks," office canteens and vending machines traditionally deliver the most disgusting food imaginable,

although many are trying to upgrade their wares. You may be able to purchase the occasional apple, but most of the quick-service food offered is of very low standard. And the price is most definitely *not* right either!

I suggest that you invest in one of those round, sectionalized, airtight, plastic Tupperware bowls, with a press-down top. Then you can take your snacks to work or school with you. The airtight container will keep everything fresh, and the variety of healthful foods you can take is endless—slices of cold cuts (but avoiding those containing nitrites), cheese, tuna, salmon. There will be room for celery, carrots, tomatoes, cabbage, lettuce, and more.

Many Tupperware dishes have three sections. I would use one for protein foods such as sliced eggs or egg salad, meat, cheese, nuts, or fish; the second section for vegetables such as lettuce, cucumber, tomatoes, cabbage salad, spinach salad, alfalfa sprouts; and the third section for fruits—orange sections, grapefruit sections, melon or peach slices, etc.

One of the all-time favorite foods of bodybuilders is tuna. In fact, nutrition expert Bill Dobbins once joked, "If you are what you eat, then most bodybuilders must be made of tuna."

Personally, I find that tuna can become a very boring food. Ideally, it should be blended somehow with other foods. However, many bodybuilders don't want the additional calories from other foods, especially when preparing for a contest, so you will see them eating tuna direct from a can, with no other foods whatsoever.

There are many varieties of tuna. Most of us prefer the white tuna; others don't mind the dark. But the main difference to take into consideration is the dissimilarity between tuna packed in water and in oil. Beware! Oil contains loads of calories. Just a tablespoon of oil (or butter or margarine) provides about 100 calories. It comes down to this: If you want to gain weight rapidly, then tuna packed in oil makes sense, not just because of the added calories, but because oil-packed tuna also contains more nourishment— the protein content, for example, is considerably higher. On the other hand, if you are cutting up for a contest, there is only one tuna for you, the water-packed variety.

Here's looking at two 12½-ounce cans of

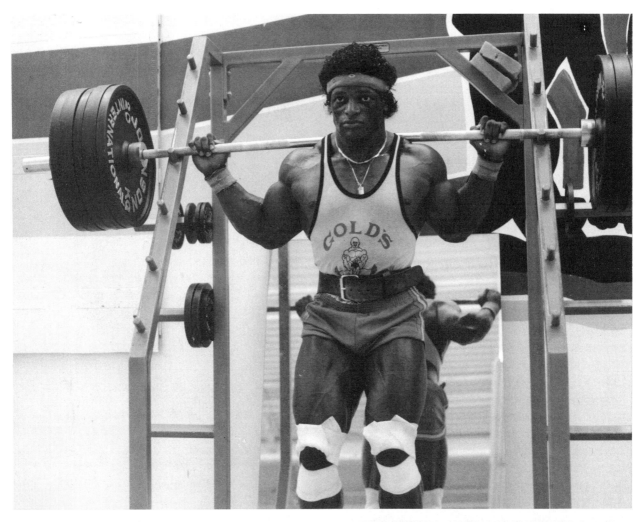

Mr. America Tony Pearson, an advocate of tuna as a protein snack.

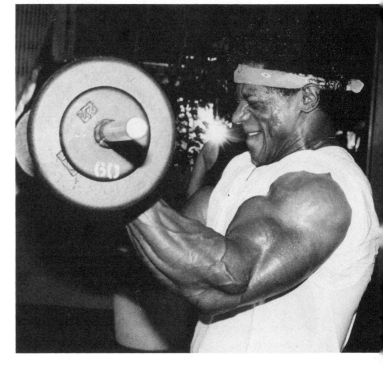

tuna, identically priced, so you can compare the water- and oil-packed varieties:

	Calories	Protein	Fat
Oil-packed	490	60 grams	32 grams
Water-packed	242	42 grams	5 grams

It's a good idea to check the labels on tuna (and everything else). You wouldn't take a chance of tossing the contents of any old gasoline can into your car's fuel tank would you? Tuna quality varies greatly. Check it out. But remember to check out *all* the variables. You can't easily compare an eight-ounce can with a ten-ounce can unless you are a mathematical whiz kid. Compare apples with apples, as they say.

When Tony Pearson was a young up-and-coming bodybuilder, he had very little money indeed. He hitchhiked to California to train at Gold's Gym, the Mecca of bodybuilding. Tony would sleep on the beach and when manager Kent Keuhn opened the door at 6 A.M., there was Tony on the doorstep. "He was the most enthusiastic bodybuilder around," says Kent. "He used to bring a can of tuna to eat in the gym. We didn't mind at first, but then everyone started copying him, and pretty soon the whole gym stank of tuna! So we had to put our foot down."

Yes sir, Tony Pearson made some good progress with his tuna. It's the bodybuilder's favorite fish food.

Another favorite snack food is cheese. True, it is high in fat—two-thirds is fat—but it has its uses as an extraordinary muscle builder, even though it contains virtually no carbohydrates. Cheese is high in protein, calcium, and vitamin A.

Cheese is *not* a food to be eaten on a low-fat diet, nor will it help you in the countdown period when preparing for a bodybuilding contest. "Make sure that you use only aged or properly cured cheese, not processed cheese spreads," says Dr. Michael Walczak, who has been nutrition counselor to many top California and international bodybuilders. There are a number of fat-reduced cheeses on the market. Some are made from part skim milk. If you are on a low-fat diet, which is in line with my general recommendations in this book, then don't have meat at the same meal if you have cheese.

Poultry also makes an ideal snack. Happily, there is a trend toward eating more chicken, turkey, and lean unmarbled meats. They have less fat than hamburger meat, which in turn has less fat than beef steaks, roasts, chops, ham, and pork. If limiting yourself to lean meats sounds restricting, then remember that trimming all visible fat from the high-fat meats can also cut the amount of fat per serving by as much as 50 percent.

The ideal snacks, especially for those of us trying to lose weight, are probably vegetables.

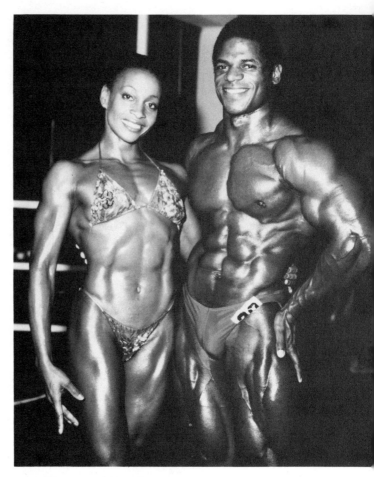

Carla Dunlap and Tony Pearson.

They are handy to transport and make for satisfying nourishment in themselves, while keeping overall calorie intake to a minimum. Celery, tomatoes, and carrots mix suitably with cottage cheese or whole-wheat bread (or both) to make a suitably balanced mini-meal.

See the snack recipes offered in the recipe section at the back of this book for other suggestions that offer good nutritional value.

18
BODY FAT LEVELS
How Low?

The demands of bodybuilding are unique. On one hand, you are required to build *muscle mass*—a lot of muscle mass—a feat that requires an abundance of calories. On the other hand, you are expected to display a *low body fat* percentage, considerably below average. Since bodybuilding training is done in short, intense bursts, it is not an activity that burns huge amounts of calories. Consequently, one has to follow a tight, calorie-restricted diet. Talk about a sport of contradictions. You have to *eat* to build muscle, yet *not eat* to lose fat.

Most bodybuilders fail to maintain maximum mass with minimum fat. A few, like "Mr. Ripped," Clarence Bass, come pretty close.

A person is said to be obese (excessively overweight) when body weight is 20 percent greater than ideal or normal weight. This normal weight invariably comes from statistics compiled by life insurance companies or from charts supplied by your doctor's office. These charts are totally meaningless to the bodybuilder, because a physical culturist is dealing with muscle mass, which weighs more than fat but is less of a burden on the individual than rolls of pure human lard. A five-foot-seven-inch male bodybuilder may well weigh a healthy 200 pounds with just 10 percent body fat, while a totally untrained person at the same height and weight will be carrying a not unusual 25 percent body fat and may be on the verge of a heart attack. The same comparison, albeit on a lesser scale, holds true for women. Your overall body weight does *not* indicate how fat you are—or, more correctly, what percentage of your weight is body fat.

Many people miscalculate their own degree of fatness. High fashion models often think that they are too fat when in fact they are too skinny. Meanwhile a laborer may feel he's really "built" when actually he's carrying rolls of unhealthy adipose around his middle.

The level of fat is best identified by percentages in relation to total body composition. The accepted maximum level—although perhaps

Susie Green has trimmed body fat to the max!

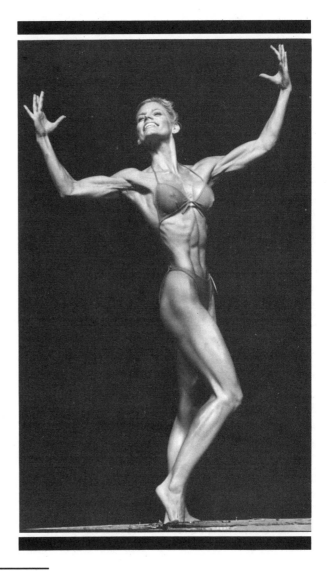

meaningless to a bodybuilder whose goal is to keep body fat to a healthy minimum—is very significant with regard to appearance and, of course, overall wellness and vitality. Generally speaking, a man should have about 15 percent of his total weight as fat. A woman should have no more than 22 percent. Holding these levels while exercising vigorously to maintain tone and shape will pretty much guarantee a good appearance. Hardcore bodybuilders perhaps could strive for somewhat better off-season percentages of 12 percent body fat for men and 18 percent for women. Coming into a contest, of course, is a whole new ball game. Fat levels must then come down to an all-time low, at least for a day or two.

Make no mistake about it, fat is your enemy. Too much of it causes ill health, and to the body culturist fat is detrimental to vital good looks.

One of the most attractive things about the human body is the configuration of the muscles that nature has provided us. Whether you go to the most northern or southern parts of our planet, visit a huge metropolis or the most distant desert island, the anatomy of the human body is fundamentally the same. We all have deltoids and biceps, triceps, lats, and glutes. A pygmy's pectorals have the same muscle origins and insertions as those of an Eskimo.

Male and female, we all have muscles, and whether partially or fully developed, they are beautiful. More than that, they are beguiling, especially to the opposite sex.

Fat destroys this muscular attractiveness. Fat destroys shape. It fills in the valleys between different muscles and robs them of their attractive curves. When a bodybuilder is overweight by more than ten pounds, he or she starts to look like a shapeless blob. The size is there, but the definition that makes for impressiveness has scooted out of sight. First the delineation between those chunky abdominals disappears. What was once a series of firmly set abdominal muscle rows now becomes a bed of rippled, dimply fat. The peak on your arms shallows; the fat rounds off the biceps mound, and your arms look rotund and...drab city. The lower pec line fades into obscurity; the thighs lose their curve. Knees thicken—you say good-bye to that neat boniness that contrasted so well with those swell-

ing diamond-shaped calves. The backs of your thighs look flat as a pancake—fat has stolen away that super hamstring bulge. Your shoulders flow into your arms. Remember when they used to "pop out" like two melons? And your back! What was once a veritable nest of squirming serpents now more resembles a rained-upon sea of mashed potatoes. Yes, *fat is your enemy!*

Nobody wants to be fat, but it often creeps up on us when we least expect it. Many people are concerned about being fat. They yearn to be lean, with all the attendant social, physical, and emotional advantages. You don't just look better, more attractive; you *feel* better and *are* healthier.

"The war on fat can be won," says Clarence Bass in his best-selling *The Lean Advantage* (Ripped Enterprises). "I believe it can be won without making yourself miserable in the process." (In the next chapter I will deal at length with the how-to aspect of losing weight, and I'll cover more severe "cutting-up" for bodybuilding contests in chapter 25.)

Is being lean healthy? Yes, so long as the body receives its proper nutrients. Dr. Thomas J. Bassler, a prominent runner-pathologist who studies the things that kill (bit of a morbid job, eh?), says the day you use up all your body fat is the day you die. So what does this tell us? That Clarence Bass is eternally on the verge of death? No! In fact, Clarence Bass looks good, feels good, and is extremely fit and healthy. He never lets his body fat level go above 6 percent, and each year he takes it to below 3 percent. Once he had it at an amazing 2.4 percent. Other athletes have been tested at very low levels, too. World class marathon runners generally range from 4 to 8 percent. Frank Shorter, 1972 Olympic marathon champ (and runner-up in 1976), was measured at 2 percent. When players on the New York Jets football team had their body composition measured, one man (a three-time All-American) had 3.1 percent body fat. Two other players had 4 percent fat.

Women tend to have more body fat than men, mainly because the breasts are largely fat. Other organs and the female hormonal setup demand a higher overall body fat percentage than for men. For years scientists claimed that not even the leanest women could reduce their essential fat levels to less than 10 to 12 percent.

But in 1980, at the American Women's Body-building Championships, Body Accounting, a fitness testing facility with headquarters in Irvine, California, tested most of the contestants and disclosed that Kay Baxter had 11.8 percent body fat, Claudia Wilbourn had 11.2 percent, and the winner, Laura Combes, measured 7.1 percent—a surprise to the scientists.

But Body Accounting was not surprised at all. Prior to the American Championships, its technicians had already recorded a bodybuilder with even lower body fat levels. Susie Green, a successful model turned bodybuilder, had been measured at an amazingly low 5.6 percent!

When women take their body fat levels below 10 to 12 percent they often develop menstrual irregularity. Many don't have periods for months and months. This absence of monthly menstruation (amenorrhea) is not harmful and apparently does not harm health. Of course bodybuilding women are not the only ones to suffer from amenorrhea. Many female athletes encounter the condition because of their intensive training habits. In 1979 the American College of Sports Medicine issued the following statment: "Disruption of the menstrual cycle is a common problem for female athletes. While it is important to recognize this problem and discover its etiology, no evidence exists to indicate that this is harmful to the female reproductive system."

I suspect that many women who achieve unusually low body fat levels, whether we are talking about bodybuilders, track athletes, tennis players, or weight lifters, owe the extreme lack of body fat to chemical usage. The various hormonoids help maintain body mass and reduce body fat. Now, whether these chemicals are harmful to the reproductive system has not yet been conclusively determined.

It is clear that a bodybuilder, for reasons both of health and peace of mind, should strive to keep body fat levels under control—and this is best done by controlling diet. Most other athletes who need strength for their sports (hammer and discus throwers, shot putters, weight lifters, wrestlers) do not have to rid themselves of anywhere near as much body fat as the bodybuilder. Many ignore the fundamentals of good nutrition. They tend to junk-out, eating excessively to keep their calorie intake high.

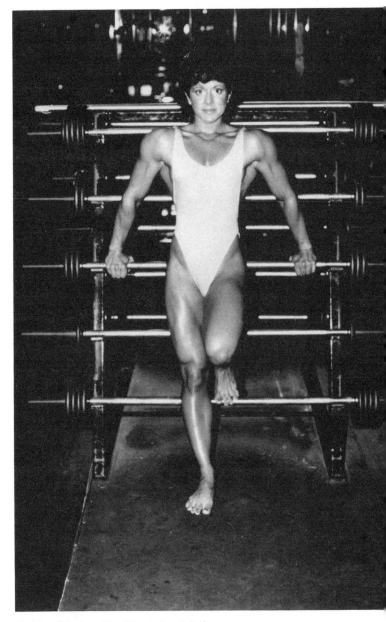

Donna Oliveira: Check out the delts!

Bodybuilders cannot afford the luxury of haphazard nutrition. When a bodybuilder steps on stage, an experienced judge is usually able to assess his or her condition in a matter of seconds. There's no hiding body fat.

It takes us back to the basic uniqueness of our sport. We simply must feed our muscles correctly, giving our body adequate protein, carbohydrates, fats, vitamins, and minerals, yet we must at the same time restrict calorie intake to prevent the enemy coming aboard. We have to be forever vigilant.

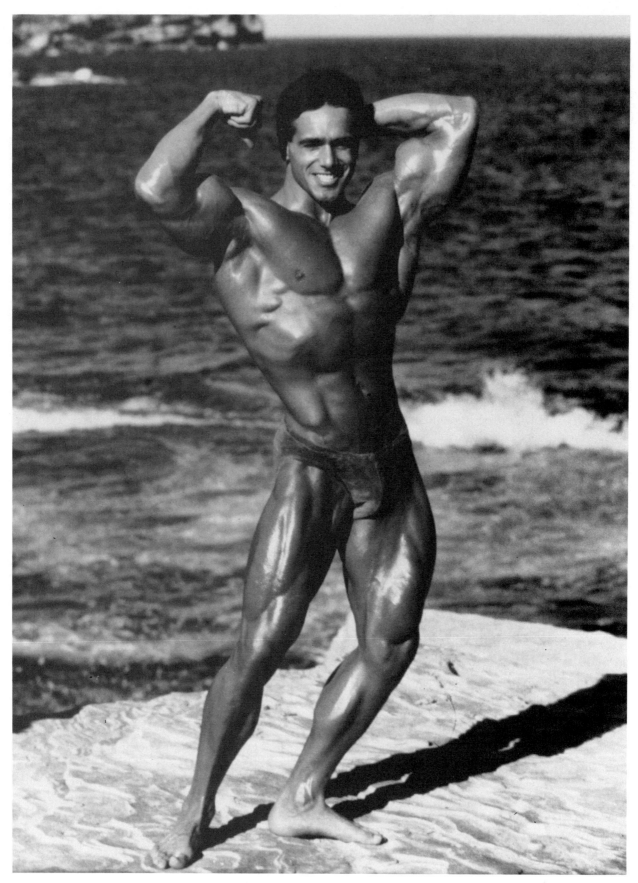

Australia's John Terilli, symmetry plus.

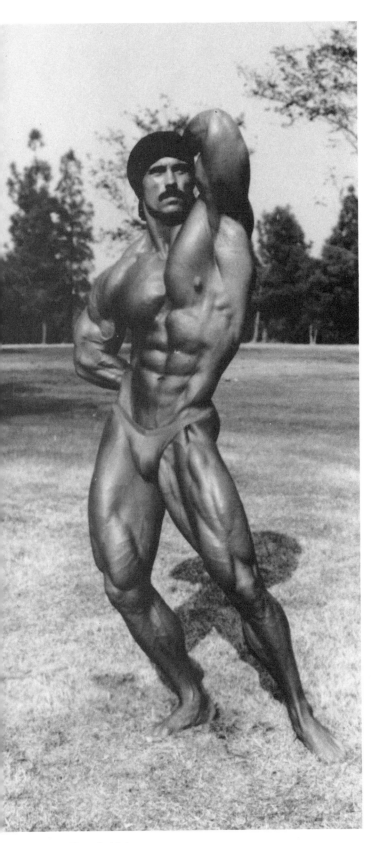

Rory Leidelmeyer.

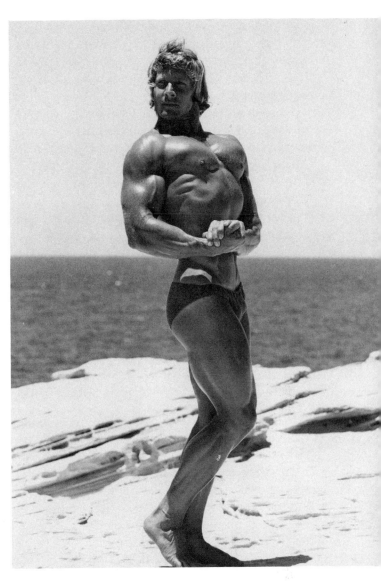

Ted Matush, Mr. Australia.

There are several ways to monitor your body fat. Probably the most accurate method is immersion in a water tank. You are weighed first on a standard scale and then weighed while immersed in water in a specially constructed tank. The only snag to total accuracy in measuring body density is that a research assistant must determine how much air is in your lungs, since that makes your body more buoyant. This can be both costly and time-consuming. Expect to pay $60 to $160 at fitness centers and university laboratories for this test. Some of the larger commercial gyms also offer this service.

A far simpler way of measuring how much fat you have on your body is the "pinch test." I first wrote about this in 1959 and may even have been responsible for naming it—a dubious achievement, admittedly.

More than half of all your fat is on the surface of your body—under the skin but over the muscles. You can measure it with the pinch test, which can be done in the privacy of your own home. (I can hear that sigh of relief from all you overweights.)

There are several sites at which you should pinch test yourself:

1. **Back of the upper arm** (midway between the shoulder and the elbow)
2. **The side of the waist** (just above the hipbone at the level of the navel)
3. **The upper back** (just below the shoulder blade)
4. **Back of the thigh** (midway between the hip and knee)

While the pinch test does give you a good idea about your fat percentage, it is still only an estimate. It cannot be exact because fat distribution varies and the pinch test measures only four specific body sites. A more accurate reading can be obtained by the use of medical calipers. (These spring-loaded pinchers are relatively inexpensive—some cost as little as $19.95 —and they are available at pharmacies, chemists, medical supply outfits, or from mail order sources through various fitness and health periodicals.)

It is better to obtain the help of a partner to take the pinch test, whether you are using fingers or calipers. To ensure accuracy have your partner take each measurement several times, then record the average for each test site. Do the test standing up. Get your friend to grab between thumb and forefinger as much tissue as possible at the designated site. Lift and pull it away from the muscle underneath. Don't allow the pinched area to extend beyond the tips of the fingers—it should fold and rest in line with your friend's fingers so that the measurement can be made accurately. When you are sure that

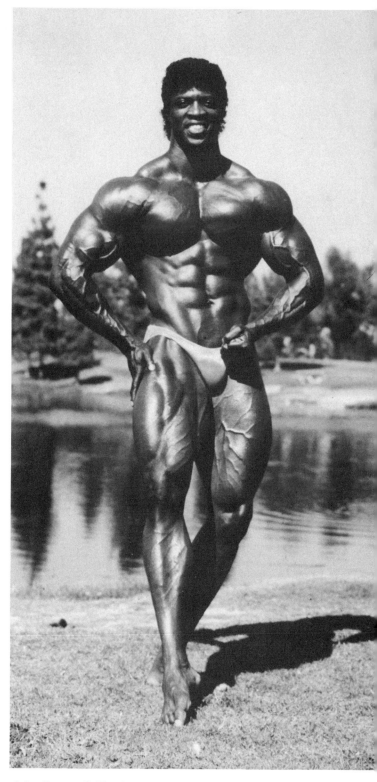

John Brown, California.

128

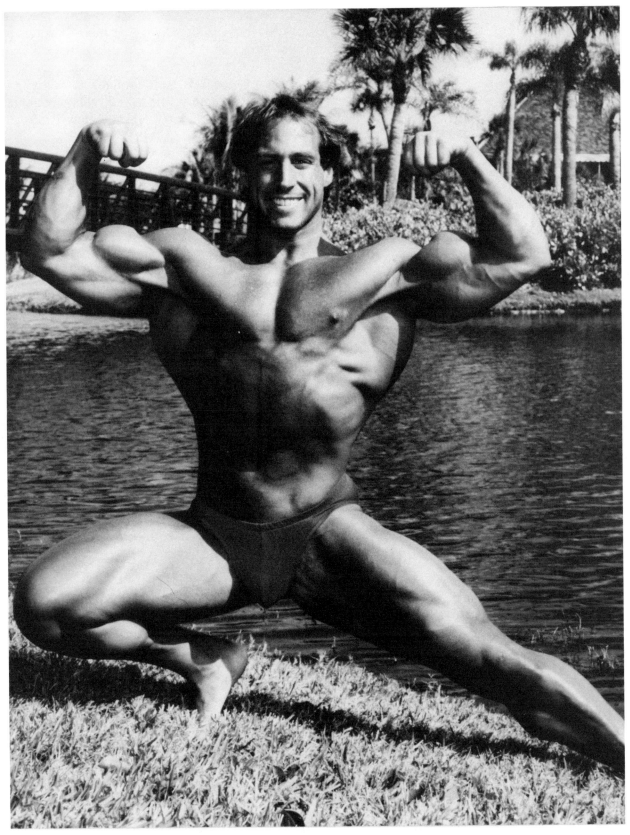

John DeFendis, USA.

your friend is pinching pure fat (and not the muscle underneath), have him or her take a ruler and measure the distance across the top of the skin, between the thumb and forefinger. Write down the measurement for the four test sites.

Compare your measurements to the following skin fold thicknesses for normal adults:

- Arm   ½ inch
- Waist 1 inch
- Back   ¾ inch
- Thigh ¾ inch

For each ¼ inch in excess of normal measurements you can conclude that there is approximately 5 percent excess fat. The thicker the pinch, the more fat you are carrying.

Most bodybuilders do not resort to having their fat percentage measured, although there was somewhat of a craze in the early 1980s to have regular tests.

Today a bodybuilder will be guided more by the mirror and by casual self pinch-testing in and around the waist area. With experience you soon learn whether you are a Pillsbury doughboy or a veritable lean machine.

Ideal weight is the single most sought-after goal pursued by those of us living in North America. It even supersedes the yearning for wealth, and—hard as it is to believe—the desire for health follows in a distant third place.

As a result of all this, dieting is both an obsession and a major industry with us. Weight reducing products crowd the drugstore shelves. Hardly an issue of a women's magazine is published that doesn't contain a "new" way to lose weight. Even *Reader's Digest* jumps on the diet bandwagon regularly—it helps sales. And books on weight loss are so numerous that they merit their own section in most bookstores. And still no diet seems satisfactory; millions of us continue to search for the ultimate answer in a never-ending quest to shed pounds.

In this chapter I will tell you the answers. It is not my intention to blind you with science or psychology or anything else. I could fill this book with a million theories about why people are fat. I could tell you that, because your mother stuck a pacifier in your mouth when you cried as a baby, gave you a candy whenever you fell and hurt yourself, or rewarded you with a cookie for being good, you have ever since regarded food as being synonymous with love. But I won't.

I could tell you that it doesn't matter what foods you eat, as long as you reduce overall calories (recommended by Dr. Irwin Maxwell Stillman, M.D., who authored a million-copy best-seller on the subject). But I won't.

The truth is that some of us were born fat, with more fat cells than the average. Others of us were so overfed as young children that we developed more fat cells, which are now with us permanently, thanks to our doting, misguided parents.

As for the rest of us, we are overweight for one, two, or all three of the following reasons:

1. We eat too much food.
2. We eat the wrong food.
3. We do not exercise enough.

John Terilli training triceps.

19
LOSING WEIGHT
Going Down

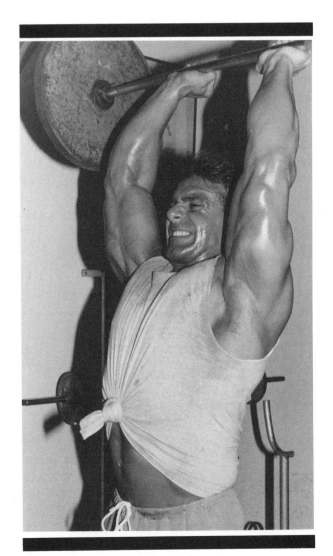

And don't ever let anyone kid you that you don't need willpower to lose weight! Willpower, whether it comes from insecurity, inferiority, or has to be consciously drummed up, is the priceless ingredient that makes us *act* to lose weight—or do anything else that requires positive effort.

I suppose it's fair to say that many diets seem to work. Most people lose some weight if they limit their calorie intake or lower their consumption of certain foods. The problem is that when a sticking point is reached, the diet is often discarded from boredom and through frustration. Or else one simply gives in to the temptation to eat more.

Overweight people should do whatever it takes to lose their fat, and then adopt a life-style nutrition plan that they can easily follow for the rest of their lives. There's nothing more ludricious than being on the diet treadmill, losing weight for a special event (a pool party, a wedding, a vacation) only to fatten up again afterwards. One statistic indicates that the average North American has dieted over sixty times and lost a total in excess of 300 pounds.

It is important to realize that you should not have as your goal merely losing pounds. Your objective should be to lose fat. Fat is your enemy. Weigh scales are incapable of distinguishing between pounds of fat and pounds of muscle. One is unhealthy; one is healthy. Your body has to carry around excess fat, but muscle carries you!

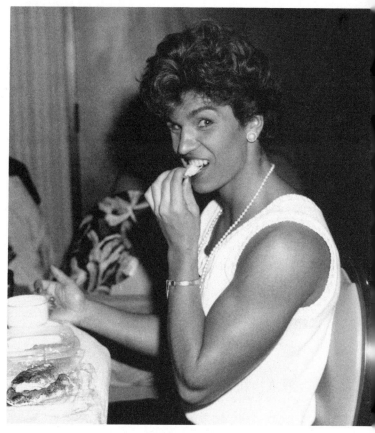

Chicken: That's the ticket for Finland's Marjo Selin.

FACING PAGE: *Kevin Lawrence.*

EATING TOO MUCH OF THE WRONG STUFF

Yes, all food has calories; calories make us fat. At least, when we eat more calories than we require for maintaining lean body weight, we become fat. Food energy (calories) is needed to keep us alive. It enables us to train, work, and play—and even to sleep and breathe. But if we ingest more than we use up, then those extra calories are stored on the body as fat.

When your body takes in as many calories as it burns up, you are in a state of *thermodynamic balance.* One way of simplifying thermodynamics is to look at it like a bank account. You start with a given amount of money in the bank (fat on your body). Eating corresponds to making deposits. Exercise (walking, breathing, weight training) can be regarded as writing a check. If your deposits equal your withdrawals your balance (weight) will stay the same. Burn more calories than you consume and your body will start losing weight. If you eliminate just one pat of butter a day, that is 3,780 calories less deposited each month! This is approximately one pound of fat "burned off"—twelve pounds a year. Eliminate two pats of butter a day and that's a difference of about half a pound a week—twenty-five pounds a year.

Any diet should be balanced nutritionally. To simply choose low-calorie foods is not satisfactory. Foods should never be evaluated strictly on their calorie count.

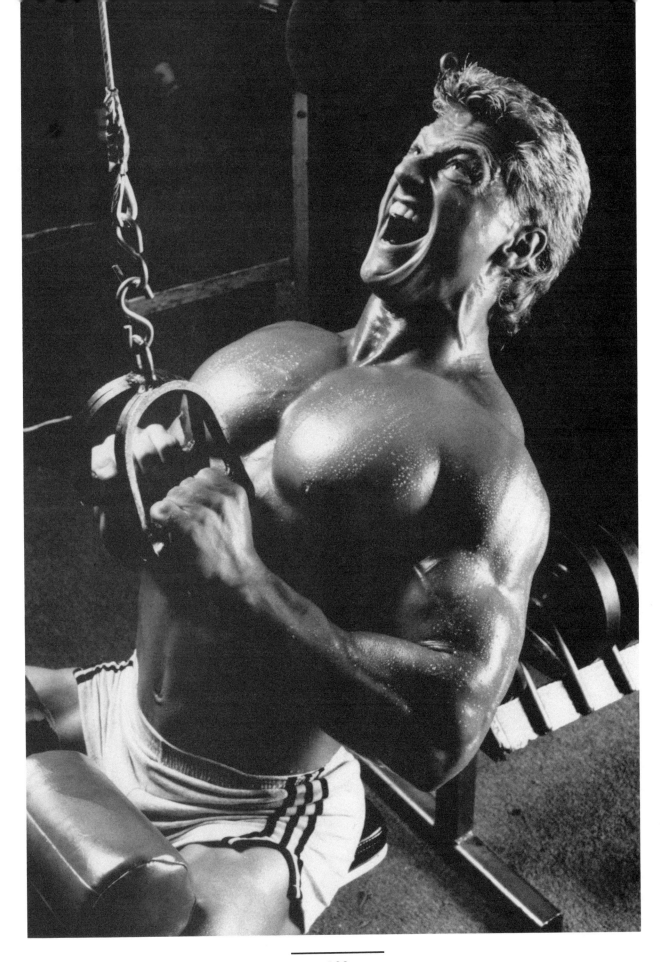

Opinions vary about how much and what kind of food we require for a balanced eating program. But generally speaking, one should select foods from each of the five main groups:

1. **Milk group**—milk, cheese, yogurt
2. **Animal protein**—beef, veal, lamb, poultry, eggs, fish
3. **Vegetable/fruit group**—the fresher the better
4. **Bread/grain group**—with emphasis on unprocessed whole grains
5. **Fats/oil group**—margarine, butter, seed and fish oils (usually only in small amounts)

When you want to lose weight (fat) you should always start cutting down gradually, reducing intake a little more every few days. Do not throw your body into shock by suddenly dropping from a 4,000-calorie intake to 1,500. Cut down slowly in 500-calorie steps. For example, during the first week you should be ingesting 3,500 calories per day, the second week 3,000 per day, and the third week 2,500 per day, and so on.

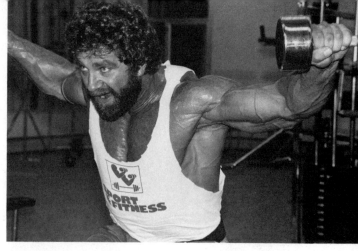

Jusup Wilcosz of West Germany, working the delts.

Balance your nutritional intake by selecting foods from the five basic groups, but be sensible: Keep away from most calorie-dense foods—fruits canned in sugar or syrup, colas or soft drinks, bleached white bread, cakes, chocolate, candy bars, commercial cereals, hot dogs, cream, butter, pretzels, potato chips, pastries, alcohol, salted nuts, pies, ice cream, ketchup, salad dressings, jam, sugar, and all fried foods.

Lee Haney works the shoulders with lateral raises.

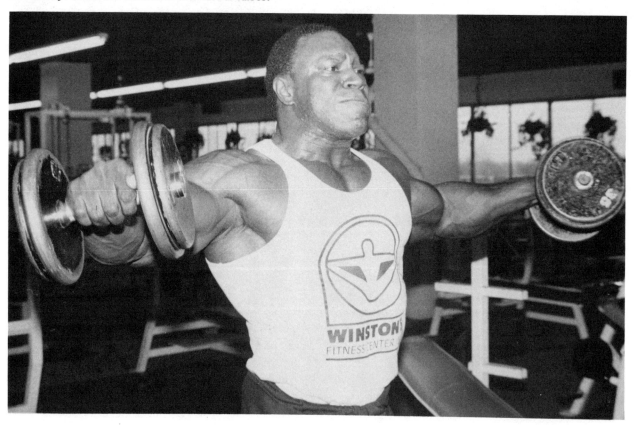

You should also somewhat restrict proteins (meats) and fats because both are very high-calorie items. You'll need some, of course, but you'll do far better by making complex carbohydrates (fruits, vegetables, whole grains) your main food sources.

Does this take willpower? You bet it does! Especially when you are dining out, visiting friends, or partying. And then, of course, there's the inevitable diet saboteur—you know, the "friend" who cajoles, "Oh come on, spoilsport, just one piece of chocolate cake!" or "You have to try this ice cream; it's delicious!" or "Mother will be hurt if you don't eat it all." Yes sir, people will try to sabotage your diet efforts whenever they get the chance. They love to test your willpower, and when you give in they experience a sinister moment of joy at having initiated your momentary weakness. Yes, dieting takes willpower!

Do not try to rush things. If you cut your calories too drastically, your body will retaliate by slowing its metabolic rate. While 2,000 calories a day might take off fat, 1,000 calories or less could cause your body to hold on to fat stubbornly. If your body thinks that it's in for a famine, it will become amazingly efficient; your basic metabolic rate will slow down and no more weight will be lost.

THE IMPORTANCE OF EXERCISE

Read the average diet book and you wouldn't think there was such a thing as exercise. But *exercise is vital* when you're dieting to lose weight. It keeps you toned, builds energy, maintains lean muscle mass, promotes internal health and well-being, builds strong ligaments and bones, strengthens the heart, benefits the circulatory system, improves cardiovascular efficiency, combats stress, and enhances self-image . . . and confidence.

Of course, the dieter specifically needs exercise to promote weight loss. Exercise burns calories and can double fat loss when combined

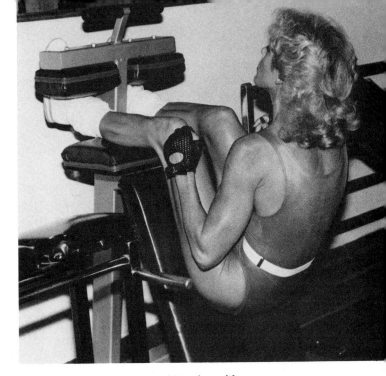

Georgia Miller defines her midsection with inverted sit-ups.

with calorie-reduced diet. Exercise also stimulates the metabolism (your BMR) so that you burn more calories even when resting.

In actuality, the only successful way to lose weight and keep it off is a planned program of exercise with moderate dietary restrictions. The best kinds of exercises for burning fat are aerobic—those that use large amounts of oxygen, causing a fast rate of breathing and an elevated heart rate. Running, fast walking, mountaineering, rowing, swimming, skipping, skating, cross-country skiing, cycling, stair climbing, dancing, or formal aerobic classes at a gym are all good weight loss exercises. You should exercise aerobically for twenty minutes or so three to five times a week. Twelve minutes of aerobics is the minimum time recommended.

Typically, aerobic exercise is performed by groups of people to the beat of loud music at gyms and health clubs. However, thousands of enthusiasts perform aerobic routines in the privacy of their homes. But before starting an aerobic routine, take the following precaution (if it applies to you): If you are over forty or have (or are concerned about) heart problems, have an electrocardiogram taken to make certain the routine will not overstress your heart. Once you have your doctor's okay, you will be able to exercise with renewed confidence and joy.

Aerobic exercise elevates your heart rate, but *do not exceed 80 percent of your maximum heart rate.* Subtract your age from 220 to estimate your maximum heart rate. For example, a person who is thirty years old has a maximum heart rate of 190 (220 minus 30). Eighty percent of 190 is 152. Accordingly this person should try to exercise to a point where his or her heart rate is elevated but does not exceed 152. The following chart will guide you in ascertaining your recommended heart rate during aerobic activity:

Age	Maximum Heart Rate	80% of Maximum
20	200	160
22	198	158
24	196	157
26	194	155
28	192	154
30	190	152
32	189	151
34	187	150
36	186	149
38	184	147
40	182	146
45	179	143
50	175	140
55	171	137
60	160	128
65	150	120

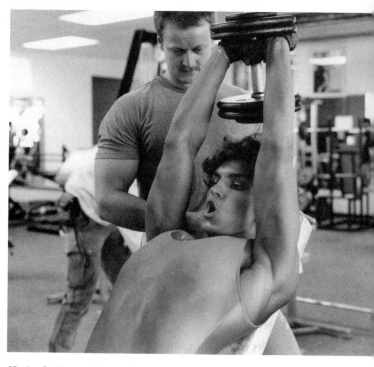

Marjo Selin performs triceps curls while husband Hanu looks on.

DIETING TIPS TO AID WEIGHT LOSS

- Eat breast of chicken without the skin. Peel the skin off before eating.
- Avoid extra salt. Sodium encourages water retention. Pass up salt-cured foods such as ham, salami, kippers, olives, and pickles.
- Cook with spices, herbs, and lemon, orange, or lime juice for seasonings. You can make otherwise very bland meals taste great.
- Steam vegetables rather than boil them. Boiling takes out valuable micronutrients. Do not add butter or margarine to steamed vegetables.
- For salad dressings use vinegar and lemon or lime juice rather than vinegar and oil or commercial salad dressings.
- Eat potatoes and bread without the regular accoutrements—no butter, sour cream, jams, peanut butter, or margarine. Good, whole-grain bread and ungarnished potatoes are fine, but the diet effect is spoiled by adding high-calorie extras.
- Broil, steam, or poach meat and fish. Never fry anything. Trim meats before cooking. Stick to lean meats, chicken, and lamb—limit ham or pork.
- Eat high-fiber foods. Fiber is great for the entire system and has no caloric value. It even absorbs some of the calories that would otherwise enter the bloodstream.
- If you must have milk, make sure it is the nonfat variety. This goes for all milk-based products.
- Eat fresh fruits in their natural, raw form rather than drinking juices. The fiber slows up calorie assimilation.

W hen a skinny person wants to gain weight—I mean *really* gain weight—the concern can be all-consuming, the desire can burn red hot. It can cause you to worry, lose sleep, and, curses of all curses, lose even more weight.

Almost every bodybuilder alive, male or female, wants to gain a little more muscle somewhere. "I'd like an extra inch or two on my arms." "It would be nice to have a little more size in the lower legs." "If only my shoulders carried more muscle!" You've heard it. Heck! You've probably said it!

Ideally, any gains you make should be pure muscle. This is the best kind of weight; yet, ironically, many super skinny people don't care what kind of flesh they add to their bones. They merely want to fill out, to gain weight, no matter what it is.

"Most experts agree," says Pat Neve, Mr. International, "that approximately five to seven pounds of pure muscle can be gained in one year. So the young athlete who gains twenty pounds in two months on junk foods can be assured that a large percentage of extra body weight is fat, not muscle."

But the really thin person is justified in not minding some gains in fat, as long as it isn't so excessive as to add rolls around the hips and midsection, or anywhere else. Mike Mentzer, Mr. Universe, puts it this way in his course *Heavy Duty Nutrition*. "For those who might be grossly underweight, the addition of a little fat along with the muscle may not be a bad thing. While pure muscle gains will obviously be the slowest, they should be a priority as you gain experience and start to add on pounds."

There are four types of weight gain:

1. Gaining pure muscle
2. Gaining muscle with some fat
3. Gaining bulk
4. Gaining muscle while losing fat

20
GAINING WEIGHT
Filling Out the Frame

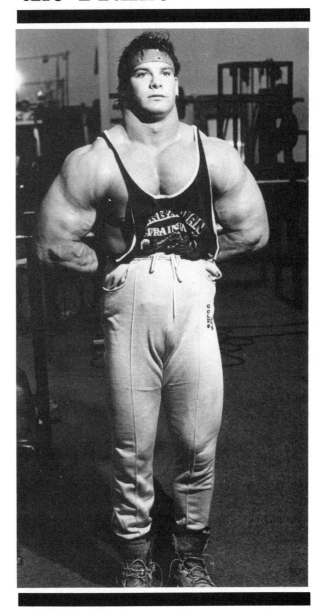

A Barbarian. Massive!

GAINING MUSCLE MASS WHILE LOSING FAT

Adding pure muscle while losing fat is the most difficult thing of all, but it can be accomplished. You have to train with an increased awareness of intensity while decreasing your calorie intake. The strategy is to coax the body into feeding off its own fat reserves.

Vince Gironda, incidentally, believes that an overweight bodybuilder should first reduce the excess fat right down with a severe calorie-restricted diet, after which he or she can press on with the muscle building aspect of training. This is in contrast with Mentzer, who states that the best way to reduce fat while building muscle is merely to eat slightly less calories than needed for maintenance while training with high intensity. I guess both methods work—there is more than one way to skin a cat! The same result can be arrived at via different techniques. Choose the method that suits your temperament or seems the most workable in your case.

In following Gironda's method of losing fat, you would cut large chunks of calories out of your diet. Aim to lose two to three pounds a week and include aerobic exercise to burn calories. Your objective is to shed body fat only. Forget heavy workouts and concentrate solely on shedding that rolypoly look. When you have succeeded, *then* get back to muscle building, being careful to eat only enough to add muscle size, not fat.

Mentzer's method incorporates the following well-defined rules: 1. Train with maximum intensity to stimulate growth. 2. Follow a well-balanced, calorie-reduced diet—try to consume the normal 60 percent complex carbohydrates, 25 percent protein, and 15 percent fats.

GAINING MUSCLE WITH SOME FAT

This is easier to do than gaining pure muscle and can be accomplished far quicker. It is therefore a favorite method of those super skinny people who have abdominals bursting through their skins and are ashamed that their ribs show not only from the front, but from the back, too.

Gaining muscle mass with some fat is not quite the same as bulking up. You still have to watch your diet, to rely as much as possible on wholesome natural foods that are good for your overall health, well-being, and high energy levels. You can include organ meats, fish, lean red meat, nuts, cheese, poultry, vegetables, whole grains, fruits, and leafy greens.

Super skinny people can accelerate their weight gain by drinking milk. At least, many claim that bodybuilders will make tremendous weight gains if they resort to milk. Bear in mind, however, that many people cannot tolerate the stuff. Nutrition

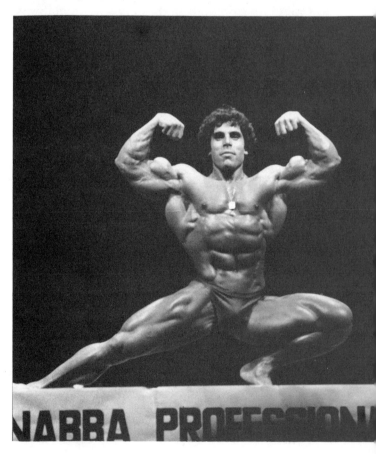

Ed Kawak.

138

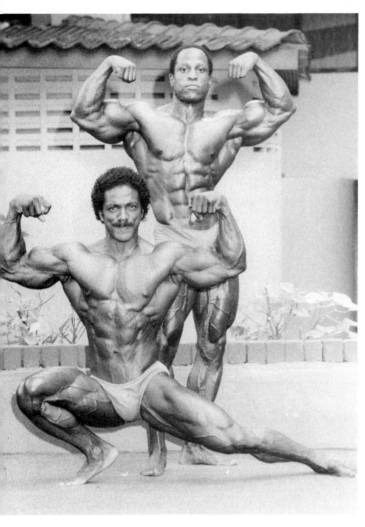

Chuck Williams and Charles Glass.

can blacks, Ashkenazi Jews and North American Indians."

Lactase deficiency in the intestine is responsible for the intolerance to milk, and the affected individual will suffer cramps, gas pains, bloating, and diarrhea—all unpleasant conditions to contend with—as a result of drinking milk. However, now there are lactase pills that an individual can obtain so that milk digestion can take place without these unsettling side effects. A visit to your local drugstore or chemist will lead you to the right product. There is also a milk product available with enzymes added to it.

If you are a skinny person who is able to digest milk, then you couldn't wish for a finer weight-gain product. As you know, all mammals spend their first months drinking nothing but milk. It is the greatest bodybuilder of all, although it is not quite the perfect food it has been touted as by the milk marketing professionals. While it does contain all the necessary basic nutrients, including protein, it is deficient in iron, vitamin D, and copper.

The right amount of milk in your diet can help you gain weight faster than any other natural food. Too much, however, will give you a thick layer of fat over your entire body. If this begins to happen, you should adopt the use of skim milk in preference to a product higher in fat. Those who don't mind a little excess weight may find that a high-quality milk and egg powder supplement will help keep gains coming at a steady level. (See the protein shakes given at the end of this chapter.)

expert Armand Tanny has a thing or two to say about that. "Lactase deficiency is common in adults. A great part of the world's adult population cannot digest milk easily. It has now been determined that an insufficient supply or a total lack of lactase in the small intestine is the main cause." Lactase is the enzyme necessary for digesting lactose, a carbohydrate component of milk.

Tanny goes on: "For the most part, those who can properly digest lactose come from the cultural groups that have traditionally raised cattle and drunk milk—i.e., Caucasians living in northwestern Europe and their American descendants. On the other hand, there is a high lactase deficiency (and therefore lactose intolerance) among Orientals, Greek Cypriots, Arabs, Ameri-

GAINING PURE MUSCLE

Never will the word *balance* mean more. Those people who want to look terrific all the time simply cannot afford to have any fat at all covering their external muscles. These people want to gain mass, yes, but they also want that gain to be pure muscle, nothing else.

"After stimulating muscle growth with high intensity exercise," says Mike Mentzer, "we must provide adequate nutrition along with just enough calories to supply our daily maintenance needs along with a tiny bit extra to allow for stimulated muscle growth." That's it!

When you want only muscle you can not afford to overeat. Your meals (four to six a day) should be small, and the nutritional value should be of the highest quality. Many of those who strive for "muscle only" gains take desiccated liver tablets and free amino acid pills to supplement their food intake. Juliette Bergman, Holland's wonder woman, feels that since she is a natural she must watch her diet closely: "Yes, I want to add muscle without fat. This means that I have to balance my nutrition so that I gain slowly in mass without encouraging fat accumulation. I never go on food binges. Small, regular meals are what give me regular improvement."

GAINING BULK

Bulk is really another name for fat. Well, to put it in perspective, bulk does include *some* muscle, but the greater percentage, probably about 80 percent, is fat.

A bulked-up condition is only useful to sumo wrestlers, super heavyweight power lifters, or those who just have to fill out in a short period of time. It is neither attractive to look at nor healthy.

Bulk results from force feeding, eating when not hungry. One eats anything at any time with an emphasis on milk and other calorie-dense foods. Often beer is consumed in large quantities. Few people on a bulk diet bother about the quality of their nutrition. More often than not junk food forms the main part of the diet. Cakes, doughnuts, candy, soft drinks, alcohol, pies, gravies, French fries, dairy products, processed foods, white bread, sugar-loaded products, hamburgers, sundaes, hot dogs, fried chicken…you name it, the bulk freak will eat it. Surprisingly a few top name bodybuilders are bulk freaks. They binge shamelessly for size at any cost.

Paul Anderson, a former heavyweight Olympic

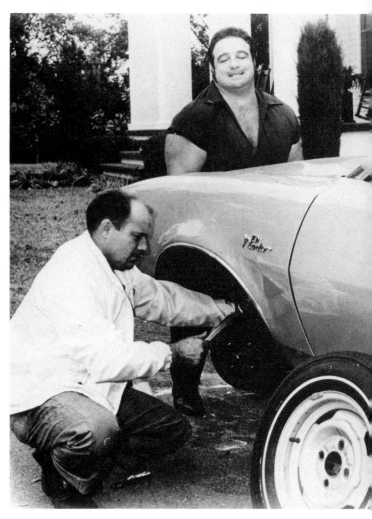

Strongman Paul Anderson gives a friend a helping hand.

lifter, bulked up to over 400 pounds using milk almost exclusively. Paul didn't care about looking trim or athletic. He just wanted to be strong, and *that* he was. He could raise over 400 pounds above his head in a lean back press and was particularly famous for his enormous squatting ability. He could in fact squat with 1,000 pounds any time and was reported to have done a couple of reps with 1,200 pounds. Needless to say, he won an Olympic gold medal before turning professional.

Another huge man, but not a naturally big-boned man like Anderson, is Bruce Randall. Whilst an ambulance driver in the Army, Bruce had time on his hands and decided to take advantage of the canteen facilities, which were open to him 24 hours a day. Well, to cut a long story short, Bruce trained and ate and ate and trained. He visited the canteen every hour or two. The man wanted to gain size and strength and took advantage of an inexhaustible supply of food to do it. He went from 170 pounds to 401 pounds, more than doubling his body weight within fourteen months. "I remember one time," says Bruce, "I was getting a bit of a name for myself as an eater. For a bet, I filled up my entire tray [note: he said tray, *not* plate] with rice and proceeded to eat every last grain. About three quarters of the way through I was beginning to feel full, so I resorted to eating a mouthful of rice followed by a gulp of water to help it down. Well, I won my bet, but that night as I lay in my bunk I thought I was going to die. The water was causing the rice to swell and I just lay on my back sweating and panting for breath, convinced that I would meet a ghastly death by bursting."

Somehow Bruce survived the night. Not long after that he decided to cut down his diet and get into Mr. Universe shape. His transformation was documented in *Iron Man* magazine, which ran a month-by-month account of his progress with pictures. Within eight months Bruce Randall was down to 189 pounds of lean muscle mass. He entered and won the Mr. Universe contest in London, England.

The Bruce Randall story is rare. Few people can halve their body weight in eight months; it's not the most healthy thing to do either. But he did it, and you can see his rapid weight reduction recorded in the pages of *Iron Man*. At his heaviest he could do a bent-leg good morning exercise with over 800 pounds and standing press 400. Because he trained with heavy weights, he had a substantial amount of muscle along with his fat. When I saw him at the Mr. Universe contest after his mammoth feat of weight reduction, there was not a millimeter of loose skin anywhere on his body. This is all the more unbelievable when you realize that he lost a total of more than 200 pounds.

Other bodybuilders to try the bulk route include six-foot-four-inch Lou Ferrigno, who went to 305 pounds; five-foot-eight-inch John Terilli, who went up to 260 pounds; and five-foot-ten-inch Scott Wilson, who went to 270 pounds;

Bruce Randall, before and after.

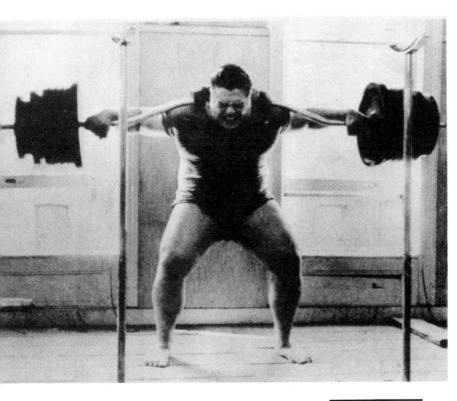
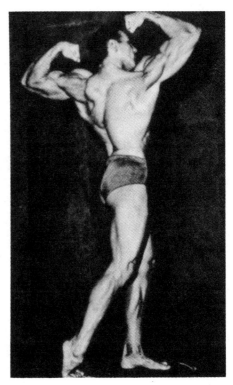

even six-foot-one-inch Arnold Schwarzenegger took his weight to 280 pounds in his early twenties. Each in turn learned that bulking up to a very high body weight in order to cut down to contest condition is not the best route to a physique title (but isn't it curious how each had to learn the lesson for himself!). Far better to train and eat with quality muscle in mind so that contest-winning condition can be achieved without undue months of prolonged heavy dieting.

The difference between men and women often shows itself in the area of body on which one puts fat. Women invariably gain fat first on their hips and upper thighs. Men, on the other hand, often have quite well-muscled (and fat-free) legs, while gaining rolls and rolls of fat around their waistlines.

To sum up then, gaining weight should really involve gaining muscle, although very thin bodybuilders need not worry about adding a little fat. Bulking up is generally considered an undesirable way to bodybuild, because you end up gaining more fat than muscle. Remember that fat does not add to attractiveness nor to the impressiveness of a physique. Fat fills in the valleys between the muscles and softens the separation. Fat detracts from the curves of a feminine physique and from the cuts of a masculine physique.

If you need weight quickly, nothing will do the job better than milk. People who don't want to go the milk route can try cheese or red meat. Gladys Portugues, who always had trouble gaining weight, found that eating red meat several times a day gave her the high amount of calories and first-class protein to gain weight. I should mention that Gladys' favorite food, which she also eats regularly when wanting more body weight, is pasta—always, I might add with Prego sauce.

Exercise routines while gaining weight should not be long, nor should you do much aerobic exercise, which will burn off valuable calories.

The usual theme of a weight-gaining plan is to ingest more calories. This is best done by

Gladys Portugues and Tom Terwilliger.   FACING PAGE: *John Terilli.*

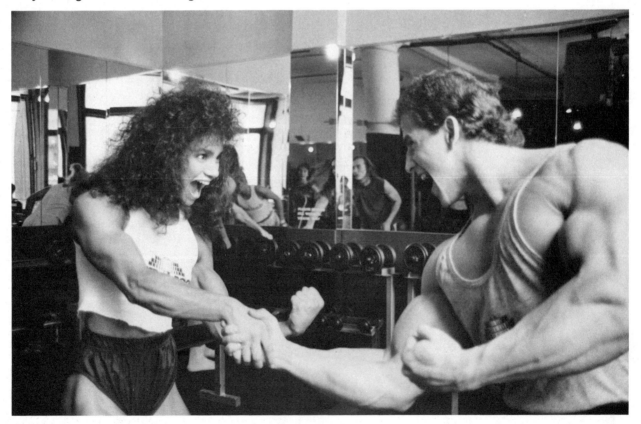

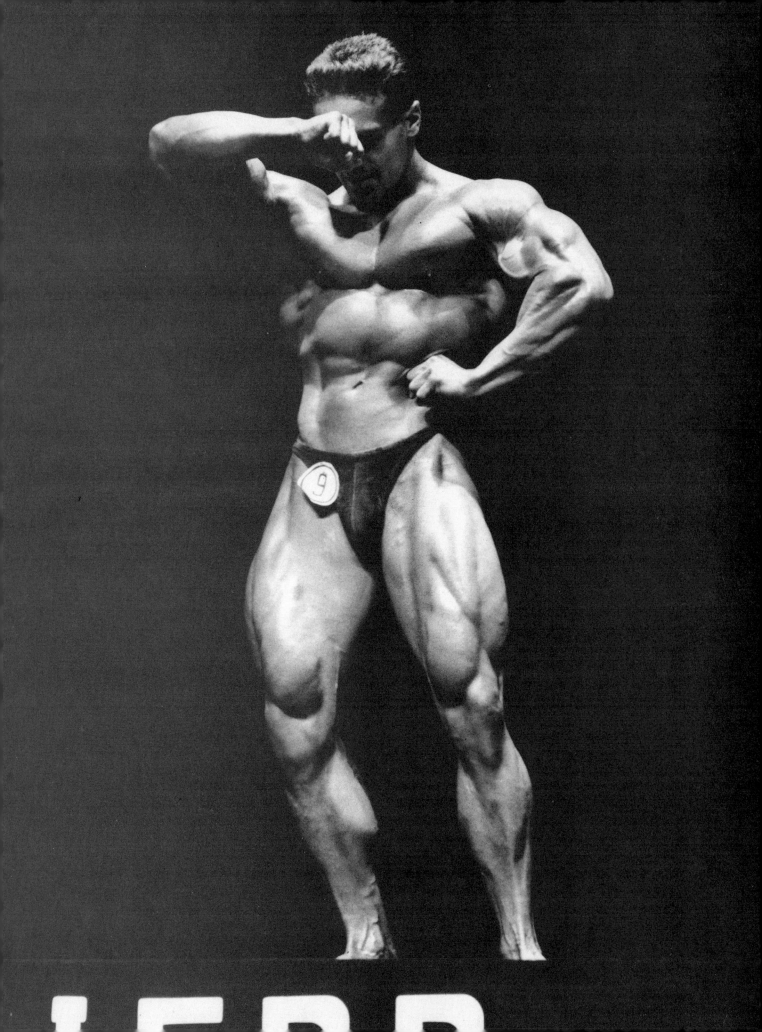

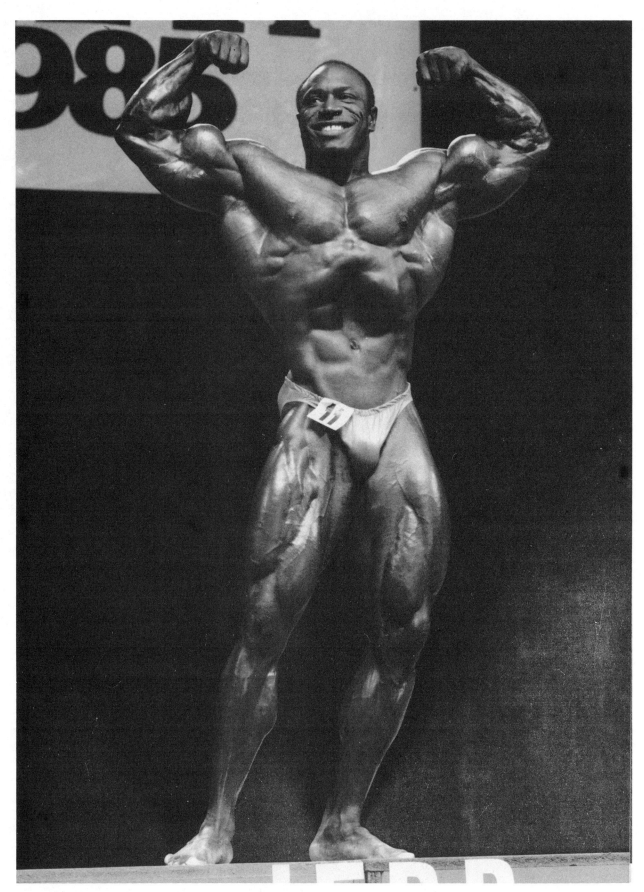

The King! Lee Haney.

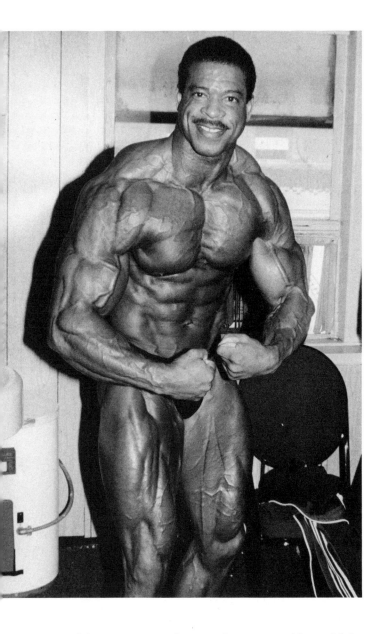

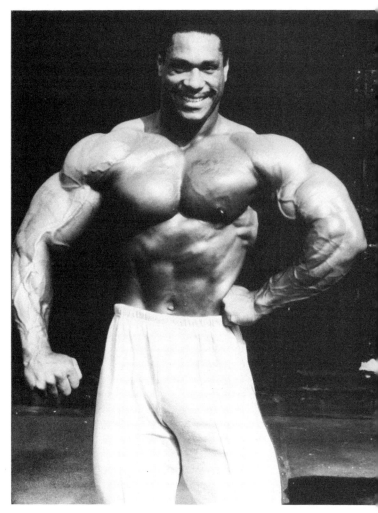

Goliath! Mike Christian.

Bill Grant, Mr. World.

taking extra meals, snacks, or nutritious high-protein milk shakes rather than by increasing the amount eaten at any one meal.

Protein shakes are best mixed in a blender, since items like fruit and protein powders are not easy to mix in a glass with a spoon. Always remember to put the liquid in first, then add the more solid items while the blender is operating. After mixing you may chill the shake further in the fridge. You can then remove at any time, shake or mix briefly, and enjoy!

Protein drinks mixed with milk should never be part of a precontest diet during the last few weeks. (However, amino acid capsules may be taken right up to competing.)

Here are some good high-protein shake variations:

High-Protein Shake #1

1 pint cold whole milk
2 scoops natural ice cream
½ cup evaporated milk

Mix and chill.

High-Protein Shake #2

1 pint whole milk
2 scoops natural ice cream
1 whole banana

Mix and chill.

High-Protein Shake #3

1 pint whole milk
1 tablespoon honey
1 banana

Mix well and chill.

High-Protein Shake #4

1 pint whole milk
½ cup evaporated milk
1 tablespoon peanut butter
1 tablespoon wheat germ oil

Beat or mix thoroughly and chill.

High-Protein Shake #5

1 pint whole milk
1 raw egg
½ banana
1 scoop natural ice cream
1 tablespoon peanut butter
1 teaspoon of wheat germ oil

Mix well and chill.

High-Protein Shake #6

1 pint whole milk
3 ounces natural yogurt
6 strawberries
1 tablespoon honey

Mix well and chill.

High-Protein Shake #7

1 pint whole milk
1 cup evaporated milk
1 tablespoon honey
1 scoop ice cream

Mix well and chill.

High-Protein Shake #8

1 pint whole milk
2 scoops natural ice cream
½ cup evaporated milk
1 whole egg

Beat well and chill.

High-Protein Shake #9

1 pint skimmed milk
5 tablespoons skim milk powder
6 strawberries

Blend well and chill.

High-Protein Shake #10

1 pint 2 percent milk
½ cup milk-and-egg protein powder
1 cup blueberries

Blend well and chill.

High-Protein Shake #11

1 pint skim milk
1 cup low-fat yogurt
½ cup blueberries
4 tablespoons milk-and-egg protein powder

Blend well and chill.

High-Protein Shake #12

1 pint whole raw milk
½ cup powdered egg whites
½ cup sliced kiwi
Shaved ice

Mix and drink.

High-Protein Shake #13

1 pint skim milk
½ cup milk protein powder
½ cup low-fat yogurt
½ cup sliced bananas and strawberries

Mix and drink.

High-Protein Shake #14

½ cup 2 percent milk
½ cup coconut milk
½ cup pineapple chunks
4 tablespoons milk-and-egg protein powder

Mix and drink.

High-Protein Shake #15

1 cup 2 percent milk
½ cup applesauce
¼ teaspoon cinnamon
4 tablespoons milk-and-egg protein powder
Shaved ice

Blend and serve.

21
FASTING
Down-Sizing Nutrition

Fasting is as old as humankind, but no doubt in prehistoric days cave dwellers didn't choose to go without food. It simply happened now and again because hunters couldn't outsmart their prey, or else weather and climatic changes caused prolonged food shortages.

Among the ancient Greeks, Hippocrates, "the father of medicine," recommended fasting for health, and both Plato and Socrates fasted to heighten their mental awareness and physical well-being. Fasting has also been practiced by the Indians and Orientals over the past twenty centuries, give or take a few.

There is little doubt that fasting heightens the body's sensitivity and helps to clear out waste products and debris that can otherwise clog up the system. Here's what Canadian health expert Hans Selye says: "A person is as young or old as his smallest vital component . . . the cell." It stands to reason, therefore, that to retain health and vitality, our body must be constantly replacing dead cells with new cells, and both dead and old cells should be cleared from the body efficiently. A controlled fast can do this.

A note of caution, however: Fasting does not suit everybody. In fact, if you are thinking of going on a fast, it is essential that you check with your doctor beforehand. Tell him why you are doing it and for how long. Get his unqualified approval before you begin.

Fasting, especially modified fasting, whereby you still take fruit juices and vegetable liquids, can work some pretty efficient and healthful body changes because the lack of food virtually forces the body to feed on itself, clearing out first and foremost cellular waste materials. That in turn provides a healthy environment for new cells to grow.

Andreas Cahling, Mr. International, has this to say: "The *secret* of fasting's effectiveness is that the body is selective in the use of its own cells. First, to satisfy its nourishment needs, it starts breaking down and burning the cells that are diseased, degenerated, old, or dead. During a fast, the system feeds on the most unclean,

Dave Hawk.

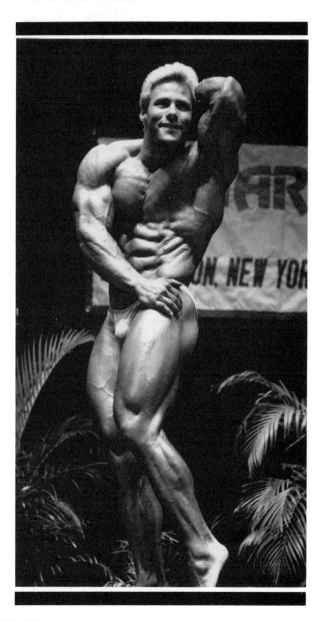

inferior material in the body, such as fat deposits, tumors, etc. Cells from vital body organs, the nervous system, and the brain will not be used."

Waste products clog your body and reduce overall efficiency. When you fast, lungs, kidneys, liver, and other internal organs are relieved of their toxic waste.

There are three negative things that may happen when you fast:

1. You may get light-headed.
2. You may develop a headache.
3. You could notice variations in energy levels.

These side effects can be minimized if you make a point of beginning a fast correctly. It is best to gear down to your first day of fasting by taking fruits and vegetables only for a few days prior to starting. In addition, curtail the severity of the fast by allowing yourself juices rather than plain water. Many health-conscious people, especially the fringe or borderline fanatics, may cynically claim that a fast on juices rather than water is not a "real" fast. The fact is such a fast could be considered superior in that chopped or pureed fruit and vegetable juices (mixed with water) can accelerate the body's cleansing capacity by supplying essential minerals and ionic charges.

MODIFIED FASTING FOR BODYBUILDERS

I suggest that you go on a fast (with your doctor's approval) about fifteen weeks prior to competing in a bodybuilding contest.

Day #1
Cut down on your regular eating to half portions.

Day #2
Eat only raw vegetables and fruits; drink water and juices.

Day #3
Continue with a variety of raw vegetables and fruits, water and juices.

Day #4 to end
Begin your juice-only diet (vegetables and fruits) and remain on it for three to five days. You may drink as much juice as you wish. Hunger will be subdued and the cleansing action will go into high gear. Include carrot, celery, apple, orange, lemon, watermelon, and any other naturally prepared juices. Do *not* ingest artificial or processed juices of any kind. This will defeat the purpose of the fast completely.

BREAKING A FAST

Muscle and Fitness magazine quotes famous health doctor Otto F. Buchinger as saying, "Even an idiot can fast, but only a wise man knows how to break a fast." Do not sabotage your efforts by returning to solid foods in full force. Bernarr McFadden, the father of modern physical culture, was said to have become very ill when he broke a long fast by eating a huge three-pound steak.

When you break a fast, first return to peeled fruit in small amounts. Eat slowly and chew everything thoroughly. Gradually add new foods during the next three days until you are back on a normal diet. Do not shock your system by eating large amounts of hard-to-digest foods that traditionally cause indigestion in people, or at the very least stomach irritation. A fast highly sensitizes your body to undesirable foods—coffee, alcohol, and drugs are just three. Do not break a fast with any of these items or with any other potential irritants.

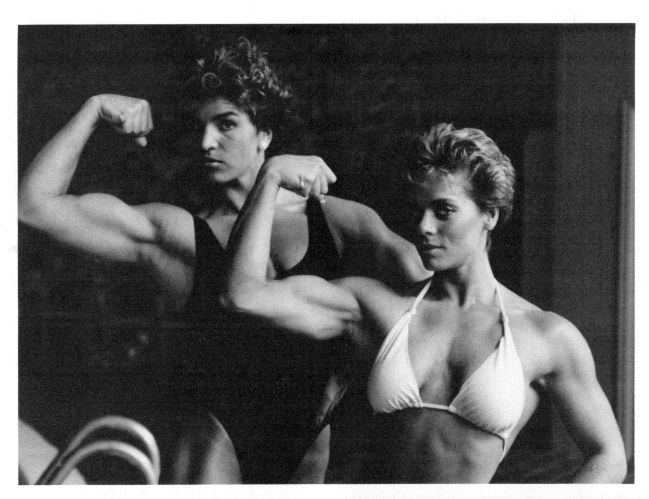

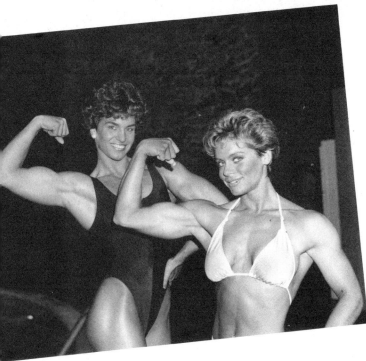

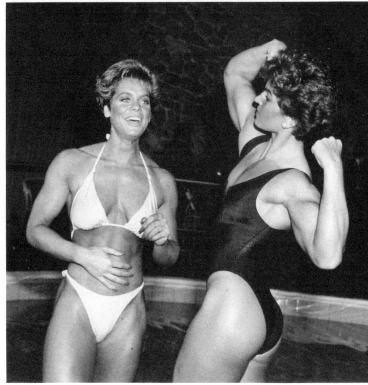

Marjo Selin (Finland) and Carla Temple (Canada).

THE GAINS

A fast may do more to rejuvenate you than anything else, but it must be carried out correctly. Your first fast will teach you more than you ever dreamed about your body and mind. There's no need to stop training while on a fast. Simply cut down slightly on the length of your workouts. Your energy level may dip at first, but when you are well and truly into the fast you will notice an *increase* in energy, plus an increase in mind perception. *You will be more in tune with your body than ever before in your lifetime.*

Rather than maintaining a body composed of diseased and worn-out cells and toxins, you'll be on the road to having a body consisting of pure, natural nutrients and fresh tissue. Finally, lean muscle gains will come quicker after a fast. Martin Katahn, Ph.D., author of *Beyond Diet: The 28-Day Metabolic Breakthrough Plan,* conducted fasting experiments with rats and found that rats subjected to fasts actually "learned" to assimilate food more efficiently than rats that were kept on a consistent diet. They also gained weight more easily.

If the results of Katahn's experiments with rodents can be translated into human reactions, then you may well find that a timely period devoted to fasting can help you add more muscle to your body. At the very least, you will detoxify your system and ready yourself for ultimate health and vitality, both of which you need for super gains.

"**A**s a practicing physician," says Dr. Robert C. Atkins in his *Super Energy Cookbook* (New American Library), "I can assure you that the most common complaint for which a patient walks into a doctor's office is fatigue."

Yes, there are millions of us in the Western world who are lacking vitality. Our energy levels are totally depleted. What is the cause? Yes, some of us could be suffering from anemia, a sluggish thyroid, a chronic infection, or even some serious heart or other ailment, but most of us who lack vitality owe our drained feelings to problems in our life-style, and more often than not the trouble is rooted in our eating habits.

Are you a victim of the human energy crisis? Are you drained at the end of the day, when you should be all fired up for your workout? Perhaps you don't feel 100 percent at the beginning of the day either?

Physical energy. The words bring to mind movement, vitality, and enthusiasm. All achievers have energy. Where does it come from? Is it inherited? Is it natural? Or does it have to be earned?

In reality, vitality is our inherited birthright. It's natural to a person in normal robust health. When we feel good we enjoy movement and effort. We *spend* energy recklessly and in doing so rebuild our capacity to generate greater and greater amounts of energy.

To understand how physical energy is generated, think of your body as a power plant. Nutrition is your fuel, oxygen the agent that keeps the energy fire burning. As oxygen is transported to body cells, the fire is ignited, burning consumed food and thereby releasing energy.

Basically, what you eat determines your energy levels, but there are thieves that can rob you of energy quicker than you can say "Arnold Schwarzenegger"!

To keep your energy at a maximum pitch, you have to live a holistic life-style. Pay attention not only to diet, but to exercise and relaxation, and stay alert to negative habits that can quickly drain you of every last ounce of energy and make life seem barely worth living.

Corinna Everson.

22
ENERGY
Recharging the Batteries

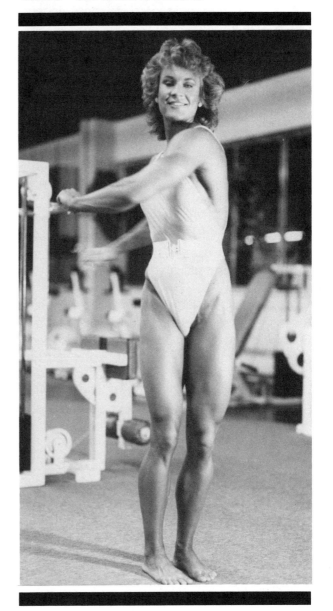

You need energy just to survive, but more than that, you require it for everyday work, walking, talking, writing, you name it. For the bodybuilder it is required in abundance right when you need it most, at workout time. For that reason it is a good idea to train at approximately the same time each day. That prompts the body to set its internal clock, to ready its energy levels so that at the appointed hour you are rarin' to go!

Michael Durocher, a lab technician at the University of Toronto's fitness laboratory, assesses training programs of a variety of athletes. He says, "Energy doesn't increase; the ability to produce it does. Everyone has that ability. The degree to which you can create more depends on how fit you become."

There is no doubt that regular formal exercise, especially when it stimulates the heart and lungs, increases the blood's oxygen-carrying capacity. More oxygen is transported faster and more efficiently to where it is urgently required. You can rejuvenate your body energy by stressing yourself physically on a regular basis. All things being equal, we become efficient and good at what we show nature we want by actively striving for it. If we rest, we rust. "Life is movement," said the first modern bodybuilder, Eugene Sandow, almost a century ago. Failing to exercise is unhealthy because the pumping power of your heart drops dramatically when you do not exert yourself regularly.

On the other hand overexercise can bring about identical low-energy symptoms. If you overtrain and under-rest, you will not fully recuperate from your workouts. This also leaves you tired and listless—you have been robbed of energy by your own doing. Many bodybuilders are almost constantly overtrained; and often they don't know that this is the reason for their constant tiredness.

BEWARE THE ENERGY THIEVES

Coffee

Many bodybuilders drink coffee because it seems to provide a perk-up effect. But unfortunately, if it is consumed in large quantities, it actually drains you of energy. The culprit is caffeine. Too much of this drug can cause heart palpitations (irregular beat), insomnia, increased gastric acid secretion, and high blood pressure.

In some cases coffee can trigger a flow of insulin and precipitate a hypoglycemic "attack." The symptoms of hypoglycemia are easy to recognize. They are also easy to imagine. At first you will experience a feeling of emptiness (not hunger), fatigue, irritability, shallow breathing, and tightness in the chest. There may be some sweating and dizziness with heart palpitations. Some people have headaches, too.

These symptoms usually occur about three hours after a meal and are relieved by eating. But eat starch (whole-grain bread, muffins, cereal) or proteins (cheese, meat, beans, eggs), which will normalize your insulin flow, rather than try to "cure" the condition with sugar candies or soft drinks, all of which will relieve the symptoms, but only temporarily.

Hypoglycemics should never miss meals. Try decaffeinated coffee or tea. Although the medical establishment currently pays little attention to hypoglycemia, the condition is recognized as an energy drain.

Cigarettes

We all know the dangers of cigarette smoking, although we may not want to believe them. There are diseases associated with tobacco that defy the imagination; they are too horrific to describe. Fortunately, not all heavy smokers are victims of these diseases. The same cannot be said for shortness of breath or lack of energy. There all heavy smokers are victims to some degree.

The ultimate smoker, of course, is so debilitated by the 200-plus poisons in each cigarette that he or she is usually felled in the prime of life, unable to think straight or breathe easily. Walking, our most natural movement, becomes difficult and can only be carried out with discomfort. Robert C. Atkins (*Dr. Atkins' Super Energy Diet,* Bantam Books) says, "Smoking causes a fall in blood sugar by stimulating the adrenal gland. By joining the millions of people who have become non-smokers, you may find considerably more energy." Nothing negates the endurance-building benefits of super nutrition more than the poisons we take into our lungs.

Alcohol

For hypoglycemics or those hoping to lose fat, any alcohol is undesirable. For those who are trying to maximize energy output, alcohol consumption should be limited to small quantities with meals. Even then there may be a quick onslaught of tiredness.

Alcohol has calories, but poor-quality "empty" calories. It is an energy destroyer par exellence. Ned Bayrd and Chris Quilter, authors of *Food for Champions* (Berkley Books), write, "There is some evidence that a couple of drinks a day may be good for us, because such moderate drinking is associated with a lower risk of heart disease. But a couple of additional drinks will probably affect our training and performance and a couple beyond that definitely will."

There is no doubt—and it has been known for hundreds of years—that excessive drinking can ruin your health. Alcohol has no real nutritional value and often replaces food containing the protein, vitamins, and minerals that bodybuilders need to function and progress efficiently. Alcohol also interferes with the absorption of several B vitamins and often deprives our bodies of these vitamins even when we are ingesting them through an otherwise high-quality diet. Furthermore, alcohol can disrupt life-style, relationships, sleep, and exercise patterns. Taken in excess it slowly interferes with normal functions of the brain and over time can lead to fatal liver disease. It's an energy drain with dangerous potential.

Stress

Despite the fact that many cases of fatigue, depression, and related symptoms are correctable by diet, there are other considerations. For example, an individual may be suffering from emotional problems, some so serious that they require psychiatric help.

If you've had a recent infection or other physical or emotional stress, it is important that you take the recommended dosages of vitamins and minerals and maintain a balanced diet. It's natural, when suffering from emotional problems or some personal worry, to pay little attention to your diet. In moments of crisis you may pass up meals, live on junk food eaten at irregular intervals, even resort to alcohol, cigarettes, and coffee.

Try not to fall into these habits. No one is immune to emotional stress. You may be a successful business person, own a couple of mansions and a fleet of Cadillacs, and have a seven-figure bank account...then find it all counts for nought when your husband or wife ups and leaves you for the "charms" of someone else half your age. It happens. And expect to suffer emotionally if it does! When love gets battered around and our egos get bruised, we can hit the bottom of the barrel. We experience feelings of worthlessness and exhaustion. Nothing is tougher to overcome than an emotional clobbering.

But simple, everyday worry can cause low energy levels, too. In most cases worry doesn't solve anything. More often than not, the things we worry about never materialize, whether they be money problems, health concerns, or political or work-related anxieties. Our worrying only works to affect our own physical and mental health negatively.

Drugs

All drugs have undesirable side effects, so it is better to avoid them if at all possible. The medical profession is bombarded with an ongoing release of new drugs on a daily basis; doctors cannot keep up with all the advances. No doctor

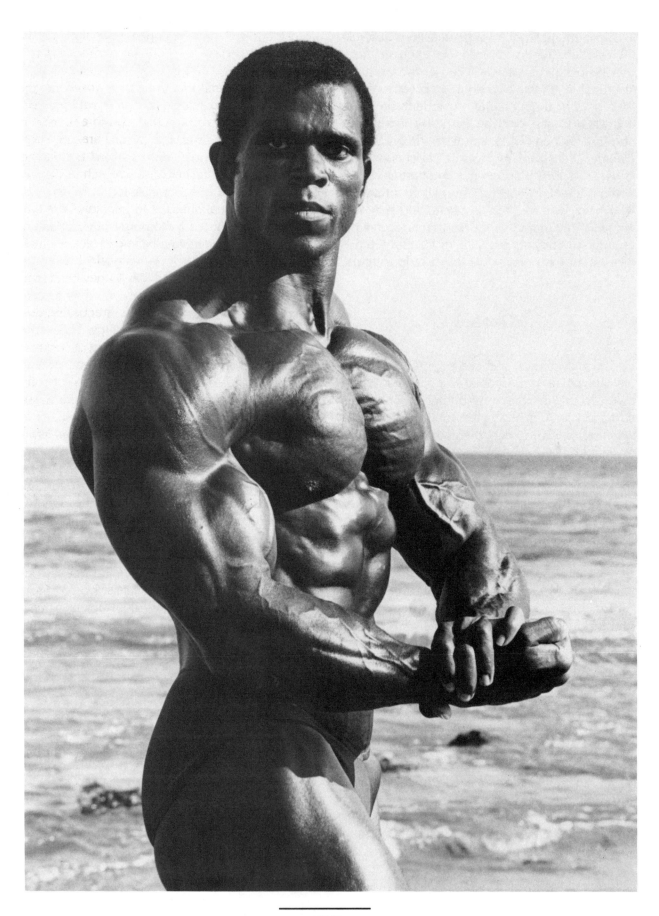

knows all about each and every drug—there are too many.

Today we have drugs that calm you (e.g., Valium) and drugs that rev you up (e.g., caffeine pills). Both tranquilizers and antidepressants can be bad for your natural energy levels. If you take a pill to *give* you energy, you will quickly reach a peak and burn out, returning to an energy level far below that which you experienced in the first place. Tranquilizers rob you of life-giving energy by slowing you down until you lose all relationship with natural true vigor. Hard, so-called recreational drugs need not be discussed here. Their destructive debilitating effect is widely known.

Poor Nutrition

I remember seeing Serge Nubret, Mr. Universe, fall asleep between sets of leg presses. This type of thing happened regularly when Serge was on a low-carbohydrate diet prior to competing. He just plain ran out of energy and fell asleep.

Today most bodybuilders eat some carbs every day, even when they are only a week or two from competition. They seldom fall asleep in the gym. Most have abundant energy even when ripping up for an important event.

Carole Alcorn, a nutritionist at the Toronto Health Education Center, says, "What you eat determines the flow of your energy. Your body's cells will be formed from either high octane fuel or cheap stuff. Positive foods and beverages are life-creating. Negative ones drain the alkalines from the body."

Eliminating energy-robbing foods from the diet is the first step toward an energy-producing regimen. Complex carbohydrates found in starchy foods such as whole-grain bread, cereal grains, and fruits and vegetables are vital to health and energy. Simple carbohydrates (sugars) in the form of soft drinks, pastries, and candy may give a quick energy boost, but all too soon they leave you running on "empty." Stay away from these as much as possible.

Some people with low energy owe their condition to iron deficiency. Iron is a primary ingredient in hemoglobin, the blood's oxygen carrier. A lack of iron in the diet will cause your oxygen-deficient body to tire easily, and you will feel short of breath. You will find iron in abundance in foods like liver, dried fruits, asparagus, spinach, and beef. It has been observed that eating iron-rich foods together with food rich in vitamin C improves the iron absorption.

Do not make the mistake of thinking that nutrition alone is the answer. You can eat a perfect diet and still your energy levels can be low. The best nutrition in the world has to be used by mobilizing your body to get the blood circulating.

Vitamins and minerals do not directly energize the body, but they are vital to energy. They work with food to keep the system running correctly. If there is any doubt about your present level of vitamin and minerals consumption, consider taking a one-a-day supplement as a form of insurance.

Protein has been denigrated recently, especially by those who have jumped on the carbohydrate bandwagon. But listen to this: "Protein is important to endurance," says Bill Evans, Ph.D., of Tufts University. "We once thought of protein as having a trivial role in bodybuilding and energy levels. We now know it has a significant place." Peter Lemon, at Kent State University's laboratory in Ohio, suggests that the level of activity will determine an athlete's protein need. For the recreational athlete 1.0 gram of protein per kilogram (2.2 pounds) of body weight is sufficient. A training athlete should take 1.5 grams per kilogram per day, and a bodybuilder who makes extraordinary demands on his or her muscles should take up to 2.0 grams of protein per kilogram per day. For the carbo-generation this may sound like an awful lot of protein, but a bodybuilder must pay homage to two requirements: a need for abundant energy and protein-to-spare for the muscle-building process. (See chapter 6.)

Serge Nubret, Mr. Universe.

Sugar

This is the big enemy of energy, yet ironically the man in the street feels that sugar is energy-plus. The truth is, we don't need sugar if we have starch. But we are so accustomed to the taste of sugar that none of us does without it, except some diabetics, who may have to in order to stay healthy. Check the labels of soups, condiments, cereals, ketchup, canned foods, breads, or most any other processed food; sugar's in it! Most North Americans, Britons, Australians, and South Africans consume around 100 pounds of sugar annually. A teaspoon of sugar contains 25 calories. When you finish off a meal with chocolate cake instead of an apple you are eating far more calories but far less nutrition. Learn to say no, and say it with authority when your family tries to "sweet-talk" you into having one more brownie. Sugar and sugar-loaded products are lethal, not only to our energy levels but to life itself.

Sugar was not part of mankind's diet until relatively recently. It became important around the nineteenth century, when Napoleon set up sugar factories in Europe. In 1815 the average Englishman was consuming about seven and a half pounds a year. By 1850 world sugar production was 1.5 million tons a year. Today world sugar production is 70 million tons and growing fast!

Dr. Robert Atkins says, "My practice has taught me one basic thing. If a person is tired, and you take away his sugar and give him vitamins and minerals, you can usually get him to feel better."

Sugar is the chief initiator of hypoglycemia (low blood sugar). Sugar overstimulates the pancreas to produce too much insulin, which then eats up all the sugar in the blood and leaves you with low blood sugar. You're out of gas!

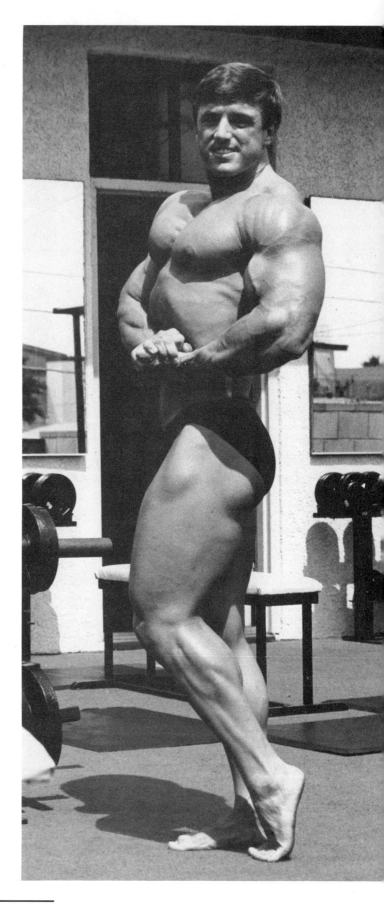

Canadian champion Andre Maille.

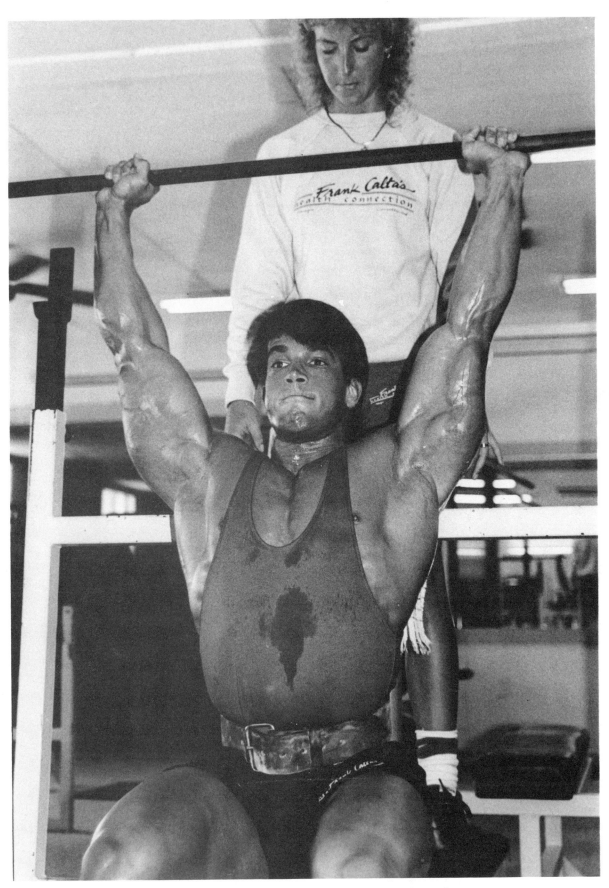

Brian Silk of Florida completes a press behind the neck.

HIGH-ENERGY DRINKS

I have two high-energy drinks for you, neither of which I invented personally, but both of which I can vouch for sincerely.

1. The High-Energy Drink (with raw liver), given by Dr. Michael Walczak in his book *Nutrition and Well Being* (Mojave Books).

Take good-quality calf or beef liver (the fresher the better) and freeze it. Take the equivalent of two tablespoons of the frozen liver and put it in a blender with a glass of tomato juice. Add a little Tabasco to taste. Set the blender to chop or grate, not blend.

Walczak believes that this drink is a superior source of energy and nutrition. "You are getting nucleic acids, which are potent proteins. It is high in nitrogen. The nucleic acids affect chromosonal activity which make up the DNA and RNA." For those who do not have access to a blender, grate the frozen liver on a metal cheese grater and then add to a glass of tomato juice.

2. The Dynamite Energy Milkshake formulated by the scintillating Naura Hayden. Naura is author of the best-selling *Everything You've Always Wanted to Know About Energy, But Were Too Weak to Ask* (Pocket Books).

Into a blender pour two cups skimmed milk, one tablespoon safflower oil, two packets (or the equivalent) sugar substitute, and one teaspoon vanilla extract.

Start the blender and add a teaspoon of yeast and a teaspoon of lecithin. Add to these each week so that after a month you are using ten teaspoons of both powdered yeast and lecithin.

Ms. Hayden suggests that after you have blended this concoction you cover it and put it in the fridge overnight. Apparently the overnight cold greatly benefits the taste. Next morning blend again for twenty seconds until frothy, and drink. Prepare the next day's batch the night before.

It doesn't take a whole lot of intelligence to conclude that the person who wakes up to a cigarette, a jelly doughnut, a cup of coffee with three lumps of sugar and then lunches on hot dogs, French fries, and a cola...who also swamps his or her system with coffee, smoke, or candy morning, noon, and night...does not have a great chance of ready access to natural energy.

True, you may feel well some of the time, but now's your chance to change all that. You can feel like a million bucks *all* of the time.

23
OFF-SEASON NUTRITION
Quality Eating

When you first start training with weights there's no such thing as an off-season period. It's gung-ho all the way. But as time goes on and you start entering contests, you begin to categorize each part of your training year.

The off-season is the time of general all-round training and basic nutrition. During this period you are not trying to define your body and get ripped for a contest. You are merely trying to build quality muscle. Perhaps you will use this time to specialize somewhat on some of your weak points.

People who enter four or five contests a year don't have an off-season. They simply ride up and down like a yo-yo. Making steady gains under these conditions is difficult. Ideally, you should enter only one or two shows a year while you are still striving for added size and symmetry.

The off-season period (when no contest date is in sight) is the time to make progress. Your nutritional intake tends to be more relaxed. Few people count calories during the off-season. It is a time when you need a constant, steady supply of energy. The calorie content of your meals will tend to be generous.

But be warned. It is not a good idea to eat so much that you gain excess fat. According to Arnold Schwarzenegger, "Male bodybuilders should keep their body weight within six to eight pounds of their competition weight; women within four or five pounds." Actually, I have noticed that many men put on from fifteen to twenty pounds between contests, and quite a few women add ten to twelve pounds. This, of course, makes dieting all the more difficult when you have to get in shape for an exhibition, a contest, or a photo session. Besides that, an overweight bodybuilder is not a good endorsement for our sport. What's the use of training all year round if you only look acceptable for one week of the fifty-two and like a fat slob for the rest of the time?

The fact is that many bodybuilders get so heavy between shows that they end up fat all the time; finally they *never* get back in shape, *never*

Steve Davis.

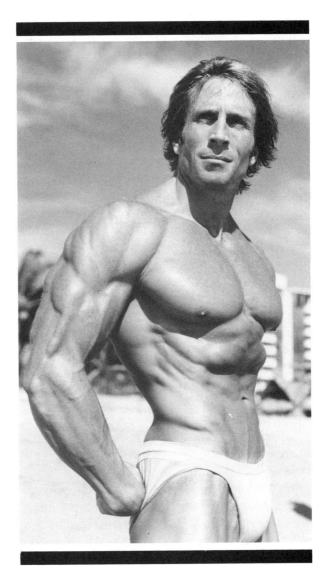

enter another show, and *never* look good again. In or out of clothes, they are fatsos. In his book *Gaining Muscle Size and Density* (Valencia Books), competitive bodybuilder Steve Davis of California says, "The off-season is a time for constructive training, not a time to get fat. But at this time when you are trying to add size you will have to lose some muscularity, but never to the point where your abdominals disappear."

Mr. Olympia Samir Bannout agrees that bulking up for the sake of merely weighing more is foolish. "It's garbage. For most bodybuilders, bulking up is simply an excuse to eat like a pig for three or four months." Diana Dennis feels the same way. "Why get fat in the off-season? You only have to work like a dog to get it all off again."

For almost a century bodybuilders have been recorded as having huge appetites. Well, most of them anyway. Some of the old-time Austrian strongmen would think nothing of downing several pounds of ham or beef and chasing that with a gallon of beer! John Grimek, a prewar Mr. America, could really put food away. Six-pound steaks, chicken, you name it. Then there was Mr. Universe Ken Waller. Did he ever eat less than three chickens at one meal? According to Bill Reynolds, some of the off-season gastronomical feats of champion bodybuilders are worthy of inclusion in the *Guinness Book of World Records.* He cites bodybuilder Larry Gordon (a Mr. America finalist), who once ate thirty-seven pieces of chicken in one sitting in little more than an hour. The restaurant at which Larry recorded this "feat" had an "all the chicken you can eat" invitation. After his mammoth eating session, the restaurant realized the folly of its ways and promptly rescinded the "all you can eat" policy, fearing it might lead to bankruptcy.

I can recall eating with French bodybuilder Serge Nubret. Even during his precontest period, he would eat several pounds of meat at one sitting, but no vegetables save for a few lettuce leaves. The meat was invariably horse meat (unlike North Americans the French eat horse meat), and he would eat as much as ten pounds daily. Bill Reynolds, who translated Nubret's chest course into English, corroborates the Frenchman's penchant for horse meat in *Supercut: Nutrition for the Ultimate Physique* (Contemporary Books),

penned with successful author and bodybuilder Joyce Vedral, Ph.D.

To some the term *off-season* may seem a little negative. It is not meant to be. The off-season is actually the most positive (and longest) period of your training year. It is the time when your workouts and nutrition habits should link up to help you make the best gains of your life.

Off-season eating has to be the most nutritious and beneficial possible. It must serve your every dietary need. There's no excuse for deficiencies of vitamins or minerals. Virtually every meal should contain 15 to 25 grams of high-quality protein; whole-grain products are a must, as are fruits and vegetables.

Getting back to Steve Davis: "There is definitely a special method of adding muscle density. During this endeavor, the muscle (sarcoplast) and the muscle environment (sarcoplasm) ratio must be nearly equal. This means you must keep your ingestion of high-quality, muscle-building protein and complex carbohydrates at a higher than precontest level. Prior to a contest, when the diet is almost void of carbohydrate for a while, the quantity of sarcoplasm is greatly diminished, which obviously causes muscle girth to decrease proportionately."

The off-season is a time for *correct* nutrition. Proper nutrition can make a striking difference in the way you look and feel. It does not require superhuman effort or megadoses of vitamins. You do not have to seek out rare and expensive foods. Neither does it mean eliminating many foods from your diet.

Proper nutrition simply means supplying your body with the nutrients it requires in the approximate quantities needed in assimilable form. In previous chapters, I have reviewed some of the best health and muscle-building foods, but I should remind you that nutrition is not the total answer. In truth, exercise is the most important factor in bodybuilding. Your food intake merely helps it along. You cannot hope to follow a slipshod training routine and make up for it by following an optimum diet; you cannot eat your way to muscular size. Correct nutrition merely helps you reach your goals by supplying your body with the nutrients it needs to allow muscle growth to occur at the quickest possible rate, without storing excess fat.

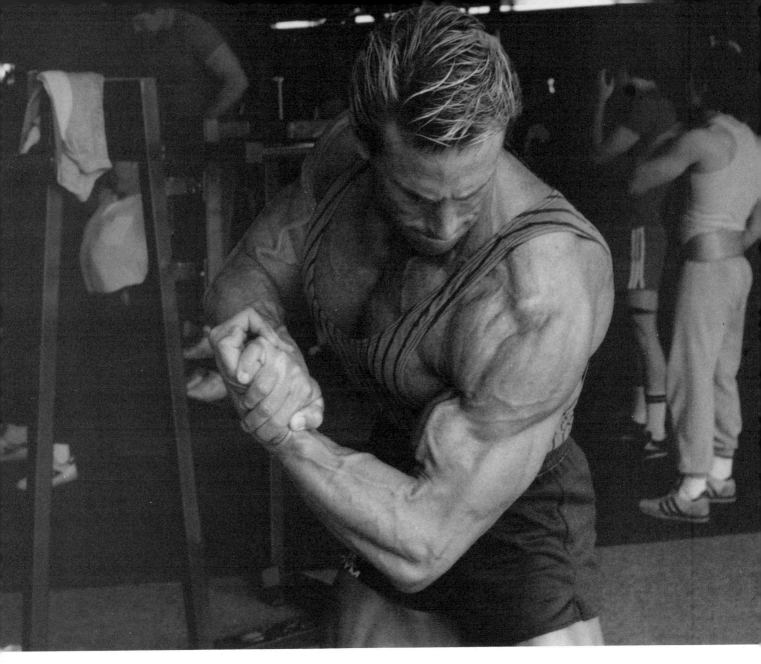

Steve Davis, California.

Through trial and error I have found that it's easy to get careless with one's nutrition. A slip here and there can lead to *frequent* slips here and there. Pretty soon you're back to eating junk, refined foods, or high-fat dishes. You have to pull yourself up now and again. An occasional departure from the straight-and-narrow is okay, but if it becomes a habit, you're no better than anyone else. And the point of this book is to *feed* you better in order to *make* you superior. It all begins with the off-season diet.

Many people rely on their instincts when it comes to off-season eating. Quite often if we have a high-carbohydrate, low-protein breakfast we will instinctively feel like having a high-protein, low-carbohydrate lunch. This *instinctive training principle* works to an extent when applied to food, just as only eating when we're hungry works. But in this day and age of hustle and bustle, of school, job or family-related stress, not everyone can rely on instinct for accurate feedback. I feel it is better to *plan* your nutrition intake as much as possible. Feelings about nutrition often signal us too late, and if we have something else on our mind we may not get the message at all. Use the information in this book to make your off-season diet the best it can be. That's what *Rock Hard!* eating is all about.

Y es, this is a nutrition book, but a chapter on the other aspects of bodybuilding will not go amiss. I have recorded my specialized training philosophy in two previous books, *Reps!* and *Beef It!* (Sterling Publishing Company), for those who want advanced training advice that goes into great detail. But the following digest information will help keep you on track as far as general bodybuilding advice is concerned.

GOAL SETTING

You will not become a Mr. or Ms. Olympia after training for six months, nor probably after even three years of pumping iron. You have to be realistic.

Achievement in anything starts with wanting. The next step is to set *small achievable goals.* Do not aim to win the Mr. America title by the end of your first year in bodybuilding. The target is too hard to hit. Set a realistic goal. Tell yourself that you will put an extra inch on your arms in eight weeks. Of course, if you do it in six weeks, all the better, but at least you set an achievable target in the first place. When you have reached your goal, set a new one. Again, it must be something that you can achieve by your self-imposed deadline.

It is well known that we can more easily succeed if we have something concrete to aim at, but if it's farfetched or virtually impossible, then the prospect of failure will kill off enthusiasm. On the other hand, success breeds success.

SETS AND REPS

There is no exact system of sets and reps, no "average" that *always* works. Most successful bodybuilders perform three to six sets of an

24
THE WORKOUT
Training and Attitudes

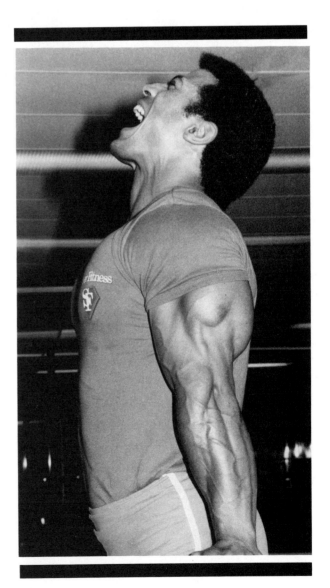

Mohamed Makkawy completes a set of dips.

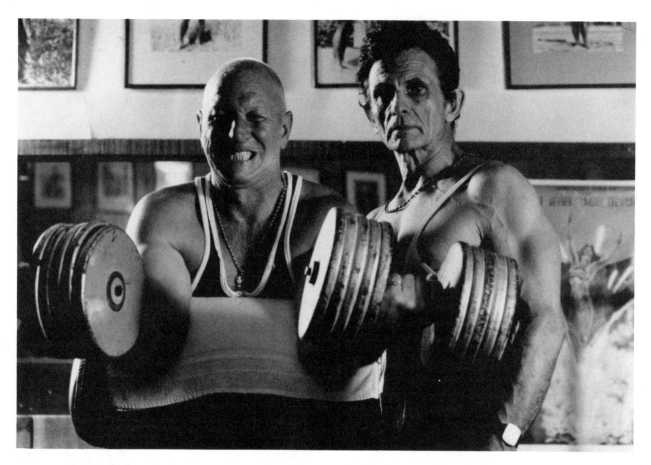

exercise for eight to twelve reps, but that doesn't mean this will work for you.

The truth is that most bodybuilders use a variety of sets and reps in their training. It is quite common, for example, to use eight sets of bench presses (a popular exercise) but only four sets of squats, rowing, curls, or abs.

Likewise with repetitions: High-rep muscle groups such as forearms, calves, and abdominals are frequently trained with a system of fifteen to twenty repetitions, whereas other areas such as the chest, back, and shoulders may be worked with a system of six to eight reps.

Are high reps better than low reps, or vice versa? No, but there are general parameters that experience has taught us to keep in mind. Generally, bodybuilders will *not* make their best gains using less than six reps per set. Nor, except for the aforementioned high-rep muscle groups, will there be significant benefit in using more than twelve to fifteen reps, except perhaps in squats. Several bodybuilders—Tom Platz is one example—have made remarkable progress by performing high-rep squats (thirty to fifty per set).

Bob Tessier and Vince Gironda.

Women differ slightly from men in their rep requirements. Because most women have lighter bone structures than men, the joints, especially in the elbows and shoulders, could become sore or damaged from prolonged heavy-duty low-rep, high-weight workouts. The main workout reps from men are usually eight to twelve (fifteen to twenty for high-rep muscles). Women should never do less than eight reps if they want to remain injury free.

EXERCISE STYLE

There is no doubt that your muscles "feel it" more if the weight is lifted and lowered slowly. On the other hand, quick movements, once mastered, enable the trainer to perform several more reps than a person using slow, concentrated form. Both ways build muscle. There is no reason why you shouldn't chop and change. Just as there is more than one way to skin a cat, there is more than one way to fatigue muscle cells. Listen to Vince Gironda: "The object of bodybuilding workouts is to hit the muscle hard in the quickest possible time; destroy it...and then move on to the next muscle area."

Cheating, swinging the weight up and down or using momentum to raise a weight, has its own variations. The bench press, for example, can be performed in many different ways. You can raise and lower the weight slowly, pausing at but not touching the chest, holding the elbows well back (in line with the bar). This is the ultrastrict style. Other, less strict methods would involve fast lowering of the weight, bouncing the bar lightly on the chest, drawing elbows in to the sides, heaving the hips up from the bench, arching the back during lift off, etc.

Creative cheating is using your intuition and inventiveness to direct more pressure to a specific area of the body that you want to concentrate on.

GENETICS

It is unlikely that a tall six-foot-plus person will ever become an Olympic gymnast, nor will a big-framed 300-pound man ever win an Olympic gold in the marathon. A short barrel-chested individual with small feet will not win a swimming gold, and a skinny small-framed person will not win the Olympic medal for shotput. We are all limited to some extent by our genetics with respect to what we can achieve physically. You will not make it to the very top of the bodybuilding ladder if you are not genetically predisposed to carry a lot of muscle mass.

Not all men can obtain a muscular twenty-one-inch arm, and not all women can build the dynamic proportions necessary to win a Ms. Olympia title. Nature has already drawn the line.

It's hard, I know, but none of us can exceed the limitations laid down by Mother Nature.

WHERE TO TRAIN

Most of us have only two alternatives when it comes to where to train. We can either do it at home or at a commercial gym. There are pros and cons for both. If you become a member of a gym, you may find that it is overcrowded on the nights when you want to train (especially on Monday nights). Also the gym may be a long way from your home, which could prove awkward during inclement weather or if you are pressed for time. However, progress is often greater for those who train at a gym, because the atmosphere there is usually conducive to making you train harder. Everyone tries a little bit more. Finally, a commercial gym invariably has a wider variety of apparatus than home gyms.

Home training has its great advantage in always being available. There are no hassles from others, and never any waiting in line to use apparatus. But you do need strong willpower and singleness of purpose to keep hitting hard at your workouts. Most bodybuilders have, during their careers, alternated their workouts between home and commercial gym training.

INCREASING INTENSITY

To an extent, the more weight you use the bigger your muscles will grow. But it doesn't *always* apply. Your muscles can't "see" what weight you are using. They can only "feel." So the weight itself doesn't matter. It's how you make your muscles feel the weight that counts.

The simple-minded among us can only relate increased *intensity* to increased *resistance*. There's more to it than that. The whole object is to involve as many cells as possible during a set. (A cell either contracts 100 percent or not at all, so the object is always to involve as many cells as you can.)

You can get normally dormant cells to contract by using added resistance, more reps (either while maintaining or increasing weight), additional sets, extra concentration, less rest between sets, stricter style, looser style, extra squeezing of the muscle being worked, half reps, super sets, giant sets, pre-exhaustion, pyramid training, compound sets, forced reps, rest pause. All these techniques are explained in detail in other books dealing with hardcore bodybuilding including *Mass!* (Contemporary Books) and *Flex Appeal* by Rachel McLish (Warner Books).

REST AND SLEEP

It's no good applying regular effort to your workouts if you don't recuperate properly between each exercise session. Of course, as explained earlier, nutrition has a great deal to do with muscle recuperation. But there is also the matter of rest. The body builds up when in a relaxed state, especially during sleep. You certainly cannot reasonably expect to build volumes of muscle if you play several sets of tennis before your workout and go dancing afterwards.

Bodybuilders usually require hours more sleep than nonbodybuilders. That means eight hours per night as an average. Some professional bodybuilders actually sleep ten hours each night, and not a few take an additional nap (muscle sleep) during the day.

Men and women who do manual labor seldom build to their maximum size, although men like Chuck Sipes, Lou Ferrigno, Sergio Oliva, and Frank Richards have all combined hard physical jobs with their training and built title-winning physiques. It is always ideal if after your training you can go home, have a meal, and put your feet up for an hour or two. Office jobs or other sedentary work are better for the aspiring bodybuilder than physical labor, which can drain

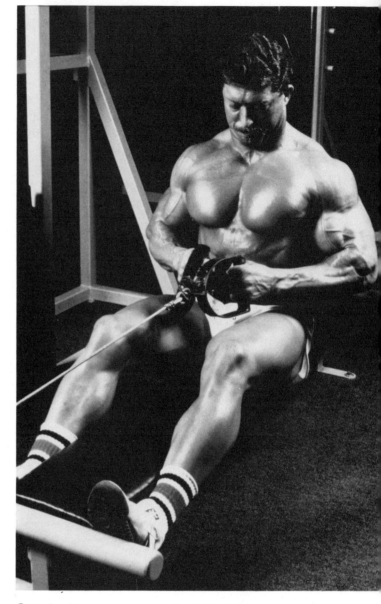

Seated cable rows, as shown by Kal Szkalak.

important energy and even rob your muscles of their size-giving protein.

Weight training is a great companion and help to achievement in other sports, but the *competitive* bodybuilder cannot afford the luxury of participating in other activities—they prevent the achievement of maximum size. By all means, take off the summer to enjoy outdoor activities. You can always get back to where you were after a month or two's training. But remember, if your *sole* ambition is to compete in bodybuilding contests and to win, then you just cannot afford to miss this training time. While you're taking the summer off, someone else is not!

No, I'm not saying you should be downright lazy when you're not actually training. The garbage still has to be taken out. But relaxation periods during the day will definitely help your progress, and a good night's sleep is essential. If you must party, do it on a weekend, so you can make up for your late hours by sleeping in the next morning.

TRAINING FREQUENCY

You can get good results by training the whole body three days a week. Most people choose to train on Mondays, Wednesdays, and Fridays because this leaves at least a day's rest between your workouts and your weekends are free to be with your family or friends.

More serious bodybuilders find that training the complete body in one workout is too difficult. "You just cannot do justice to every muscle group," says seven-time Mr. Olympia Arnold Schwarzenegger. "It is far better to split your routine in two and perform half your workout one day and the second half the next day." When professionals do this they usually train for two days in a row, and then take the next day off. Others like to split their workouts into three parts and train over a three-day period. After that they take a one-day rest and then begin the cycle over again. Frank Richards, for example, trains his legs and triceps on Day One. Then on Day Two he exercises his chest and biceps, and Day Three sees him working shoulders and back. Day Four is a rest day, except sometimes for a few weeks before a contest, when he trains six days straight before taking a day off.

Another variation of training frequency is the *every-other-day split.* The workout routine is split in half. You perform the first half of your routine on Day One. Day Two is a rest day. On Day Three you go through the second half of your routine, and Day Four is a rest day. The process is repeated. Quite simply, you train half your body parts every other day.

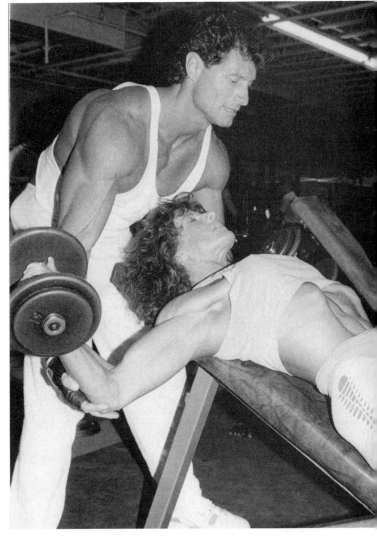

Kevin Lawrence and Diana Dennis.

Incidentally, when I interviewed most of the top professional women for *Superpump!* (Sterling Publishing Company), a book I wrote with Ben Weider, the great majority told me that they trained three days on and one day off; most split their workouts into three parts.

CONSISTENCY

Rachel McLish says that consistent training is one of the most important aspects of bodybuilding success. It's true. Every workout is "one in the

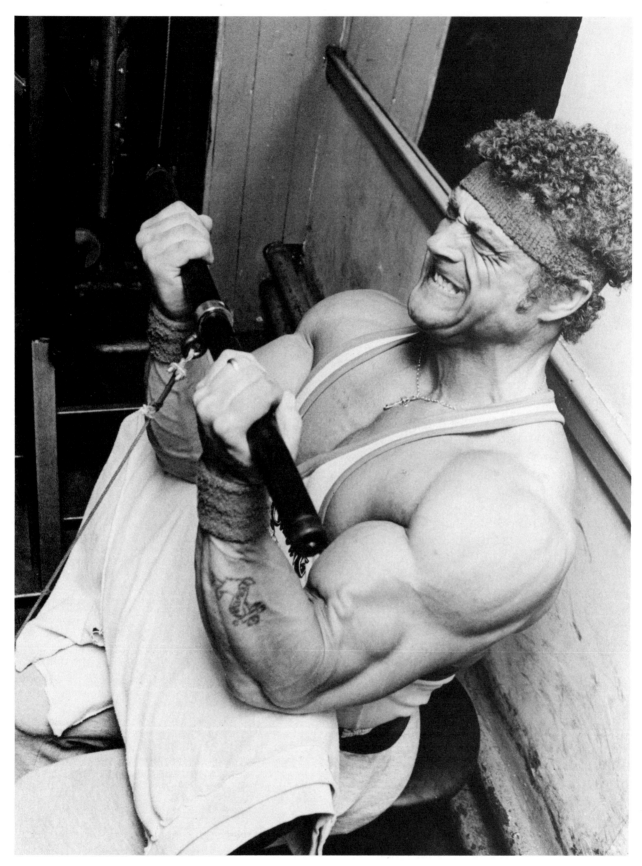

Frank Richards works his biceps with Scott curls...

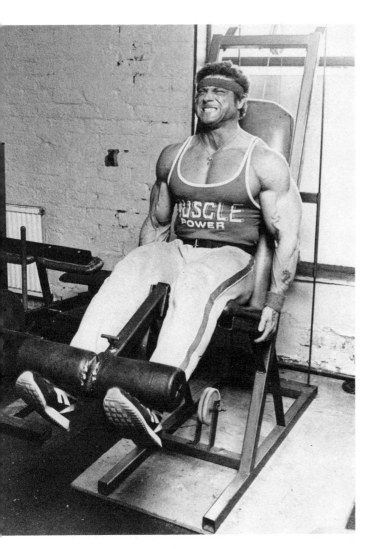

and gives everything to his thigh extensions.

bank," so to speak, and just as money accumulates, so will your muscle size and shape. Very few on again—off again bodybuilders succeed. When you feel like missing a workout, ask yourself if it is because you are just too tired or sick, in which case you *should* miss it, or is it because of laziness? The occasional bodybuilder is never a consistent winner. Determination and a desire for muscles is important, but it is the consistent trainer who is rewarded with the best results.

SAMPLE ROUTINES

There is no magic routine that works for everyone. No single routine can truthfully be called "the best." Too many bodybuilders are waiting for *one* routine to surface that can be acclaimed as the all-time "result getter." Such a routine just does not exist. Bodybuilders are pretty well willing to do almost anything to speed up their muscle growth, but they won't find a perfect routine that will do it for them simply because as you progress your needs can change. It's a good idea to swap around exercises from time to time to *shock* the body into responding. A change is better than a rest.

Yes, it's true. You have to find out what's best for you personally, but there *are* guidelines. A routine of thirty different exercises, for example, is not going to do much for a beginner, except cause rapid burnout. In the same vein, an advanced bodybuilder training for the Olympia will not get in shape by performing a basic routine of squats, bench presses, and curls.

The following are some sample routines for men and women that can act as guidelines for you to follow. Remember, if you are short of time (or energy), you can split these routines into two or three parts.

Beginners' Routine

Rope jumping (warm-up)	1½ minutes	
Crunches	3 sets × 10	reps
Broomstick twists	3 sets × 100	reps
Bench press	3 sets × 8	reps
Incline dumbbell bench press	3 sets × 12	reps
Upright row	3 sets × 10	reps
Lat-machine pulldowns	3 sets × 10	reps
Squats	3 sets × 10	reps
Thigh curls	3 sets × 12	reps
Calf raise	3 sets × 20	reps
Barbell curls	3 sets × 8	reps
Triceps extensions	3 sets × 10	reps

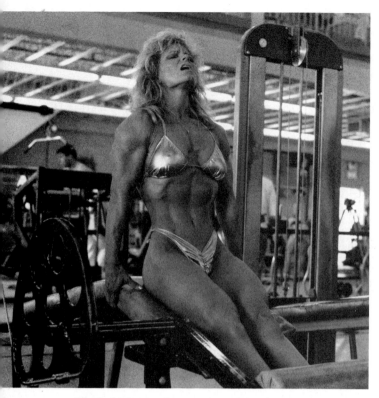

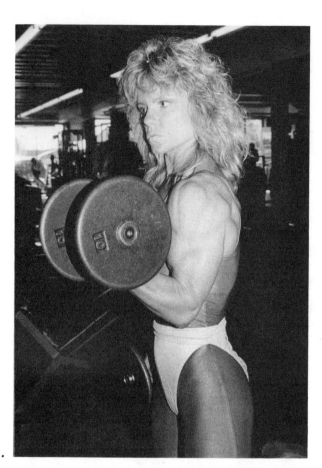

Dinah Anderson demonstrates leg extensions...

dumbbell curls...

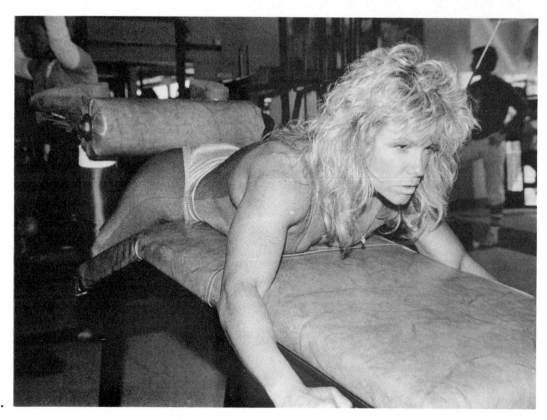

thigh curls...

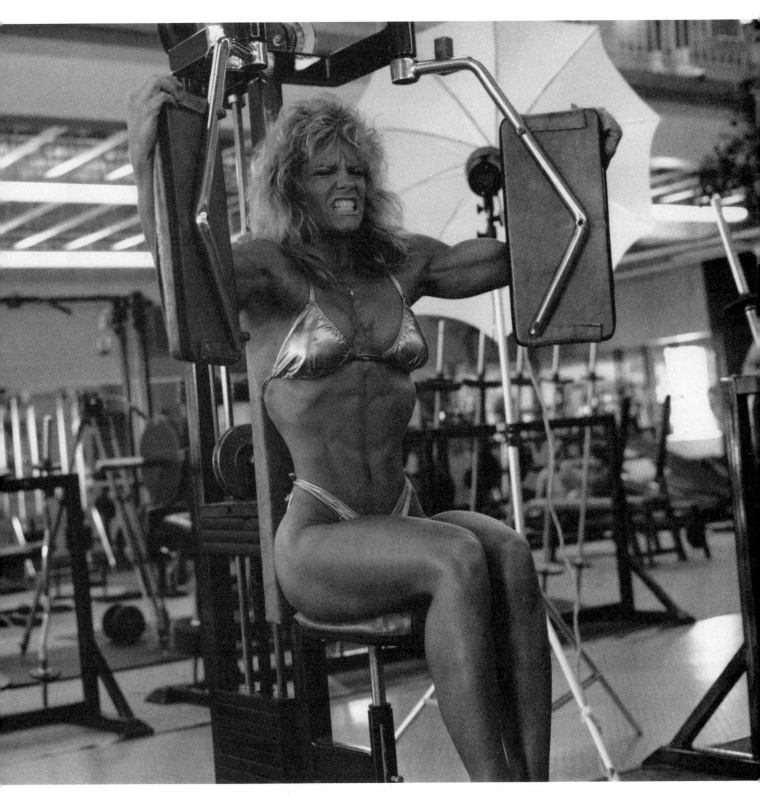

chest exercises on the Pek-Dek machine.

Intermediate Routine

Rope jumping (warm-up)	2½ minutes	
Crunches	4 sets × 20	reps
Hanging knee raise	4 sets × 20	reps
Bench press	5 sets × 8	reps
Incline dumbbell flyes	4 sets × 12	reps
Press behind neck	5 sets × 8	reps
Dumbbell lateral raise	5 sets × 10	reps
Lat-machine pulldowns	4 sets × 10	reps
T-bar row	4 sets × 10	reps
Squats	5 sets × 10	reps
Thigh extensions	5 sets × 10	reps
Thigh curls	5 sets × 12	reps
Calf raise	5 sets × 25	reps
Incline dumbbell curls	4 sets × 8	reps
Scott curls	4 sets × 8	reps
Closer-grip triceps bench press	4 sets × 10	reps
Lat-machine pressdowns	4 sets × 10	reps

Advanced Routine

Rope jumping (warm-up)	3 minutes	
Hanging knee raise	3 sets × 20	reps
Crunches	3 sets × 15	reps
Prone hyperextensions	3 sets × 20	reps
Bench press	8 sets × 8	reps
Incline dumbbell bench press	5 sets × 8	reps
Supine dumbbell flyes	5 sets × 10	reps
Seated press behind neck	5 sets × 8	reps
Seated dumbbell press	5 sets × 8	reps
Lateral raise	5 sets × 10	reps
Bent-over lateral raise	5 sets × 10	reps
Chin behind neck	5 sets × 12	reps
T-bar row	5 sets × 10	reps
Seated pulley cable row	5 sets × 12	reps
Hack squats	6 sets × 12	reps
Thigh extensions	6 sets × 12	reps
Leg press	5 sets × 12	reps
Thigh curls	5 sets × 12	reps
Standing calf raise	6 sets × 20	reps
Seated calf raise	6 sets × 20	reps
Barbell curls	5 sets × 8	reps
Scott curls	5 sets × 10	reps
Single-arm cable curls	5 sets × 12	reps
Close-grip triceps bench press	5 sets × 8	reps
Lying triceps curls	5 sets × 10	reps
Lat-machine pressdowns	5 sets × 12	reps

When bodybuilding contests were first started almost a hundred years ago, there was absolutely no preparation whatsoever. One simply heard about a contest and entered there and then. It wasn't until annual contests became popular—the Mr. Britain (started in 1930) and the Mr. America (first held in 1938)—that contestants began to train specially for the event. Even so, training for an upcoming national title involved little more than added effort in the workouts. If changes in food intake were made, it usually involved eating more sausages and drinking more beer. Even Steve Reeves, who competed up until 1950, never changed his food intake prior to a contest. The only thing he did was increase his training intensity by reducing rest time between sets.

How times have changed. Today contest preparation is a scientific art. True, each individual must first find his or her own specific formula, but there are certain rules of the game that can help maximize your chances.

They laughed at Samir Bannout's annual attempts to cut up his physique. He always appeared a tad off form, a little bloated as a result of holding water. Well, the early adversity paid off. With his back against the wall he *tried* harder. Today Samir is one of the best-informed bodybuilders on all matters of contest preparation. He has mastered the technique of peaking for the day of the contest. He gets ripped to the bone! "Low-calorie dieting is more in tune with the biochemical makeup of most bodybuilders than is low-carbohydrate dieting," says Bannout in his *Mr. Olympia's Muscle Mastery* book (New American Library). "A low-calorie diet must be low in fats. Each gram of fat is more than twice as rich a source of calories as is a gram of either protein or carbohydrate, so reducing fat consumption is far more effective in limiting calorie intake than is lowering your consumption of carbohydrate or protein."

Once you have decided to enter a specific contest, you have to plan both your training and your diet. Actually, not too much change will

---

Frank Richards shows off his delts.

25
RIPPING UP
Contest Preparation

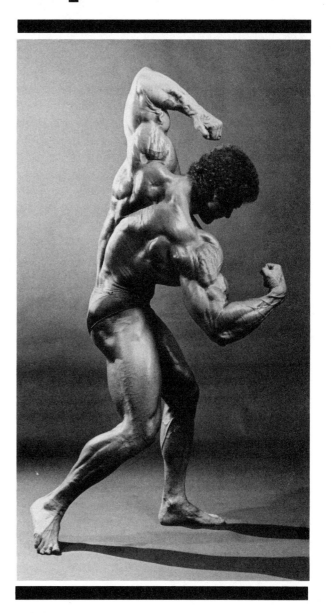

take place in your training. It is advised that you increase intensity gradually so that your muscles hold on to as much mass as possible. Use more isolation exercises (concentration curls, thigh extensions, crossover pulleys, etc.) than combination movements (rowing, benching, squatting). Increase your workout frequency from the normal training of each body part twice weekly to two and a half to three times weekly. Gradually reduce rest time between sets and use more principles such as the Weider iso-tension technique (squeezing and flexing the muscles during exercise and between sets).

But diet is a different matter. Some bodybuilders do not change anything about their training, but this can *never* be said about their nutrition. Diet *has* to change.

Normally a bodybuilder will start a low-calorie diet six to eight weeks prior to a show. Naturally, this period varies greatly depending on how much fat you have to lose. I have no hesitation in stating my opinion that the biggest mistake made by bodybuilders of both sexes (but more frequently by men) is that they start their diets too late. Far better to take more months to diet off your surplus painlessly than to leave the task right up to the last month, then starving yourself in the process. Chances are you won't get the fat off, and if you do you'll be left with loose skin and a flat-looking physique. Remember, if you cut your calorie intake down too low and too suddenly, your body can be thrown into panic; metabolism will slow down to compensate, preparing your body for the "coming famine."

A select few, usually bodybuilders in their early twenties, can get ripped with just a couple of weeks' hard dieting, but most need a good eight to twelve weeks, and sometimes more.

It's been said before, but I'm going to repeat myself to emphasize the point: *When you go on a diet, begin moderately. Start by gradually reducing your food intake each week or so.*

You are mistaken if you think you can suddenly drop from a daily 4,000-calorie diet to 1,500. You'll not only lose fat but muscle and energy as well. Your workouts will be a constant fight against fatigue. However, if you drop your calorie intake gradually, there is no reason why your workouts shouldn't be enjoyed right up until you stop them the week of the competition.

The general rule of thumb is to start dieting by trimming 200 calories from your total, then dropping a further 100 calories every two or three days.

The following is a typical precontest diet. The portions, of course, will depend on your basic size category and on the amount of fat you have to lose to be ultimately ripped.

Breakfast
Bran cereal with nonfat milk or soft fruit
Egg whites
Coffee, tea, or water (no sugar, but artificial sweetener is acceptable)
Supplements

Lunch
Broiled fish
One or two green vegetables
Baked potato (with no butter or sour cream)
One piece fresh fruit
Coffee, tea, or water (no sugar)

Dinner
Broiled chicken breast (white meat)—remove fatty skin before cooking
Brown rice
One green vegetable or light salad (no dressing, only lemon juice)
Coffee, tea, or water (no sugar)

Snacks
Raw vegetables

You will notice your fat gradually disappearing as you continue your diet. This is the time to become *ultra-aware* of what is happening to your physique. If you feel you are losing too much weight (muscle mass) too fast, then moderate your food intake accordingly—eat a little more, but keep to complex carbs such as fruits, grains, and vegetables. Avoid junk, even if the weight is melting off by the minute. Don't suddenly grab for doughnuts and ice cream just because you feel you are losing too fast.

On the other hand, if you suspect that your calorie-reduced diet is not helping you shed fat, then eat even less. Double-check the fat content of your daily menu. Reduce it (fat) to as low as 10 percent of your overall intake. This may mean that your protein intake is quite low, too, but don't worry. Short periods of lower protein consumption can improve your definition.

To avoid your body "shutting down" its metabolic rate (and hoarding calories), don't allow your calorie consumption to go below 1,500 (for men) or 1,200 (for women).

If things are still not coming together as you had hoped, then increase aerobic activity rather than decrease calorie consumption further. Only as a last resort, when during your last week or ten days you discover that you are still considerably overweight, should you decrease your calories to below the suggested minimum levels.

The best type of aerobic activity is stationary bike riding—only the hips and legs move, which benefits overall size in the arms, lats, and shoulders (which do not move).

Poor aerobic exercises for the bodybuilder preparing for a contest include cross-country skiing, racquetball, aerobic dance, tennis, and trampolining. Particularly bad is swimming, which thins the arms and thickens the fat under the skin (the cooling effect of the water causes the skin to insulate the body with subcutaneous fat).

Pro Mr. America Scott Wilson only does occasional aerobics during the off-season. "But during the last six to eight weeks prior to an important competition I do one or two hours on my stationary bike each day. I usually pedal at a leisurely pace while watching television. I get less bored if I have something to occupy my mind."

Probably the most critical period of contest preparation is the last ten days, particularly the final week. As you approach the seven-day countdown to competition day, cut out all salt (sodium) from the diet. This includes every food or drink that may contain sodium. You'll have to check all labels for sodium content. Do not eat at any restaurants and avoid airline food, which is nearly always super high in sodium. If you are traveling, prepare your own food beforehand. Sodium holds water under the skin, up to 180 times its own weight. Surprisingly, you'll find sodium in many seemingly innocent foods.

Scott Wilson of San Jose, California.

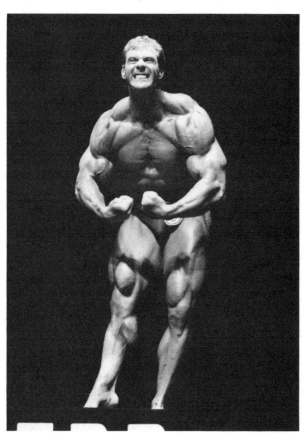
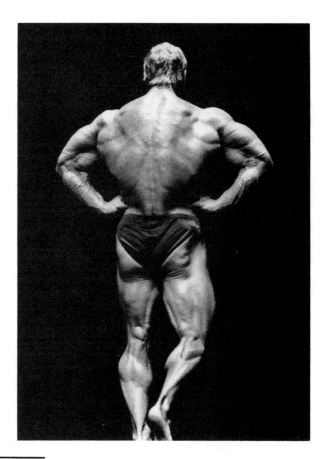

FOODS NATURALLY HIGH IN SODIUM

Cantaloupe	Turnip	Lamb
Honeydew melon	Watercress	Pork
		Turkey
Artichoke	Bagel	
Beets	Brown rice	Bass
Broccoli	Cooked oats	Canned salmon (very high)
Brussels sprouts	Cornbread (very high)	Clams
Cabbage	Corn grits	Cod
Carrots	Sunflower seeds	Flatfish
Cauliflower	Wheat germ	Haddock
Celery	Whole-wheat bread	Halibut
Celery root		Mullet
Chard (very high)	Cheddar cheese	Ocean perch
Collards	Cottage cheese (very high)	Oysters
Kale	Milk	Pike
Lettuce	Ricotta	Pink salmon
Mushrooms	Yogurt	Scallops
Parsley		Shrimp
Peas	Beef	Tuna
Spinach	Chicken	Whitefish
Tomato	Duck	

FOODS CONTAINING ONLY TRACES OF OR NO SODIUM

Fresh yellow corn	Lime juice	Crab meat
Green bulb onion	Vinegar	Octopus
Hot green pepper	Equal/NutraSweet artificial	
Squash	sweetener	Corn oil
Sweet red pepper		Olive oil
	Brook trout	Safflower oil
Dark buckwheat flour	Lake trout	Unsalted butter
Raw unhulled pumpkin seeds		

If you are absolutely forced to eat in a restaurant, have a special talk with the chef. Stick to egg whites (poached or boiled), plain baked potatoes, and fresh fruit. A good rule is, "If you don't know the sodium content, don't eat it!" This even applies to water. Drink only distilled water during the last week. When you talk to the chef about non-sodium food preparation, do not—I repeat, do *not*—tell him that you must keep your salt intake low because you don't want to hold water under your skin. Tell him that your doctor says you will *die* if he so much as uses one grain of the stuff!

During the last week of preparation you should

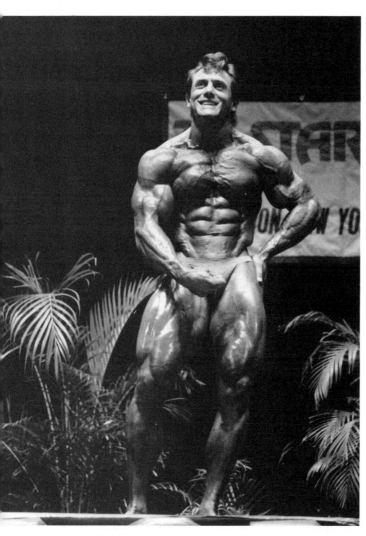

Bob Birdsong.

continue to train until the Wednesday prior to the Saturday night competition. Again, this is only a suggestion—some bodybuilders train right up to Friday night; others make their last workout on Monday. Training causes a degree of edema (water retention between the muscles). After a three-day layoff this invariably vanishes, and you get a more cut appearance. (Vince Gironda says no one should train their abdominals during the last three weeks of contest preparation.)

Remember that muscle is 70 to 75 percent water. You do not want to drain your body of fluid during the last week or so. On the other hand you do not want to appear waterlogged, or puffy. There's a fine line to follow. You have to consume enough water and carbohydrate to plump up the muscle cells yet not ingest so

much that the water in your muscles spills over into the area just under the skin, bringing about the dreaded bloated look.

Carbohydrate stored in the muscles as glycogen holds 3 grams of water per gram of carbohydrate. Too little carbohydrate, and water will flatten out the muscles; too much will give you a puffy appearance. There is an ingredient that will help you balance the water in the muscle and minimize its occurrence beneath the skin. That ingredient is potassium. During the last three days before a contest your low-sodium diet should be coordinated with potassium supplementation. Exactly how much potassium is an individual thing, but the usual rule is that a 200-pound bodybuilder should take about 100 milligrams five times daily for a total of 500 milligrams. (Take your potassium supplement with meals or snacks, not on an empty stomach.)

I should not let this important chapter proceed further without mentioning sodium loading. This is comparatively new. Bill Dobbins is the expert. Because the body is a homeostatic organism (always having to keep things in balance), when you ingest high levels of sodium it will tend to conserve potassium to keep the two in balance. Consequently, if you eat fairly high levels of sodium (but not megadoses) for a week or so prior to going on a low-sodium diet program, when you finally do reduce your sodium levels (seven days prior to competing) you will have naturally high levels of potassium, resulting in a pronounced potassium/sodium imbalance. That, in turn, will result in movement of water *into* the cells (where you want it) and *out* from under the skin (where you don't want it). Don't forget that during the last three days before a contest your low-sodium diet should be accompanied by taking potassium supplements. This further aids the desired imbalance.

One of the accepted techniques of peaking for a contest, holding maximum muscle mass with minimum body fat, is to follow a carbohydrate-deprivation/loading cycle at the conclusion of a normal low-fat–moderate-carbohydrate precontest diet. This is known as "carbing up." The technique was developed by Swedish exercise physiologist Eric Hultman as a blitz method of storing more carbohydrate (glycogen) in the muscle tissue than normal.

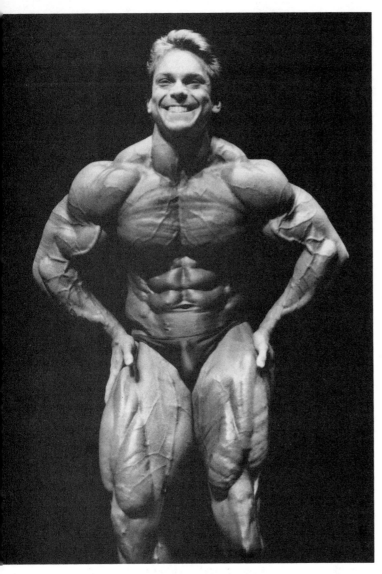

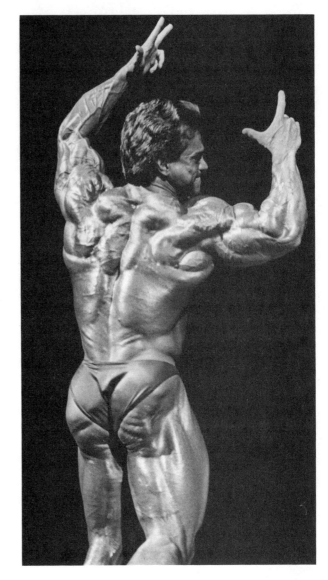

Rich Gaspari, ripped to the bone!

With this technique you follow a low-carbohydrate diet for four to six days in order to deplete the stores of carbohydrate in your body. This is a tough period—you lack workout energy, your physique will look flat and a bit smooth, and you will be a little depressed mentally.

After this phase you load up with complex carbohydrates for the last three or four days immediately preceding the contest date. As a result your muscles will appear full and shredded, and your vascularity will be prominent.

Bill Reynolds, who has studied champion bodybuilders and their contest preparations more than anyone else, says, "This low-carb stage can

be gruesome. You will feel rotten; like you're ready for the undertaker...and your mind will trick you into thinking that you have no chance of pulling off a win. Many people drop out of contests at this final stage of preparation, but if they can stick it out and carb up correctly, they will look superb."

Samir Bannout says of this stage, "I can handle my precontest diet easily, but when I reach my carbohydrate-deprivation phase about two weeks prior to competition, it almost turns me into a zombie, particularly the couple of hours after I have trained.

"Before cutting back on my carbs I eat broiled

chicken, fish, salads (without dressing), baked potatoes, and low-calorie fruit, but when I cut back on carbs (omitting the fruits, salads, and breads) I eat less than 30 grams of carbohydrate per day. It hurts like hell, but it's necessary for me to get completely ripped. Others may not have to be so severe."

After this carbohydrate-deprivation period, you load up on complex carbs, taking in small quantities every two or three hours during waking

Tom Platz displays his extraordinary ripped thighs.

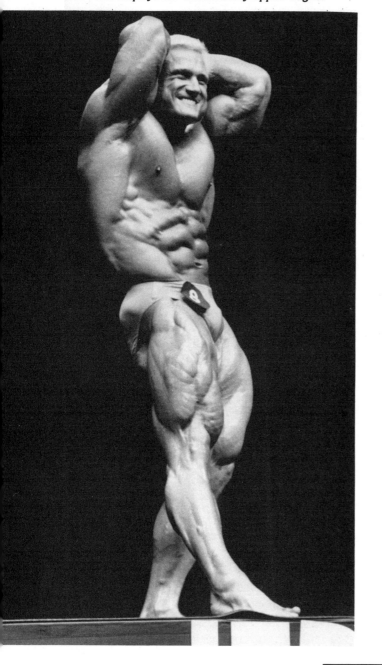

hours. It is suggested that you endeavor to keep the total carbohydrate intake down to about 1½ grams per pound of body weight per day during the carbo-loading period. Do not eat simple carbs (ice cream, sugar, sherbet, or other junk foods) during this carbing up period. They get into the bloodstream too quickly and cause excessive fluctuations in blood sugar levels. Complex carbs give you a more sustained blood sugar flow.

When you have emptied your muscles of glycogen at the end of your carbohydrate-depletion stage, you will find that the carbing up period will work almost miraculously. During those last three days you will suddenly become bigger, harder, and more shapely. Water will be pulled from under the skin into the muscle cells. Your muscles will suck up carbohydrates like a vacuum and, because of the earlier deprivation, will store 4 to 5 grams of glycogen per 100 grams of muscle weight, instead of the usual 2 to 3 grams per 100 grams of muscle weight.

The question of how many carbs to eat during a carbohydrate-loading period is difficult. The body can only accept a certain amount at any one time, so never eat big meals. The general advice is to eat small amounts regularly. Some eat every hour, others every two hours. Bill Dobbins suggests a "minimum of 25 grams of carbohydrate per hour per day," which is an average baked potato or two small oranges, either of which delivers 25 grams of carbohydrate or 100 calories. Other ideal carbing up foods are: corn, fruits, whole-wheat bread, raw green vegetables, and wild rice. But watch that sodium content! It has to be virtually zero.

During the carbing up stage (last three days), drink moderate amounts of *distilled* water. Do not take diuretics or try to dehydrate the body. You will be defeating your purpose. Saunas also dehydrate the body. They are used by bodybuilders who don't follow the new "rules" of contest preparation or by those who use excessive steroid preparations, which hold water under the skin.

When carbing up you will also have a normal need for proteins and fats. Allow yourself moderate amounts of protein and small amounts of fat. You can eat some lean beef or egg yolk at this stage.

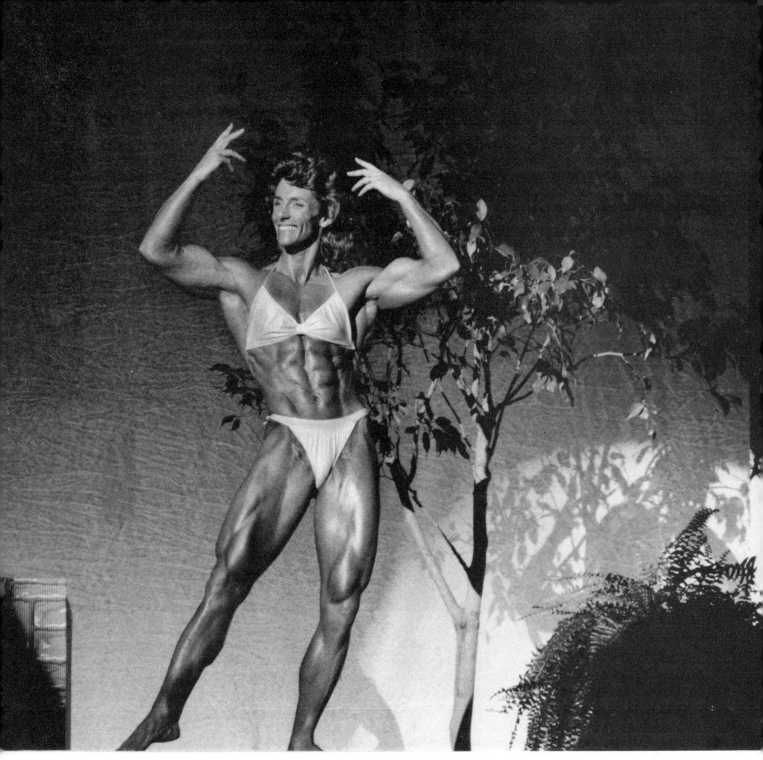

The ultimate female physique, Bev Francis.

I should warn you that use of the "carbing up" technique is predicated upon your reaching your contest weight (or slightly less) at least a week before show date. If you still have to lose weight right up to the competition, you've blown your chances. You should have begun dieting earlier.

Posing practice is a positive contributor to getting in shape. Practice for an hour a day. Your muscles will get harder and better separated. Your practice will also prepare you for the arduous prejudging sessions, in which you may be called out for comparisons or posedowns that can be very exhausting.

Arnold Schwarzenegger used to schedule pho-

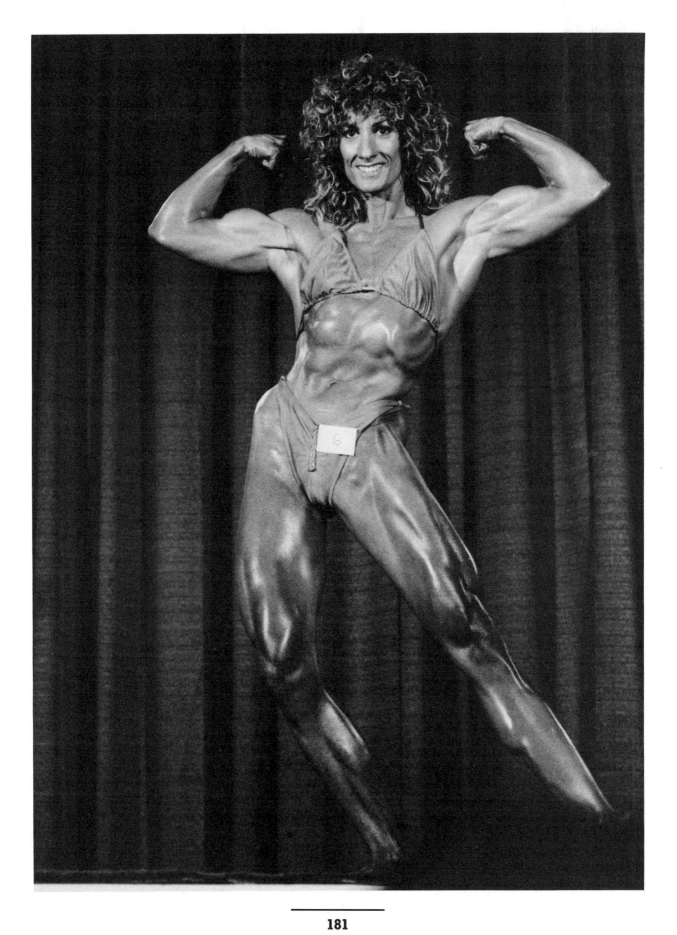

to sessions for a couple of days before a show. He claimed the constant posing for the camera always helped him sharpen up, improve muscularity, and aid his stamina for posing on the day of the contest. "I never failed to rip-up this way!" he says.

What about lipotropic or fat-burning agents? "Generally," says Dr. William N. Taylor, writing in Joe Weider's *Muscle and Fitness,* "the maximum rates of fat mobilization occur only during prolonged exercise, hormonal imbalance, prolonged reducing diets or with certain medications."

The known lipotropic medications, by no means recommended for use by healthy people, especially without a doctor's prescription, include amphetamines, caffeine, anabolic steroids, thyroid hormone, human growth hormone, glucagon, L-dopa, human chorionic gonadotrophin, and catecholamines. More acceptable, since they are not classified as drugs, are choline, inositol, and lecithin. Used in moderation in conjunction with a calorie-reduced precontest diet, these lipotropic agents may help convert body fat into energy. Certainly they do not move mountains of fat. They would make no difference to the general appearance of an obese person, but the bodybuilder looking for that competitive edge at contest time might well achieve a noticeable change in appearance. There appears to be no toxic effect from large quantities of inositol, but too much choline can be dangerous.

Boyer Coe sums up the ripping up part of bodybuilding: "Achieving peak muscularity is more than 75 percent a matter of diet. Unless you naturally have an exceedingly high rate of body metabolism (BMR), you will need to diet strictly for rather long periods of time in order to strip all fat from your body. Try dieting for four to six weeks for your first competition, keeping careful notes on how fast your body cuts up in relation to your food intake. Then when you compete a second time you can adjust the length and severity of your diet accordingly."

Daniel Duchaine, who it seems to me is a super expert on contest preparation, concurs. "It is essential to practice carbohydrate depletion and loading a few times before your contest so you know how you respond to the process. Go through a couple of trial runs to fine-tune the process."

Have I already told you that some of the top stars in our bodybuilding sport are actually poor eaters? That their diets are lousy?

Yes, it's true, but I have to admit that the vast majority do eat prudently. They balance their nutrition to ensure that adequate protein, carbohydrate, fats, vitamins, and minerals are consumed so that they get proper nourishment. Calorie consumption is invariably controlled so that an ideal body weight is maintained without too much deviation either way. And last but not least, they seldom eat junky processed foods that are loaded with sodium, sugar, or some overprocessed ingredient that virtually all of us consume too much of.

Matt Mendenhall's main concern about his food intake is that his protein percentage be high. "I am always aware of protein when I have a meal. My main concern is to make sure that I ingest 160 to 200 grams of protein each day. I do this with regular meals and snacks in between. I don't go overboard on calories, but I do try and eat only fresh foods."

Dutch champion Ellen Van Maris admits she has an occasional weak spot for sweets and other junk food, but "Most of the time my off-season diet is nutritionally sound, well balanced. But six to eight weeks before a competition I begin light dieting, gradually increasing the severity as a show approaches. I never go under 1,000 calories daily because it takes away energy from training and my workout suffers badly. When dieting for a contest, I'll eat my carbohydrates in the morning—fruit, honey, or other low-sodium complex carbohydrate foods. I'll eat a hot meal in the afternoon, any type of low-fat meat, some vegetables, and a salad. After my workout at night I have a final light meal, usually low-sodium wheat or rye crackers with unsalted cheese. I prefer *low-bulk* eating. I do not like to stretch my waistline out of shape, so I only eat small amounts at each meal."

Boyer Coe, too, feels that meals should be fairly small yet frequent. Two to three months prior to a contest Boyer recommends the follow-

Bob Paris.

26
FROM THE HORSE'S MOUTH
Talking Food with the Champs

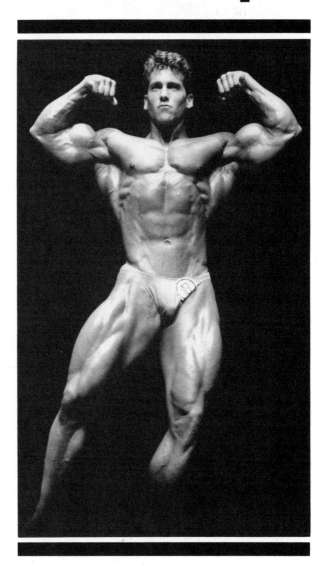

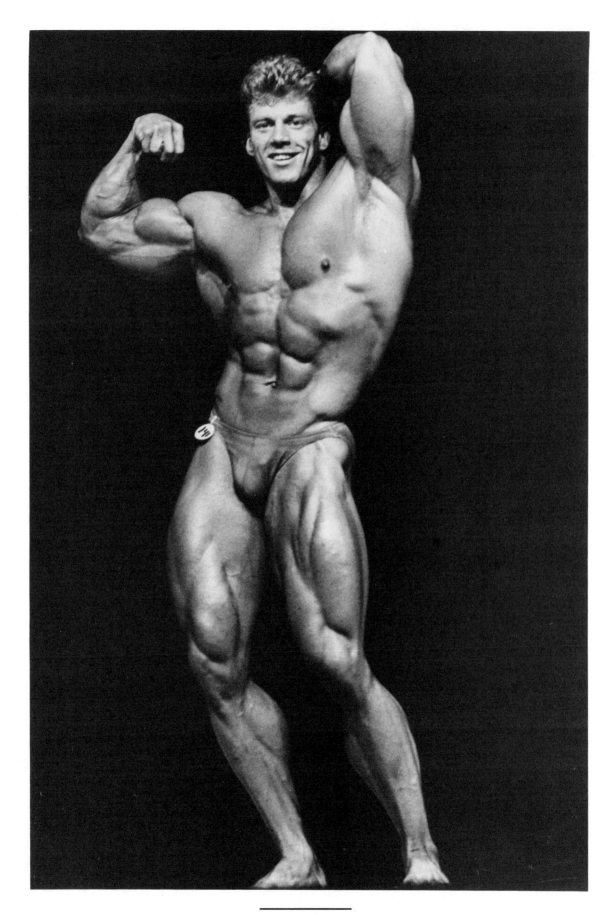

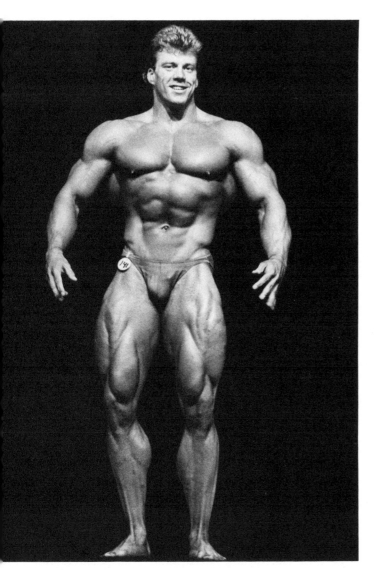

Matt Mendenhall, Mr. USA.

ing meal plan. (This is not a ripping-up plan. That comes during the last month prior to competition.)

8 A.M. Breakfast
6 eggs (boiled) and chicken breast
1 piece of whole-wheat bread

10 A.M. Snack
Chicken breast and 2 boiled eggs

12 NOON Lunch
Lean meat and salad

2 P.M. Snack
2 boiled eggs and chicken breast

5 P.M. Dinner
Liver and salad

7 P.M. Snack
2 boiled eggs

Fruit may be eaten prior to training time. No food after 7 P.M.

Boyer Coe goes on: "One of the biggest secrets in bodybuilding is the realization that no simple dietary technique will work for *every* bodybuilder. My specific diet does not work for Mike Mentzer, Rachel McLish, Roy Callender…or scores of others. It is your responsibility to determine the exact dietary philosophy that works best for you. As in developing a training pattern, this involves trying every possible food element in your diet for a few weeks at a time to decide if and how well it works for you. Monitor your body's biofeedback to determine what effect a particular food has on your body. As an example, if you ate a pint of pistachio ice cream every day for three weeks, a certain piece of biofeedback data (probably the fact that you're growing incredibly fat!) will tell you about the food's effect on the body."

Monitor everything nutritionally. Become *super aware* of what food does what. How does red meat affect your muscles? Does a certain food help or hinder your sleeping patterns? What defines you before a show—chicken, fish, egg whites? How does your system react to milk, skim milk, Tiger's Milk? What foods give you training energy? How do certain foods aid recuperation? Make notes. You'll find yourself referring to them again and again, and they will play a vital part in your winning future contests.

Rachel McLish does not believe in eating junk foods, but she admits that she will relent if she has a positive urge for something—"because a craving is usually a good indication that my body requires the nutrient I crave for, so I eat them."

In her remarkable book *Flex Appeal* (Warner Books) Rachel comments, "There are some absolutes that we must accept at one point or another, and the direct effect food has on our physical appearance is one of them. Eat for function, because the texture of your flesh will probably resemble the texture of your food (remember the jelly doughnut?)."

Rachel, incidentally, has a remarkable time-tested protein drink recipe that you can whip up in a minute in a blender:

8 ounces of raw milk (preferably nonfat)
1 tablespoon of egg white protein powder
1 piece soft fruit
1 teaspoon psyllium husk

Rachel's favorite fruits for protein drinks are fresh strawberries, peaches, and bananas.

"My mass-building maxim," says popular Tom Platz in his revealing book *Pro-Style Bodybuilding* (Sterling Publishing Company), "is: *Think mass, eat mass, train mass.*" Tom definitely believes in eating late in the evening when trying to gain maximum size. "The food seems to be assimilated much more easily late at night than earlier in the day." Here's an example of a Tom Platz weight-gain menu. He changes it frequently, but the following is an average day's eating for adding body weight:

Breakfast (8 A.M.)
Cheese omelette
2 slices whole-grain bread

Midmorning (10:30 A.M.)
Tuna salad
2 slices whole-grain bread
Square of hard cheese
Fruit juice

Lunch (1:00 P.M.)
Broiled chicken
Rice
Small salad
Iced tea
Supplements

Midafternoon (3:30 P.M.)
Protein drink
Supplements

Supper (6:00 P.M.)
Broiled steak
Baked potato
Green vegetable
Milk
Supplements

Evening Snack (8:30 P.M)
Cold cuts
2 slices whole-grain bread
Yogurt
Raw nuts and seeds
Glass of milk

Tom says, "You should eat 20 to 30 grams of complete protein each time you sit down to a meal. Those with small builds should eat around 20 grams. Larger-built people should eat 30 grams at each sitting."

One other comment that superman Platz makes is interesting. "If there's a lack of fat in my diet, I will not gain weight even when I'm consuming a high amount of calories. I just have to eat concentrated, high-fat calories, such as found in milk. Years ago I used to drink a half gallon of whole milk after every workout, and that's when I made some of my best gains."

Mike Mentzer is probably the most sane of all bodybuilders when it comes to nutrition. He has a commonsense attitude about diet because of his earlier pre-med training. "We are all unique personalities, but we are not all that different inside. We all need protein; we all require sleep; we burn carbohydrates at the rate of 4 calories per gram; we all require intense effort to stimulate growth; we all possess limited recovery abilities; and we all grow extra muscle too damned slow." Mike continues: "If I get you to understand one thing, I would like it to be this: Few people manage to gain even 10 pounds of pure muscle a year. It doesn't sound like much but a normal 170-pound man could weight 210 pounds after four years training—not bad. Actually a 10-pound annual weight gain is only .027 pound gained daily (12 grams), so believe me, you do not need much extra food to bring about this gain. Too many bodybuilders go on a calorie binge, and...get fat!"

Vince Gironda is an advocate of the importance of *Stone Age nutrition*. He believes that the quality of our diet has only regressed since the early days of humankind. It is true that most people's diet is appalling when dissected for wholesomeness and nutritional benefit. On the other hand, because of world trade today, those of us who are motivated to eat healthily can do so. More than ever before we have an abundance and huge variety of healthy bodybuilding foods. Make the right choice and gain outstanding results.

RECIPES FOR ROCK HARD NUTRITION

COOKING METHODS

The following recipes use five simple methods of cooking: broiling, poaching, steaming, stir-frying, and oven baking. I suggest that you use the same method for cooked menu items whenever possible. For example, when preparing a meat or fish dish that is to be broiled, look for a vegetable accompaniment that can also be broiled. This will reduce your preparation and clean-up time, since many of the meat and vegetable dishes can be cooked together.

The recipes have been compiled for the bodybuilder's general maintenance program, with variations for bulking up and contest preparation listed below recipes where appropriate. The approximate breakdown of protein, carbohydrates, and calories has been calculated for each version.

BROILING

Broiling is an excellent way of preparing your meat and fish dishes because it allows the food to be cooked quickly and "seals in the juices," rendering meat in particular tender and nutritious. All that is necessary to broil food is a good broiling pan with a grid that allows any fat to drain off, and you will want a spatula for turning your meat.

Foods indicated for broiling may also be prepared on an outside grill if desired. The same cooking times would apply.

Method

1. Bring meat to room temperature before broiling.
2. Preheat broiler for 10–15 minutes.

3. Heat broiling pan before placing the food on it, and spray with a nonstick vegetable coating such as PAM to prevent food sticking to the grid.
4. Trim all fat off the meat to be broiled, and score the edges to prevent the meat from curling.
5. Place broiling pan approximately 6 inches from the broiling element and follow the cooking times given in each recipe. Do not pierce the meat with a fork to turn, since this would allow juice to escape and the end result would not be as flavorful or tender.

POACHING

Poaching simply means cooking food in gently boiling water. However, beef or chicken broth can be used in place of water for extra flavor. You can further enhance the flavor of the food you're cooking by adding a complementary herb—

Canada's Marc Gagnon enjoys a precontest meal of poached fish and green beans.

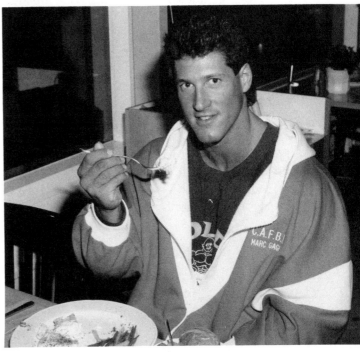

191

for example, a bay leaf or thyme—to the boiling water.

When poaching fish or chicken, always put into water or stock that is very hot.

Method

1. Heat water in a saucepan—the water should cover the food to be cooked by two to three inches.
2. Add desired herbs.
3. Add meat or fish and bring to a boil; then reduce heat and poach gently according to recipe directions.

STEAMING

Steaming is a method of cooking whereby food is placed in a steaming basket over boiling water. It is probably the healthiest cooking method of all. It preserves the color, taste, and nutritional value of vegetables and meats. Bodybuilders who are reducing weight for contest preparation will find this the best method of cooking, since there is no need to add fat and the food reaches the table in its most natural state.

Bamboo steamers are available in kitchen specialty shops and have the advantage of being stackable. If you have two steamers, the meat can be cooked in the steaming basket closest to the heat, and a second steaming basket containing the vegetables can be stacked on top.

To give your food extra flavor, add a clove of garlic or a few spring onions to the steaming water.

Method

1. Fill a pan with water and bring to a boil.
2. Add herbs, if desired.

3. Place food in a bamboo steamer and place over the boiling water.
4. Cover and steam according to recipe directions.

STIR-FRYING

Stir-frying has the advantage of being a very fast cooking method. All that is needed to stir-fry is a Chinese wok or a shallow frying pan. Meat to be stir-fried should be sliced very thin across the grain, and vegetables should be thinly sliced or shredded so that the cooking time is minimal. Since stir-frying is such a fast method of cooking, make sure to prepare *all* of your food beforehand.

Method

1. Prepare meat and vegetables for stir-frying.
2. Heat oil in a wok or shallow frying pan until very hot.
3. Follow the cooking instructions in each recipe, using a large spoon or spatula to toss the meat and vegetables.

OVEN BAKING

Oven baking is a traditional cooking method. It is a convenient way to prepare food, since many recipes can be assembled in a casserole and left to bake without additional attention. Baking in a casserole is an efficient method of cooking, as you will discover when preparing the one-dish recipes included in this book.

Method

1. Brown meat to be cooked in hot oil.
2. Add vegetables.
3. Add broth.
4. Bake as directed in each recipe.

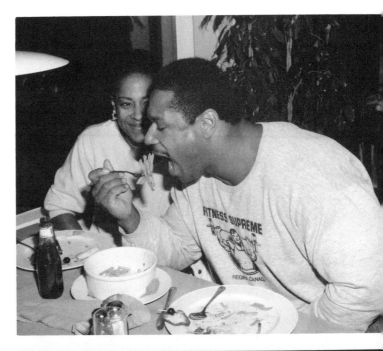

Apres contest! Mike Christian indulges in French fries.

Mr. America Casey Viator and friend.

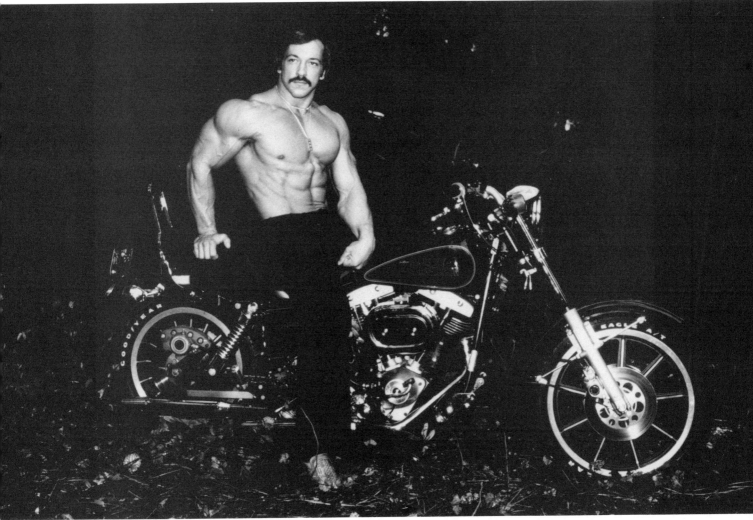

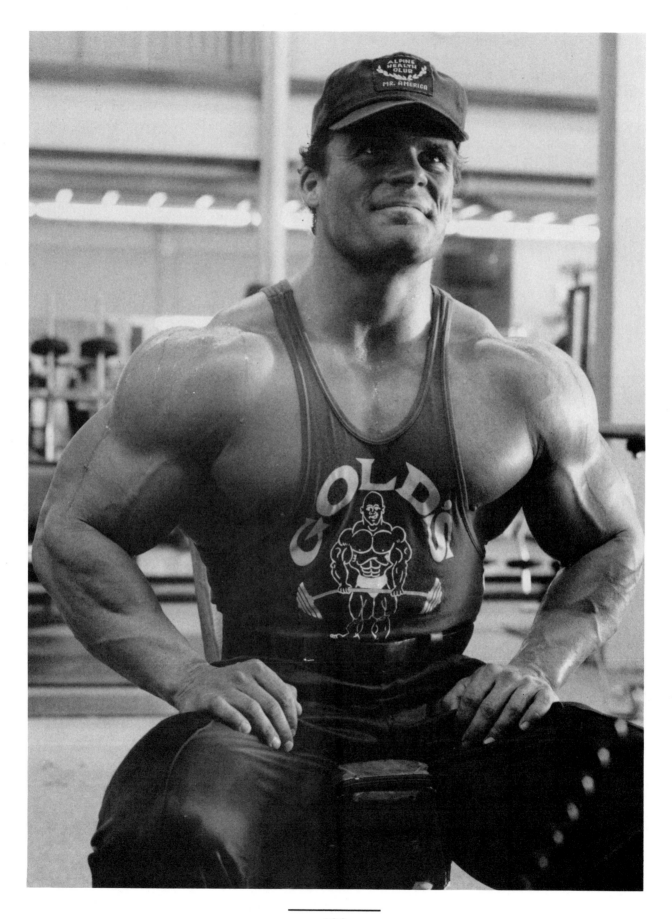

BREAKFASTS

BAKED EGGS

2 slices whole-wheat toast
1 teaspoon safflower oil
2 eggs
2 teaspoons skim milk
½ teaspoon thyme

Preheat oven to 350°. Spray two custard cups with a nonstick coating. Remove the crusts from slices of whole-wheat bread and press into custard cups. Brush with safflower oil. Break an egg into the center of each slice of bread. Sprinkle skim milk over the top of the eggs, and sprinkle with thyme.

VARIATIONS
Precontest: Use egg whites only.
Bulking up: Top with 2 tablespoons of grated cheddar cheese.

	Calories	Protein	Carbo-hydrate	Fat
Maintenance	350	18 grams	30 grams	18 grams
Precontest	220	14 grams	30 grams	6 grams
Bulking up	410	22 grams	30 grams	22 grams

OATMEAL WITH DRIED FRUITS

  Juice of ½ lemon
½ cup orange juice
1 teaspoon honey
¼ teaspoon cinnamon
¼ teaspoon vanilla
2 ounces dried apricots
1 ounce dried apples
1 ounce raisins
1 cup hot, cooked oatmeal

Mr. America Gary Leonard of Fresno, California.

In a medium saucepan heat orange juice, honey, and lemon juice. Add cinnamon and vanilla and bring to a boil. Add the apricots, apples, and raisins. Reduce heat, cover, and simmer for 5–10 minutes. Prepare oatmeal. Spoon stewed fruit over hot oatmeal and serve with ½ cup milk.

VARIATIONS
Precontest: Serve ½ cup oatmeal with fruit and ½ cup skim milk. Omit honey and raisins from stewed fruit.
Bulking up: Sprinkle with tablespoon wheat germ and serve with ½ cup whole milk.

	Calories	Protein	Carbo-hydrate	Fat
Maintenance	448	12.5 grams	93 grams	5.0 grams
Precontest	297	10 grams	64 grams	4.5 grams
Bulking up	519	16 grams	99 grams	7.3 grams

BANANA EGG NOG

Too rushed for breakfast? Whirl this in a blender and drink on the run.

1 egg
1 banana, sliced
2 tablespoons milk-and-egg powder
1 cup low-fat (2%) milk
1 packet sugar substitute

Mix all ingredients in a blender and blend until frothy.

VARIATIONS
Precontest: Use 1 egg white instead of whole egg and 1 cup skim milk in place of low-fat (2%) milk.
Bulking up: Use 1 tablespoon honey instead of sugar substitute.

	Calories	Proteins	Carbo-hydrate	Fat
Maintenance	403	33 grams	45.7 grams	11.2 grams
Precontest	305	17 grams	46.7 grams	.16 gram
Bulking up	468	33 grams	62.7 grams	11.2 grams

NUT MUFFINS

1 egg
½ cup milk
¼ cup safflower oil
1½ cups whole-wheat flour
¼ cup wheat germ
¼ cup honey
¼ cup chopped walnuts
¼ cup sunflower seeds
¼ cup chopped pecans
2 teaspoons baking powder
½ teaspoon baking soda

Preheat oven to 400°. Spray muffin tins with a nonstick vegetable coating. Beat egg, using an electric mixer. Stir in the milk and oil. Combine remaining ingredients in another bowl and mix well. Make a well in the dry ingredients and stir in the egg mixture until just blended, then spoon into muffin pan. Bake for 20–25 minutes. Makes 12 muffins.

	Calories	Protein	Carbo-hydrate	Fat
Per muffin	192	6.9 grams	17 grams	11 grams

COTTAGE CHEESE "DANISH"

2 slices whole-wheat bread
½ cup low-fat cottage cheese
1 fresh peach, peeled and sliced into sections
½ teaspoon cinnamon

Preheat broiler for 10 minutes. Spread cottage cheese over whole-wheat bread, arrange peach slices on top, and sprinkle with cinnamon. Broil for 4–5 minutes. Makes 1 serving.

VARIATIONS
Precontest: Limit whole-wheat bread to one slice and use sodium-reduced cottage cheese, available from health food stores.
Bulking up: Top cottage cheese and peaches with 1½ tablespoons raisins.

	Calories	Protein	Carbo-hydrate	Fat
Maintenance	264	24 grams	42.5 grams	2.5 grams
Precontest	192	21 grams	27.5 grams	1.5 grams
Bulking up	304	24 grams	53.5 grams	2.5 grams

ENGLISH MUFFIN WITH EGGS 'N BEEF

3 ounces lean ground beef
¼ teaspoon sage
  Pinch of cloves
  Pinch of nutmeg
¼ teaspoon pepper
½ teaspoon lemon juice
½ teaspoon parsley
1 whole-wheat English muffin, halved
1 egg, beaten
2 slices tomato

Preheat broiler for 10 minutes. Combine the ground beef, sage, cloves, nutmeg, pepper, lemon juice, and parsley. Shape into a patty and broil for 3 minutes on each side. Meanwhile spray a skillet with a nonstick coating and cook egg to desired doneness. Toast English muffin, and "sandwich" around beef patty, egg, and tomato slices.

VARIATIONS
Precontest: Serve sandwich "open-face" style, using only half an English muffin. Use egg white instead of whole egg (add ¼ teaspoon of turmeric to color egg if desired).
Bulking up: Add 1 tablespoon grated cheddar cheese to beef patty during last 2 minutes of broiling.

	Calories	Protein	Carbo-hydrate	Fat
Maintenance	364	37 grams	32 grams	6.5 grams
Precontest	246	29 grams	11 grams	5 grams
Bulking up	394	39 grams	32 grams	8.5 grams

SCRAMBLED EGGS IN PITA POCKETS

2 eggs, beaten
1 teaspoon milk
1 teaspoon safflower oil
½ tomato, chopped
1 whole-wheat pita bread, halved
½ cup alfalfa sprouts

Whisk eggs with milk in a small bowl. In a skillet, heat oil. Add tomato and heat through. Stir in beaten eggs and whisk with a fork until eggs are set. Heat whole-wheat pita halves and fill with

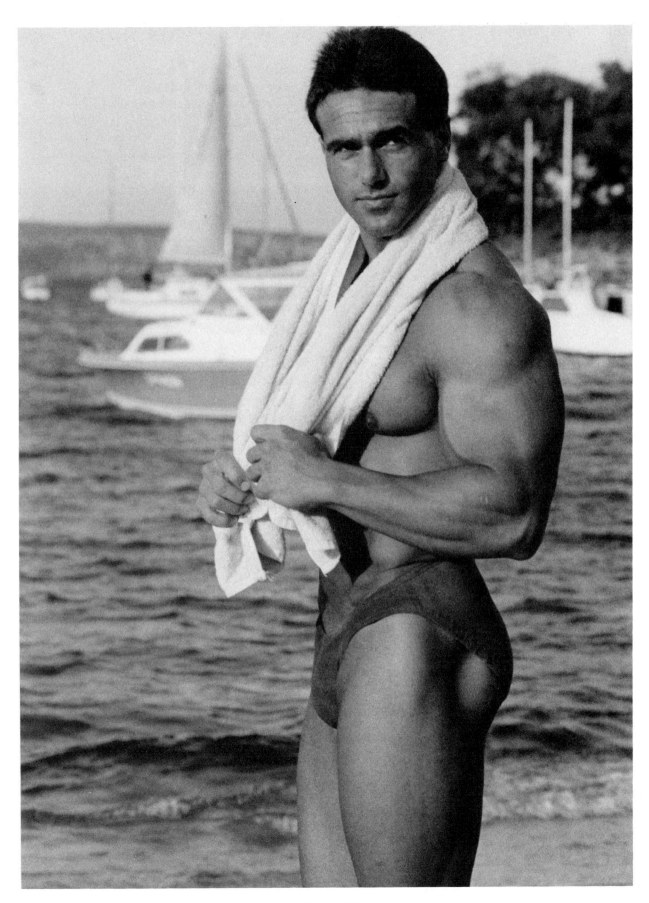

John Terilli.

alfalfa sprouts and scrambled eggs with tomatoes. Makes 1 serving.

VARIATIONS
Precontest: Use two egg whites and only one yolk. Omit safflower oil and scramble eggs in a nonstick skillet or a skillet sprayed with a nonstick vegetable coating.
Bulking up: Add 2 tablespoons grated cheddar to pita stuffing.

	Calories	Protein	Carbo-hydrate	Fat
Maintenance	346	19 grams	28 grams	19 grams
Precontest	233	17 grams	28 grams	11 grams
Bulking up	406	23 grams	28 grams	23 grams

GRANOLA

As well as making a perfect breakfast, granola can also be used as a topping for baked apples, fresh fruit salad, and yogurt.

4 cups large-flake rolled oats
½ cup wheat germ
½ cup wheat bran
½ cup hulled sunflower seeds, unsalted
¼ cup chopped walnuts
½ cup honey
¼ cup safflower oil
1 teaspoon cinnamon
¾ cup chopped dried apricots
¾ cup raisins

Preheat oven to 325°. Spray a large baking sheet with a vegetable coating. Combine oats, wheat germ, bran, sunflower seeds, and walnuts. Spread mixture on baking sheet. In a small saucepan heat honey, safflower oil, and cinnamon to boiling, then drizzle over oatmeal mixture. Bake for 30 minutes. Cool. Stir in dried apricots and raisins. Store in an airtight container. Makes 8 cups.

	Calories	Protein	Carbo-hydrate	Fat
Per 2-ounce serving	172	4.9 grams	21 grams	8.7 grams

EGG WHITE OMELETTE

1 teaspoon safflower oil
2 tablespoons chopped onion
2 tablespoons chopped celery
3 egg whites
½ teaspoon turmeric
1 tablespoon Parmesan cheese

Heat oil in a small frying pan. Add onion and celery and sauté for 5 minutes or until onion is clear. Beat egg whites until frothy. Stir in turmeric. Cook covered over low heat for eight minutes. Sprinkle with Parmesan cheese. Fold and serve. Makes 1 serving.

VARIATIONS
Precontest: Omit Parmesan cheese and safflower oil (use a nonstick vegetable coating such as PAM).
Bulking up: Add 2 ounces diced ham to beaten eggs.

	Calories	Protein	Carbo-hydrate	Fat
Maintenance	135	14.5 grams	3.5 grams	4.5 grams
Precontest	57	12.5 grams	3.5 grams	—
Bulking up	270	25 grams	3.5 grams	14.5 grams

BANANA BRAN MUFFINS

Serve a warm banana bran muffin for breakfast with a glass of milk (or a protein shake) and a piece of fresh fruit.

1⅓ cups natural bran
1 banana, mashed
⅓ cup safflower oil
⅓ cup honey
¼ cup plain yogurt
1 egg
1 teaspoon lemon juice
½ cup all-purpose flour
½ cup whole-wheat flour
2 teaspoons baking powder
½ teaspoon cinnamon
1 teaspoon baking soda
¼ cup chopped walnuts

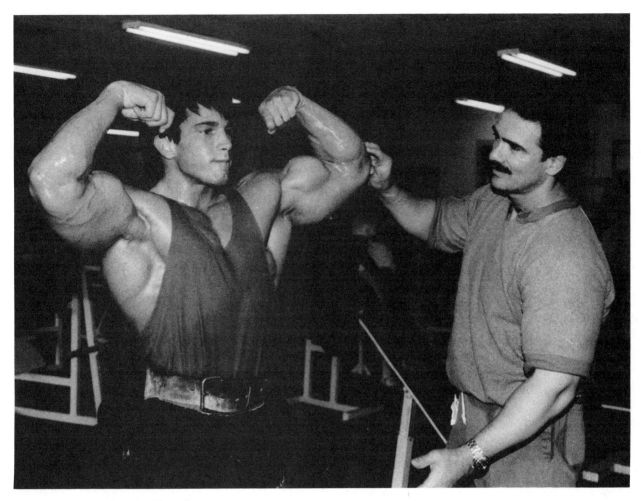

Mike Silk is appraised by his trainer.

Preheat oven to 400°. In a small mixing bowl combine the bran, banana, safflower oil, honey, yogurt, egg, and lemon juice. Beat well. In a medium-sized mixing bowl, mix together both flours, baking powder, cinnamon, baking soda, and walnuts. Make a well in the center of the dry ingredients and add the liquid mixture, stirring until just combined. (Mixture will be lumpy.) Spray muffin tins with a vegetable coating and fill ⅔ full. Bake at 400° for 20–25 minutes. Makes 12 muffins.

	Calories	Protein	Carbo-hydrate	Fat
Per muffin	156	2.7 grams	19 grams	8.5 grams

CARROT PINEAPPLE MUFFINS

¼ cup honey
½ cup oil
2 large eggs, beaten
1½ cups whole-wheat flour
2 teaspoons baking powder
1 teaspoon baking soda
1 teaspoon cinnamon
1 teaspoon vanilla
1 cup grated carrots
1 cup crushed pineapple, drained
¼ cup chopped walnuts

In a medium-sized mixing bowl, combine honey, oil, and beaten eggs. In another bowl combine flour, baking powder, baking soda, and cinnamon. Mix well and add to the liquid ingredients, stirring until blended. Add vanilla, grated carrots, pineapple, and walnuts. Spray muffin tin with a nonstick coating such as PAM and fill each cup ⅔ full. Bake at 375° for 20 minutes. Makes 12 muffins.

	Calories	Protein	Carbo-hydrate	Fat
Per muffin	190	3.5 grams	19 grams	12 grams

POACHED EGGS ON WHOLE-WHEAT TOAST

2 slices whole-wheat toast
2 eggs (at room temperature)
1 teaspoon vinegar

Poaching eggs can be made much easier with the use of an egg poacher, available through kitchen specialty shops. However, if you do not own one, the following method may be used.

Fill a skillet with 2 inches of water and add 1 teaspoon vinegar. Bring the water to a simmer. Break the eggs one at a time into a cup and gently slide into the simmering water. As soon as each egg is submerged in the water, gently push the egg white over the yolk. Repeat this procedure with the remaining egg. Simmer for 4 to 5 minutes, and remove using a slotted spoon. Serve on top of whole-wheat toast. Makes 1 serving.

VARIATIONS
Precontest: Use 2 egg whites only, and serve on 1 slice of whole-wheat toast.
Bulking up: Preheat oven to 350°. Place poached eggs on toast, and sprinkle with 2 tablespoons grated cheddar cheese. Heat in oven until cheese has melted.

	Calories	Protein	Carbo-hydrate	Fat
Maintenance	304	18 grams	30 grams	14 grams
Precontest	102	11 grams	15 grams	1 gram
Bulking up	364	22 grams	30 grams	18 grams

WHOLE-WHEAT FRENCH TOAST

French toast is best made with slightly dry bread, which is better able to absorb the custard.

2 eggs
¼ cup skim milk
2 slices whole-wheat bread
2 teaspoons safflower oil

Whisk together the eggs and skim milk. Soak bread slices in mixture one at a time. Heat oil in a skillet over medium heat. Add bread slices and brown on each side for 2–3 minutes. Makes 1 serving.

VARIATIONS
Precontest: Omit safflower oil. Use 2 egg whites and 1 yolk. Preheat oven to 350°. Place French toast on baking sheet and bake until browned.
Bulking up: Use ¼ cup whole milk in place of skim milk.

	Calories	Protein	Carbo-hydrate	Fat
Maintenance	426	20 grams	33 grams	26 grams
Precontest	261	18 grams	33 grams	8 grams
Bulking up	444	20 grams	33 grams	28 grams

CANTALOUPE WITH FRESH FRUIT AND YOGURT

½ cantaloupe, seeded
½ cup strawberries, hulled
½ orange, peeled and sectioned
¼ cup plain yogurt
1 teaspoon honey
1 teaspoon lime juice
1 egg white

Fill the cantaloupe with strawberries and orange sections. Mix together the yogurt, honey, and lime juice. Whisk the egg white until stiff and fold into yogurt mixture. Spoon onto fruit. Serve chilled. Makes 1 serving.

Bob Paris, like a Greek god.

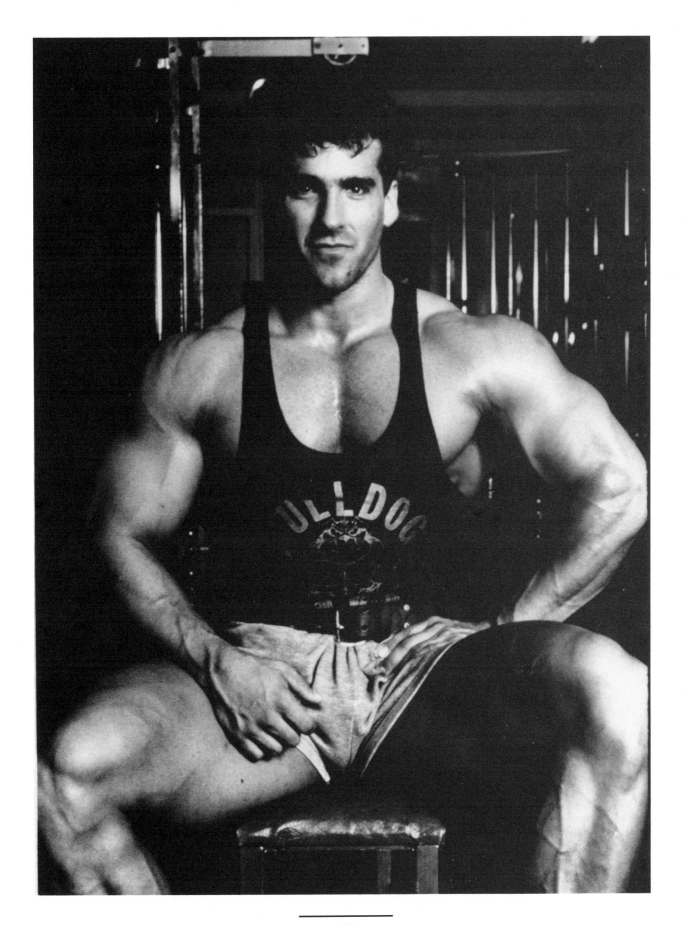

VARIATIONS

Precontest: Use ½ packet of artificial sweetener in place of honey.
Bulking up: Add ½ banana, sliced, to fruit mixture. Sprinkle with 2 tablespoons of granola.

	Calories	Protein	Carbo-hydrate	Fat
Maintenance	198	9 grams	38 grams	1.5 grams
Precontest	172	9 grams	32 grams	1.5 grams
Bulking up	334	12 grams	63 grams	6 grams

OVEN-GRILLED CHEESE SANDWICH

2 slices rye bread
2 slices Swiss cheese (2 ounces total)
1 small tomato, sliced
½ teaspoon caraway seeds

Preheat broiler for 10 minutes. Place Swiss cheese on rye bread and top with tomato slices. Sprinkle with caraway seeds and broil for 4–5 minutes. Makes 1 serving.

VARIATIONS

Precontest: Limit rye bread to 1 slice and use skim milk mozzarella cheese instead of Swiss cheese.
Bulking up: Top Swiss cheese with 2 ounces shaved ham.

	Calories	Protein	Carbo-hydrate	Fat
Maintenance	411	23 grams	41 grams	18 grams
Precontest	268	21 grams	25 grams	10 grams
Bulking up	546	34 grams	41 grams	28 grams

ORANGE APRICOT MUFFINS

⅔ cup orange juice
⅔ cup chopped dried apricots
1 egg
3 teaspoons safflower oil
2 tablespoons honey
1 cup whole-wheat flour
2 cups rolled oats
2 teaspoons baking powder

Heat orange juice and add dried apricots. Let stand for 20 minutes. Mix egg, safflower oil, and honey in a mixing bowl and add the orange juice and apricots. Mix the whole-wheat flour, rolled oats, and baking powder in another mixing bowl. Pour liquid mixture over the dry ingredients and stir until just blended. Spray muffin tin with a vegetable coating, such as PAM, fill cups ⅔ full, and bake at 400° for 20 minutes. Makes 12 muffins.

	Calories	Protein	Carbo-hydrate	Fat
Per muffin	135	3 grams	21 grams	5 grams

Dick Baldwin, Florida.

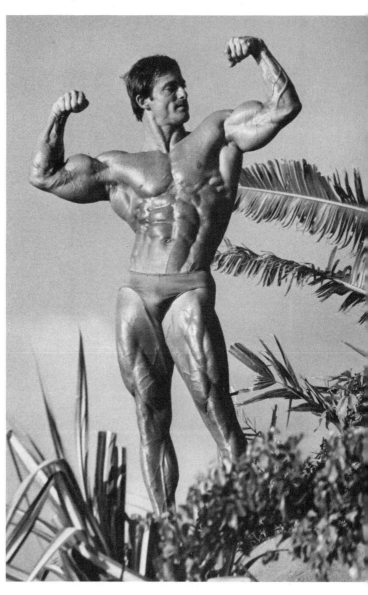

LUNCHES

CHICKEN AND PAPAYA SALAD

2 teaspoons peanut oil
1 teaspoon lime juice
¼ teaspoon ginger
3 ounces chicken, diced
½ papaya, diced
1 cup alfalfa sprouts

Mix oil, lime juice, and ginger. Stir in chicken and papaya. Line a salad plate with alfalfa sprouts and mound salad on top. Makes 1 serving.

VARIATIONS
Precontest: Use 1 teaspoon orange juice in place of oil.
Bulking up: Sprinkle salad with 2 tablespoons sunflower seeds.

	Calories	Protein	Carbo-hydrate	Fat
Maintenance	300	26 grams	15 grams	14 grams
Precontest	221	26 grams	16 grams	4 grams
Bulking up	401	30 grams	18 grams	22 grams

ROAST BEEF PITAS WITH CHUNKY TOMATO DRESSING

1 whole-wheat pita pocket, halved
3 ounces lean roast beef
½ cup shredded lettuce

DRESSING
1 tomato
¼ cup chopped green pepper
1 green onion, chopped
2 teaspoons olive oil
1 teaspoon lemon juice
1 clove garlic
Pinch of cayenne pepper

Combine all ingredients for dressing in a blender and briefly "chop." Refrigerate at least one hour. Fill pita pockets with roast beef slices, shredded lettuce, and chunky dressing. Makes 1 serving.

VARIATIONS
Precontest: Use 3 ounces sliced chicken instead of roast beef.
Bulking up: Add ¼ cup kidney beans.

	Calories	Protein	Carbo-hydrate	Fat
Maintenance	424	33 grams	32 grams	19 grams
Precontest	335	28 grams	32 grams	10 grams
Bulking up	481	36 grams	42 grams	19 grams

MINESTRONE SOUP

2 tablespoons olive oil
½ cup chopped onion
½ cup chopped carrot
½ cup chopped celery
1 garlic clove, minced
4 cups beef broth (sodium-reduced)
1 16-ounce can tomatoes, with juice
1 cup peeled, diced potatoes
1 cup zucchini, diced
1 cup green beans, sliced
2 cups shredded cabbage
1 cup canned kidney beans, drained
½ cup cooked spinach pasta
½ teaspoon basil
½ teaspoon oregano
1 tablespoon Parmesan cheese per serving

In a large pot heat the oil over medium low heat. Add the onion, carrot, celery, and garlic; cover and simmer over low heat for 5–10 minutes, stirring occasionally. Add the broth, tomatoes, potato, zucchini, and green beans. Bring to a boil, then reduce heat; cover and simmer for 1½ hours. Stir in the shredded cabbage and kidney beans, and simmer a further 10 minutes. Add the spinach pasta, basil, and oregano and simmer a further 10 minutes. Serve with grated Parmesan cheese. Makes 6 servings.

VARIATIONS
Precontest: Omit Parmesan cheese.
Bulking up: Add ½ cup diced cooked chicken to soup with the spinach pasta.

	Calories	Protein	Carbo-hydrate	Fat
Maintenance	223	12 grams	29 grams	6 grams
Precontest	200	19 grams	29 grams	5 grams
Bulking up	250	13 grams	29 grams	6 grams

BAKED EGGS IN POTATO SKINS

1 large baking potato
1 tablespoon milk
1 green onion, chopped
1 teaspoon mixed herbs
1 ounce cheddar cheese, grated
1 egg white
2 eggs
1 slice boiled ham, halved

Preheat oven to 350°. Scrub the baking potato, pierce in several places with a fork, and bake for 45–50 minutes. Cut the potato in half lengthwise and scoop out the pulp, leaving a ¼-inch ridge. Mash the potato pulp with the milk; add the chopped green onion, the mixed herbs, and grated cheese. Beat the egg white until stiff and fold gently into the potato mixture. Assemble as follows:

• Place a half slice of ham in each potato half.
• Break an egg on top of ham slices.
• Top with potato/cheese mixture.

Bake at 350° for 30 minutes. Makes 1 serving.

VARIATIONS
Precontest: Omit ham and cheese. Use egg whites only. Serve with a tossed green salad and 1 tablespoon of vinaigrette dressing.
Bulking up: Serve with ½ cup stir-fried kidney beans.

	Calories	Protein	Carbo-hydrate	Fat
Maintenance	680	39 grams	37.8 grams	22 grams
Precontest	299	17 grams	37.8 grams	.25 gram
Bulking up	795	46.2 grams	58.7 grams	22 grams

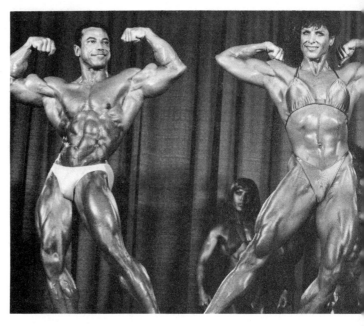

Chris Dickerson and Diana Dennis.

CUCUMBER SALAD

This salad makes a nice accompaniment to broiled meat or fish, or as part of a salad combination with tuna, chicken, or salmon.

1   English cucumber, thinly sliced
3–4   green onions, chopped
¾   cup plain yogurt
2   teaspoons safflower oil
       Juice of one lemon
1   packet sugar substitute (1-gram packet = 2 teaspoons sugar)
3   teaspoons dill weed

Put cucumber slices in a small bowl and cover with boiling water. Let stand for 2–3 minutes. Drain. Rinse with cold water. Drain. Toss green onions with cucumber slices. Mix yogurt, safflower oil, lemon juice, sugar substitute, and dill weed in a screw-top jar and shake well. Pour over salad, and mix well. Chill and serve. Makes 4 servings.

	Calories	Protein	Carbo-hydrate	Fat
Per serving	74	3.1 grams	6.8 grams	4.3 grams

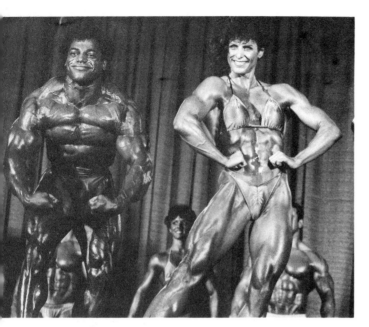

Mr. America Tony Pearson poses off against Diana Dennis (yes, they are competing against each other).

SHRIMP SALAD

Any time you're preparing to serve brown rice with a meal, make a little extra and reserve for this recipe.

½ cup cooked brown rice
⅔ cup salad shrimps, cooked
½ cup cooked peas
3 green onions, diced
1 stalk celery, diced
   Leaf lettuce for garnishing
½ orange, divided into segments
1 teaspoon capers

SALAD DRESSING
1 tablespoon lemon juice
1 tablespoon plain yogurt
1 olive oil
½ teaspoon dill weed

Mix dressing ingredients in a screw-top jar and shake well.

Combine the brown rice, salad shrimps, cooked peas, onions, and celery. Toss with dressing and arrange on leaf lettuce. Garnish with orange

slices, and sprinkle with capers. Chill and serve. Makes 1 serving.

VARIATIONS
Precontest: Omit salad dressing and sprinkle with fresh lemon juice. Omit capers.
Bulking up: Substitute ½ avocado, peeled and sliced, for the orange.

	Calories	Protein	Carbo-hydrate	Fat
Maintenance	439	27 grams	46 grams	16 grams
Precontest	294	26 grams	44 grams	1.5 grams
Bulking up	592	29 grams	44 grams	34 grams

CHICKEN SALAD WITH LIME DRESSING

1 cup tightly packed fresh spinach, stems removed
½ cup chickpeas, drained
4 ounces sliced poached chicken
6 thin slices mild red onion
½ orange, peeled and sliced
6 mushrooms, sliced thinly

DRESSING
1 tablespoon olive oil
   Juice of 1 fresh lime
1 teaspoon vinegar
1 clove garlic
¼ teaspoon ground cumin

Combine all dressing ingredients in a small bowl and whisk together. Line a salad plate with spinach. Mound chickpeas in center. Arrange slices of chicken, onion, orange, and mushrooms around chickpeas. Drizzle dressing over the salad. Makes 1 serving.

VARIATIONS
Precontest: Use 1 tablespoon orange juice in place of olive oil and omit chickpeas.
Bulking up: Add 1 hard-boiled egg, sliced, to salad.

	Calories	Protein	Carbo-hydrate	Fat
Maintenance	477	48 grams	49 grams	8 grams
Precontest	212	27 grams	22 grams	3.5 grams
Bulking up	557	54 grams	49 grams	14 grams

EGG AND BEAN FRITTATA

Eggs and beans are two items that should always be on hand in the bodybuilder's kitchen. As combined in this recipe they're just that little bit "different" and can be prepared and ready to serve in under 15 minutes.

 3 eggs
½ cup canned kidney beans, drained
½ teaspoon chili powder
 1 clove garlic, minced
¼ cup chopped onion
¼ cup chopped celery

In a medium-sized bowl, whisk the eggs. Add the kidney beans and chili powder and set aside. Sauté the garlic, onion, and celery over medium heat for a few minutes until the onion is softened. Stir this mixture into the bowl containing the eggs and beans. Spray a frying pan with a vegetable coating such as PAM and add the contents of the bowl. Cook uncovered, over medium heat, without stirring, until the underside is browned. Loosen the edge of the frittata using a spatula and turn into a second frying pan that has also been sprayed with a vegetable coating, to brown the other side. Makes 1 serving.

VARIATIONS
Precontest: Use 1 whole egg, plus 2 egg whites. Reduce safflower oil to 1 teaspoon.
Bulking up: Top with 1 ounce of grated cheddar cheese, and serve with a baked potato as an accompaniment.

	Calories	Protein	Carbo-hydrate	Fat
Maintenance	444	28 grams	27.3 grams	20 grams
Precontest	283	22.2 grams	26.4 grams	9.9 grams
Bulking up	701	39 grams	60.4 grams	29.6 grams

RATATOUILLE BURGER

 4 ounces lean ground lamb
 1 teaspoon grated onion
¼ cup heated ratatouille (see page 221)
 1 whole-wheat pita bread, halved
 1 tablespoon Parmesan cheese

In a small bowl, mix the ground lamb with grated onion. Shape into a burger and broil, 4 inches from heat source, for 8–10 minutes, turning once. Halve burger and place in pita pockets. Divide ratatouille between halves and sprinkle with Parmesan cheese. Makes 1 serving.

VARIATIONS
Precontest: Omit Parmesan cheese, and reduce lamb to 3 ounces.
Bulking up: Add 1 ounce of Swiss cheese to burger during the last 2 minutes of broiling.

	Calories	Protein	Carbo-hydrate	Fat
Maintenance	464	27 grams	33 grams	21 grams
Precontest	388	21 grams	33 grams	16 grams
Bulking up	571	35 grams	34 grams	28 grams

FRESH FRUIT AND CHEESE PLATE

½ cup fresh pineapple, peeled and sliced
½ orange, sectioned
½ cup seedless green grapes
½ cup strawberries, hulled
   Leaf lettuce

DRESSING
 2 ounces Chèvre cheese
¼ cup natural yogurt
   Juice of one lime
½ teaspoon poppy seeds

Combine ingredients for dressing and blend until smooth. Arrange slices of fruit on leaf lettuce and coat with dressing. Makes 1 serving.

VARIATIONS
Precontest: Omit grapes, and use 2 ounces partly skimmed ricotta cheese in place of Chèvre.
Bulking up: Sprinkle salad with ¼ cup chopped cashews.

	Calories	Protein	Carbo-hydrate	Fat
Maintenance	301	12 grams	40 grams	10 grams
Precontest	226	10 grams	32 grams	8 grams
Bulking up	491	18 grams	50 grams	26 grams

ONE-DISH MAIN MEALS

The following recipes are complete meals in themselves. They need no additional accompaniments other than a glass of milk and a slice of whole-wheat bread, with a piece of fresh fruit for dessert.

CHILI PIE

2 cups cooked brown rice
¼ cup grated cheddar cheese
1 teaspoon safflower oil
1 egg, beaten

FILLING
2 teaspoons safflower oil
½ cup minced onion
¼ cup minced green pepper
¼ cup minced red pepper
¼ cup minced celery
1 clove garlic, minced
6 ounces lean ground beef
½ cup canned red kidney beans
1 cup canned tomatoes, chopped
¼ teaspoon chili powder
¼ teaspoon cumin

Preheat oven to 325°. In a small bowl, mix until combined the brown rice, grated cheese, oil, and egg. Press into an 8-inch pie pan to form a crust. Heat safflower oil in a skillet and sauté onion until clear. Add green pepper, red pepper, celery, and garlic, and sauté for a further 2–3 minutes. Add ground beef and sauté until browned. Drain off fat, and add kidney beans, tomatoes, chili powder, and cumin. Spoon mixture into pie crust and bake for 30–40 minutes. Makes 4 servings.

VARIATIONS
Precontest: Omit cheddar cheese with pie crust.

Omit safflower oil from filling, and use a nonstick vegetable coating in its place. Use ground veal in place of beef.
Bulking up: Sprinkle top of pie with ½ cup grated cheddar cheese before baking.

	Calories	Protein	Carbo-hydrate	Fat
Maintenance	278	17 grams	29 grams	12 grams
Precontest	232	9 grams	29 grams	6 grams
Bulking up	353	21 grams	30 grams	17 grams

LAMB WITH BEANS AND TOMATOES

This recipe is equally as good when beef or veal is used instead of lamb. A quick version can be made by using canned white kidney beans in place of the dried navy beans.

1 cup dried navy beans, soaked overnight in cold water
1 onion, peeled
2 tablespoons olive oil
1 pound lean lamb, cut into cubes
3 cloves garlic, peeled and minced
1 onion, quartered
1 8-ounce can tomatoes, or 4 large ripe tomatoes, peeled, seeded, and chopped
½ cup beef stock (low-sodium)
½ teaspoon basil
½ teaspoon thyme
3 tablespoons bread crumbs

Drain the beans and rinse under cold water. Place in a large pot, cover with water, and add the onion. Bring to a boil, reduce heat, cover, and simmer for 45 minutes. Drain beans; discard onion and set beans aside. Meanwhile, heat oil in a large skillet and brown the lamb cubes. Add the onion to the skillet and brown, stirring constantly. Add the garlic, tomatoes, basil, and thyme and cook over low heat for 2–3 minutes. Rub an earthenware casserole with garlic and add half of the beans. Cover with the lamb and tomato mixture and top with the remaining beans. Moisten with beef stock and sprinkle with bread crumbs. Bake in a preheated oven, at 325° for 1½ hours. Makes 4 servings.

VARIATIONS

Precontest: Reduce navy beans to ¼ cup. Omit olive oil and use a nonstick vegetable coating in its place. Reduce beef broth to ¼ cup.
Bulking up: Sprinkle with 4 tablespoons Parmesan cheese during the last ½ hour of baking.

	Calories	Protein	Carbo-hydrate	Fat
Maintenance	521	31 grams	44 grams	23 grams
Precontest	335	22 grams	21 grams	16 grams
Bulking up	544	33 grams	44 grams	24 grams

Frank and Marsha Scolaro.

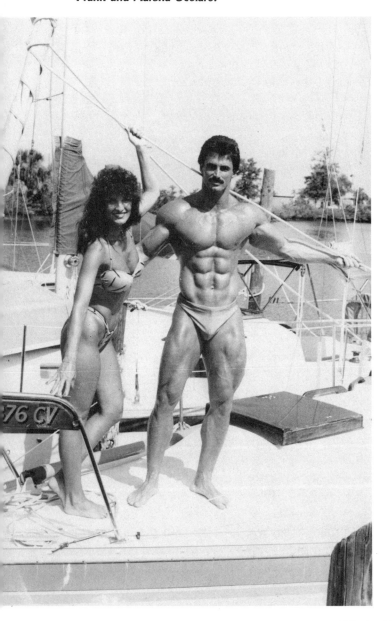

STUFFED PEPPERS

2 green peppers
½ cup onion, chopped
1 tablespoon safflower oil
6 ounces lean ground beef
¾ cup cooked brown rice
¼ teaspoon oregano
¼ teaspoon cumin
1 cup low-sodium beef broth
2 tablespoons tomato paste
1 teaspoon vinegar
1 teaspoon honey

Preheat oven to 350°. Slice tops off of green peppers and remove seeds. Rinse peppers and drain. Brown onion in safflower oil and add the ground beef, stirring until browned. Drain off fat and add the brown rice and herbs. Divide mixture between peppers. Place stuffed peppers in a small casserole. Heat beef broth, tomato paste, vinegar, and honey in the pan that was used to brown meat, and bring to a boil. Pour the broth into the casserole containing the peppers. Bake for 45 minutes. Makes 2 servings.

VARIATIONS

Precontest: Use lean veal in place of beef, and use a nonstick vegetable coating in place of oil.
Bulking up: Add ½ cup of canned red kidney beans (drained) to stuffing mixture, and sprinkle stuffed peppers with 2 tablespoons of grated cheddar.

	Calories	Protein	Carbo-hydrate	Fat
Maintenance	357	27 grams	25 grams	16 grams
Precontest	262	23 grams	25 grams	7 grams
Bulking up	443	32 grams	35 grams	18 grams

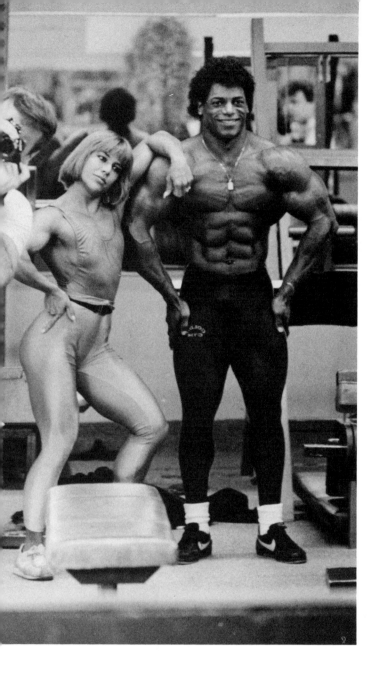

Juliette Bergman and Tony Pearson.

Preheat oven to 350°. Heat the oil in a large ovenproof pan. Add the chicken and sauté until lightly browned. Add the onions, garlic, and tomato and cook for 5 minutes. Stir in the rice, and add the chicken stock and saffron. Cover and bake for 30 minutes. Add the shrimp, green and red pepper, and lemon juice, and return to oven for a further 10–15 minutes.

VARIATIONS
Precontest: Remove skin from chicken breasts, omit safflower oil, and delete the browning process.
Bulking up: Add 2 ounces pork tenderloin, cut into 1-inch slices, with the chicken.

	Calories	Protein	Carbo-hydrate	Fat
Maintenance	436	35 grams	36 grams	19 grams
Precontest	290	34 grams	36 grams	4 grams
Bulking up	503	44 grams	36 grams	22 grams

GRILLED CHICKEN AND VEGETABLES

2 chicken breasts
6 green onions
4 small new potatoes, boiled until tender
1 small zucchini, halved and scored
1 red pepper, quartered
1 green pepper, quartered
6 mushrooms

MARINADE
2 tablespoons rice wine vinegar
½ teaspoon Dijon mustard
3 tablespoons peanut oil
3 tablespoons orange juice
1 teaspoon Chinese five-spice mixture (fennel, anise, ginger, cinnamon, and cloves)
1 clove garlic, crushed

Arrange chicken and vegetables in a glass baking dish. Mix ingredients for marinade and pour over chicken and vegetables. Marinate for ½–1

PAELLA FOR TWO

2 tablespoons safflower oil
½ pound chicken parts
½ cup chopped onion
2 cloves garlic, minced
1 large tomato, peeled and chopped
¼ cup long-grain rice
1 cup hot chicken broth
½ teaspoon saffron
¼ pound shrimps, shelled
¼ cup green pepper, chopped
¼ cup red pepper, chopped
   Juice of ½ lemon

hour. Preheat broiler for 10 minutes. Remove chicken and vegetables from marinade. Place chicken on a broiling rack and broil for 5–6 minutes. Add potatoes and zucchini and broil a further 3 minutes. Add green onion and mushrooms and broil for a further 5–7 minutes. Makes 2 servings.

VARIATIONS

Precontest: Remove skin from chicken, and omit oil and mustard from marinade. Omit potatoes.
Bulking up: Add 8 large shelled shrimp to chicken and vegetables in marinade; add to broiling rack during the last 5–7 minutes.

	Calories	Protein	Carbo-hydrate	Fat
Maintenance	405	31 grams	34 grams	15 grams
Precontest	194	24 grams	16 grams	3 grams
Bulking up	508	51 grams	35 grams	16 grams

VEAL ROLL-UPS

2 slices veal scallopini
1 teaspoon Dijon mustard
½ zucchini, cut into sticks (3″ × ½″)
1 carrot, cut into sticks (3″ × ½″)
2 green pepper rings
1 cup shredded cabbage
2 small new potatoes, quartered
1 teaspoon caraway seeds
1 tomato, quartered

Spread veal with mustard. Place half the carrot and zucchini sticks in the center of each veal slice. Roll veal around the vegetables, and secure by inserting each roll through a green pepper ring. Place the shredded cabbage in a steamer. Set the veal rolls on top of the cabbage, surround with potatoes, and sprinkle caraway seeds over all. Steam for 20 minutes, then add tomato wedges and continue steaming for a further 15 minutes. Makes 1 serving.

VARIATIONS

Precontest: Omit the mustard and potatoes.
Bulking up: Place a 1-ounce slice of mozzarella cheese on each slice of veal before rolling with vegetables.

	Calories	Protein	Carbo-hydrate	Fat
Maintenance	338	29 grams	34 grams	9 grams
Precontest	233	26 grams	11 grams	9 grams
Bulking up	419	34 grams	34 grams	15 grams

BROILED LIVER AND EGGS

Liver and eggs, two of bodybuilders' favorite muscle builders, are teamed together in this quick and tasty recipe.

2 slices calf's liver (approx. 4 ounces)
8 cherry tomatoes, halved
½ cup whole mushrooms
1 hard-boiled egg, crumbled
½ teaspoon mixed herbs

Preheat broiler for 10–15 minutes. Place calf's liver on grid of broiling pan and place under broiler for 2–3 minutes. Remove from oven and turn, using a spatula. Surround with cherry tomatoes and mushrooms and place under broiler for a further 3 minutes. Sprinkle crumbled egg and mixed herbs on top of the liver and serve. Makes 1 serving.

VARIATIONS

Precontest: Use egg white only instead of whole egg.
Bulking up: Serve three slices of liver and add a baked potato.

	Calories	Protein	Carbo-hydrate	Fat
Maintenance	272	25 grams	11 grams	6 grams
Precontest	207	23 grams	11 grams	trace
Bulking up	435	36 grams	33 grams	6 grams

BEEF TENDERLOIN STIR-FRY

2 teaspoons peanut oil
3 ounces beef tenderloin, sliced into strips
1 clove garlic, minced
6 mushrooms, halved
1 carrot, cut into 2-inch sticks
1 stalk celery, diced
6 asparagus tips
1 teaspoon sesame seeds
¼ cup low-sodium beef broth

Heat oil in a wok or shallow skillet over medium-high heat. Add beef strips and brown quickly. Remove with slotted spoon and set aside. Sauté garlic for 1–2 minutes; add vegetables and toss. Stir in beef broth and cover and cook an additional 4–5 minutes. Add browned beef strips and sesame seeds; cover and cook an additional 2–3 minutes. Makes 1 serving.

VARIATIONS
Precontest: Use a boneless veal cutlet in place of beef, and reduce oil to 1 teaspoon.
Bulking up: In a separate pan make a one-egg omelette and cut it into strips. Toss with stir-fry.

	Calories	Protein	Carbo-hydrate	Fat
Maintenance	508	25.5 grams	13.5 grams	3.9 grams
Precontest	313	28.5 grams	13.5 grams	15 grams
Bulking up	588	31.5 grams	13.5 grams	45 grams

CHICKEN COOKED IN FOIL

1 boneless 4-ounce chicken breast, skinned
1 clove garlic, minced
4 slices Spanish onion
4 slices green pepper
¼ cup chopped red pepper
1 fresh tomato, diced
1 teaspoon olive oil
2 teaspoons lemon juice
1 teaspoon parsley
1 teaspoon oregano

Preheat oven to 400°. Cut foil paper into a rectangle large enough to encase all of the ingredients. Place the chicken breast in the center of the foil; sprinkle with garlic and top with slices of onion, green pepper, red pepper, and tomato. Drizzle with olive oil and lemon juice and sprinkle with parsley and oregano. Bring the ends of the foil together and fold the edges. Next crimp the sides to make a sealed packet. Place on a baking sheet, seam side up, and bake for 30–40 minutes or until chicken is tender when pierced with a fork. Makes 1 serving.

VARIATIONS
Precontest: Spray foil with a vegetable coating, and omit the olive oil.
Bulking up: Serve with a sprinkling of 2 tablespoons Parmesan cheese.

	Calories	Protein	Carbo-hydrate	Fat
Maintenance	280	30 grams	18 grams	9.6 grams
Precontest	230	30 grams	18 grams	4 grams
Bulking up	336	34 grams	18 grams	8 grams

PASTA RATATOUILLE

If you have ratatouille on hand (see page 221), this recipe can be made in less than 10 minutes. It's ideal after a hard workout when you want something quick, but it tastes like you've slaved over it all day.

4 ounces spinach pasta (1 cup cooked)
1 cup ratatouille
2 tablespoons grated Parmesan cheese

Cook spinach pasta according to package directions. Heat ratatouille in a separate pan. Drain pasta and toss with ratatouille. Sprinkle with Parmesan cheese and serve. Makes 1 serving.

VARIATIONS
Precontest: Omit Parmesan cheese.
Bulking up: Add 1 cup cooked, cubed chicken to ratatouille before tossing with pasta.

	Calories	Protein	Carbo-hydrate	Fat
Maintenance	436	17 grams	55 grams	13 grams
Precontest	380	13 grams	55 grams	9 grams
Bulking up	551	37 grams	55 grams	16 grams

PORK TENDERLOIN WRAPPED IN CABBAGE LEAVES

2 whole cabbage leaves
1 teaspoon Dijon mustard
1 cup sliced cabbage
½ cup sliced carrots
1 small potato, halved
4 ounces boneless pork tenderloin, cut into 1-inch-thick slices
1 teaspoon lemon juice
1 teaspoon caraway seeds

Blanch the whole cabbage leaves in boiling water for 1 minute to soften. Drain. Brush the inside of the cabbage leaves with mustard and divide pork tenderloin between the two leaves. Fold the cabbage leaves around the pork slices to form a package. Place the pork packages in the center of a steamer, and surround with sliced cabbage, carrots, and potato. Set over boiling water and steam for 25 minutes. Sprinkle with lemon juice and caraway seeds. Makes 1 serving.

VARIATIONS

Precontest: Use 3 ounces boneless, skinned chicken breast in place of the pork tenderloin.
Bulking up: Add 1 whole egg to the steamer with the cabbage packages and vegetables.

	Calories	Protein	Carbo-hydrate	Fat
Maintenance	406	37 grams	35 grams	12 grams
Precontest	276	25 grams	35 grams	4 grams
Bulking up	488	43 grams	35 grams	18 grams

STEAMED LAMB WITH VEGETABLES

MEATBALLS

6 ounces lean ground lamb
1 green onion, chopped
1 small clove garlic, minced
1 teaspoon Dijon mustard
1 tablespoon ground almonds
1 teaspoon fresh mint, chopped
1 teaspoon parsley, chopped

VEGETABLES

1 new potato, halved
½ cup snow peas
8 cherry tomatoes

In a small bowl mix together all ingredients for meatballs and form into balls 2 inches in diameter. Place in a bamboo steamer with potatoes and steam over gently boiling water for 20 minutes. Add the snow peas and cherry tomatoes and steam for a further 10–15 minutes.

VARIATIONS

Precontest: Reduce lamb to 4 ounces and omit almonds from meatballs.
Bulking up: Add 1 slice of fresh pineapple to steamer during the last 15 minutes of cooking time.

	Calories	Protein	Carbo-hydrate	Fat
Maintenance	505	54 grams	30 grams	18 grams
Precontest	348	36 grams	28 grams	9 grams
Bulking up	596	54 grams	54 grams	18 grams

SPAGHETTI WITH CLAM SAUCE

1 tablespoon olive oil
1 clove garlic, minced
¼ cup green pepper, chopped
¼ cup diced celery
¼ cup chopped onion
3 ounces canned baby clams, with juice
1 6-ounce can tomatoes
½ teaspoon oregano
½ teaspoon basil
  Dash of red pepper hot sauce
1 cup cooked whole-wheat spaghetti

Heat oil in a heavy saucepan over medium-high heat. Add garlic, green pepper, celery, and onion, and sauté until onion is clear. Add clams, tomatoes, oregano, basil, and a dash of red pepper hot sauce. Simmer covered over medium-low heat for 30 minutes. Prepare spaghetti according to package directions while sauce is simmering.

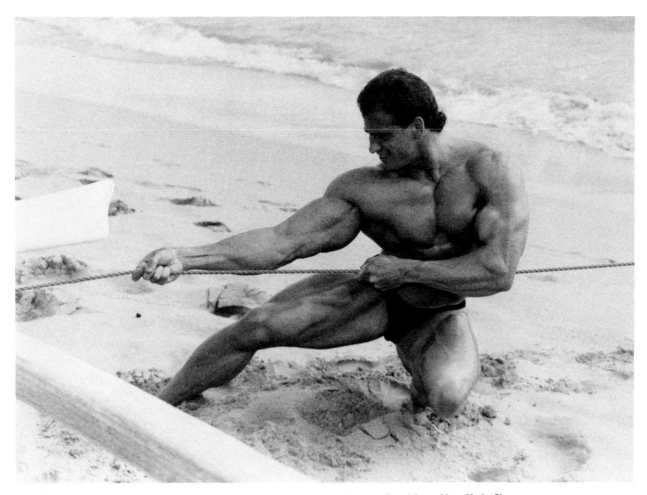

Tommy Terwilliger, New York City.

VARIATIONS

Precontest: Serve over 1 cup shredded spaghetti squash instead of over spaghetti.
Bulking up: Sprinkle with 2 tablespoons Parmesan cheese.

	Calories	Protein	Carbo-hydrate	Fat
Maintenance	391	15 grams	49 grams	17 grams
Precontest	266	12 grams	23 grams	16 grams
Bulking up	447	19 grams	49 grams	21 grams

STEAMED FISH DINNER

1 4-ounce halibut steak
1 cob of corn
1 tomato
1 new potato
½ cup snow peas
1 teaspoon fennel seed
3 slices lime

Place halibut steak in a bamboo steamer with corn, tomato, potato, and snow peas. Sprinkle with fennel seed and top halibut steak with lime slices. Cover and set over gently boiling water for 30 minutes. Makes 1 serving.

VARIATIONS

Precontest: Omit potatoes and corn and serve with tomatoes and snow peas.
Bulking up: Drizzle halibut steak and vegetables with 2 teaspoons of olive oil before steaming.

	Calories	Protein	Carbo-hydrate	Fat
Maintenance	439	36 grams	66 grams	9 grams
Precontest	219	33 grams	32 grams	8 grams
Bulking up	564	36 grams	66 grams	23 grams

STEAMED SOLE WITH CABBAGE AND CARROTS

½ cup shredded carrots
½ cup shredded cabbage
1 4-ounce fillet of sole
¼ cup chicken broth
1 teaspoon safflower oil
1 teaspoon vinegar
½ teaspoon caraway seeds
 Pinch of sugar

Combine the cabbage and carrots and steam, covered, over gently boiling water for 10 minutes or until crisp tender. Remove from steamer and set aside. Now put sole in steamer and steam for 10 minutes. Meanwhile heat chicken broth, safflower oil, vinegar, caraway, and sugar in a small saucepan. Add cabbage and carrots and toss until heated through. To serve, place sole in the center of a dish and surround with cabbage and carrots. Makes 1 serving.

VARIATIONS

Precontest: Reduce sole to 3 ounces and omit safflower oil and sugar.
Bulking up: Add ¼ cup of canned lima beans to vegetables when reheating with stock.

	Calories	Protein	Carbo-hydrate	Fat
Maintenance	315	36 grams	8 grams	9 grams
Precontest	209	28 grams	8 grams	7 grams
Bulking up	380	40 grams	20 grams	9 grams

SEAFOOD RISOTTO

1 tablespoon olive oil
1 clove garlic, minced
¼ cup chopped onion
¼ cup chopped green pepper
¼ cup short-grain Italian rice
1 cup chicken broth
3 large scallops
6 medium shrimp
¼ cup frozen peas

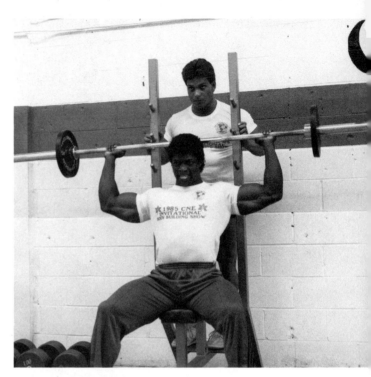

Rich Gaspari spots John Brown in the press behind the neck exercise.

4–6 mushrooms, stemmed and halved
1 tablespoon Parmesan cheese
½ teaspoon basil

Heat oil in a medium saucepan over medium heat. Add garlic, onions, and green pepper and sauté until onions are clear. Add rice and ¾ cup of chicken broth. Reduce heat to medium-low, cover, and simmer for 20 minutes, stirring occasionally. Then add the scallops, shrimp, peas, mushrooms, and remaining ¼ cup broth and simmer, covered, for a further 5–6 minutes or until the rice is creamy. Stir in the Parmesan cheese and basil. Makes 1 serving.

VARIATIONS

Precontest: Spray pan with a vegetable coating and omit the olive oil and Parmesan cheese.
Bulking up: Add 4 crab claws with the shrimp and scallops.

	Calories	Protein	Carbo-hydrate	Fat
Maintenance	530	31 grams	65 grams	16 grams
Precontest	389	28 grams	65 grams	.7 gram
Bulking up	578	38 grams	65 grams	16 grams

MAIN COURSES

LAMB KEBABS

3 ounces lean lamb, cut into 2-inch cubes
4 mushrooms
½ small zucchini, cut into cubes
½ green pepper, cut into chunks

MARINADE
2 ounces plain yogurt
1 teaspoon curry powder
1 teaspoon lemon juice
1 teaspoon safflower oil

Mix ingredients for marinade in a small bowl. Add lamb cubes and let stand for 1 hour at room temperature. Preheat broiler for 10 minutes. Thread lamb, mushrooms, zucchini, and green peppers onto skewers. Brush with marinade and broil for 15–20 minutes, turning once. Makes 1 serving.

VARIATIONS
Precontest: Omit marinade. Bring lamb to room temperature, sprinkle with 2 tablespoons of lemon juice and ½ teaspoon mint and let stand for 15 minutes before broiling.
Bulking up: Add 4 large shelled shrimp to skewers.

	Calories	Protein	Carbo-hydrate	Fat
Maintenance	275	28 grams	10 grams	13 grams
Precontest	188	26 grams	6 grams	6 grams
Bulking up	321	36 grams	11 grams	14 grams

SKEWERED SCALLOPS

¼ cup orange juice
2 teaspoons lime juice
1 clove garlic
1 bay leaf
¼ teaspoon cumin
¼ teaspoon paprika
2 teaspoons olive oil
8–10 scallops

In a glass bowl, combine all ingredients except scallops. Refrigerate for 2–3 hours or overnight. Preheat broiler for 10–15 minutes. Thread scallops onto skewers. Broil for 6 minutes, basting frequently with marinade. Serve with skewered vegetables or a crisp salad. Makes 1 serving.

VARIATIONS
Precontest: Omit marinade. Sprinkle scallops with 2 tablespoons of lemon juice and 1 teaspoon cumin. Let stand at room temperature for 15 minutes before broiling.
Bulking up: Add 2 ounces veal, cut into 2-inch by 3-inch strips, to marinade with scallops. Wrap veal strips around scallops and thread onto skewers.

	Calories	Protein	Carbo-hydrate	Fat
Maintenance	324	38.5 grams	6.5 grams	12.6 grams
Precontest	190	38.5 grams	3 grams	2 grams
Bulking up	446	53.5 grams	6.5 grams	18.5 grams

SALMON COOKED IN FOIL

1 4-ounce salmon steak, 1-inch thick
1 teaspoon safflower oil
2 carrots, sliced into julienne strips
½ zucchini, sliced into julienne strips
½ teaspoon dill
1 fresh lime, sliced
1 teaspoon water

Preheat oven to 375°. Cut a piece of aluminum foil large enough to enclose salmon and vegetables. Brush salmon steak with safflower oil and place in the center of foil. Top with carrots and zucchini strips. Sprinkle with dill. Squeeze fresh lime juice over all and drizzle with the teaspoon water. Close the foil packet and crimp edges to seal. Place packet on a heated baking sheet and bake for 20–25 minutes. Open packet and serve with fresh wedges of lime. Makes 1 serving.

VARIATIONS
Precontest: Omit safflower oil.
Bulking up: Add 6 scallops to foil packet with salmon and vegetables.

	Calories	Protein	Carbo-hydrate	Fat
Maintenance	311	33 grams	13 grams	12.6 grams
Precontest	261	33 grams	13 grams	7 grams
Bulking up	423	56 grams	13 grams	13.6 grams

VEAL SCALLOPS

4 ounces boneless veal, pounded until very thin
2 teaspoons safflower oil
¼ cup chopped onion
1 tablespoon whole-wheat flour
¼ cup chicken broth
1 teaspoon parsley
½ teaspoon grated lemon rind

Cut the veal into small pieces. Heat oil in a small skillet and add the chopped onion. Cook until lightly browned. Dredge veal scallops in whole-wheat flour and add to the pan with onion. Cook over high heat until lightly browned. Add chicken broth and cook, stirring, for a further 3–4 minutes. Sprinkle with parsley and lemon. Makes 1 serving.

VARIATIONS
Precontest: Omit safflower oil and use a nonstick vegetable spray coating in its place.
Bulking up: Omit chicken broth and add ¼ cup milk and ¼ cup grated sharp cheddar cheese, stirring until combined.

	Calories	Protein	Carbo-hydrate	Fat
Maintenance	395	32 grams	10 grams	23 grams
Precontest	285	32 grams	10 grams	11 grams
Bulking up	555	42 grams	13 grams	33 grams

CALF'S LIVER WITH APPLES

4 ounces calf's liver
¼ cup milk
1 teaspoon safflower oil
¼ cup apple juice
1 small Granny Smith apple, sliced and peeled
¼ teaspoon marjoram
2 tablespoons onion, diced

Soak liver in milk for 15 minutes. Preheat broiler for 10 minutes. Drain liver and brush with oil. Broil for 4 minutes on each side. In a small saucepan heat apple juice over medium heat; add apple slices, marjoram, and onion and simmer for 8–10 minutes or until apples are soft. To serve, place grilled liver in center of plate and top with apple slices. Makes 1 serving.

VARIATIONS
Precontest: Use skim milk. Omit oil.
Bulking up: Increase portion to 5 ounces.

	Calories	Protein	Carbo-hydrate	Fat
Maintenance	356	25 grams	36 grams	13 grams
Precontest	296	25 grams	36 grams	6.3 grams
Bulking up	392	30 grams	37 grams	14 grams

GRILLED SWORDFISH

1 6-ounce swordfish steak
1 small zucchini, halved and scored
1 orange, sliced
1 teaspoon fennel seed

Preheat broiler for 10–15 minutes. Place swordfish and zucchini on broiling rack and broil 8 inches from heat for 3–4 minutes. Using a spatula, turn fish. Top with fresh orange slices and return to broiler for a further 4–5 minutes or until fish flakes easily when pierced with a fork. Sprinkle with fennel seed and serve. Serve with ½ cup brown rice. Makes 1 serving.

VARIATIONS
Precontest: Substitute halibut steak for the sword-

fish and serve with 6 slices cucumber instead of the brown rice.

Bulking up: Serve with a baked sweet potato with a pat of polyunsaturated margarine instead of the rice.

	Calories	Protein	Carbo-hydrate	Fat
Maintenance	400	38.2 grams	45.5 grams	7.3 grams
Precontest	276	39.1 grams	24.05 grams	2.4 grams
Bulking up	489	38.2 grams	60.95 grams	12.3 grams

CHICKEN CASSEROLE

2 tablespoons safflower oil
2 chicken breasts
1 small onion, chopped
1 clove garlic, minced
1 cup halved mushrooms
1 teaspoon flour
1 cup chicken broth
2 tomatoes, peeled, seeded, and chopped
1 teaspoon paprika
1 bay leaf

Preheat oven to 350°. Heat 1 tablespoon of oil in a large casserole and brown the chicken on all sides. Remove the chicken, and set aside. Add onion, garlic, and mushrooms and sauté for 3–4 minutes. Stir in the flour and add the chicken broth. Add the tomatoes and bring to a boil. Add the chicken, paprika, and bay leaf. Cover the casserole and bake for 30–40 minutes. Makes 2 servings.

VARIATIONS
Precontest: Remove skin from chicken breasts and omit the oil and flour from the recipe. Make sure to use a sodium-reduced broth.
Bulking up: Add ½ cup chickpeas to casserole.

	Calories	Protein	Carbo-hydrate	Fat
Maintenance	360	31 grams	16 grams	19 grams
Precontest	195	26 grams	15 grams	3 grams
Bulking up	540	41 grams	46 grams	21 grams

MIXED GRILL

Mixed grill, a popular British meal, is usually served with sausages and bacon. However, due to their high fat content, these have been omitted from this recipe. Mixed grill is traditionally served with green peas and grilled tomato.

1 2–3 ounce beefsteak
1 loin lamb chop
1 slice calf's liver
1 teaspoon Dijon mustard
½ teaspoon rosemary
½ teaspoon thyme
1 tomato
6 mushrooms
1 onion, quartered

Preheat broiler for 10 minutes. Trim steak and lamb chop of all fat and make slits around edge of meat to prevent it from curling under the broiler. Place lamb chop and beef on grill and brush with ½ teaspoon mustard. Sprinkle lamb chop with rosemary and beefsteak with thyme and broil for 5 minutes. Turn the meat over and brush with remaining ½ teaspoon mustard. Add the calf's liver, the tomato, and mushrooms and grill a further 5–6 minutes, turning the liver once. Makes 1 serving.

VARIATIONS
Precontest: Omit beefsteak and lamb chop and use a 3-ounce veal chop in their place. Omit mustard.
Bulking up: Add 1½ ounces sliced kidney to grill with liver.

	Calories	Protein	Carbo-hydrate	Fat
Maintenance	353	42 grams	21 grams	10 grams
Precontest	319	32 grams	10 grams	9 grams
Bulking up	437	51 grams	22 grams	15 grams

VEGETABLES AND GRAINS

BROWN RICE CASSEROLE

- 1 cup chicken broth
- ¾ cup apricot nectar
- ¼ cup seedless raisins
- ½ cup chopped dried apricots
- 1 cup brown rice, partially cooked (20 minutes)
- ½ cup chopped celery
- ¼ cup chopped onion
- 2 cloves garlic, minced
- 1–2 teaspoons curry powder, or to taste

Preheat oven to 350°. Heat chicken broth and apricot nectar to boiling point. Remove from burner and add raisins and apricots to plump for 5 minutes. In a medium casserole, mix the brown rice, celery, onion, and garlic. Stir in the broth, fruit, and curry powder. Cover and bake for 40–50 minutes. Makes 4 servings.

VARIATIONS
Precontest: Omit raisins.
Bulking up: Sprinkle with 2 tablespoons shredded coconut and 2 tablespoons unsalted raw cashews.

	Calories	Protein	Carbohydrate	Fat
Maintenance	289	6 grams	65 grams	trace
Precontest	250	6 grams	58 grams	trace
Bulking up	421	9 grams	71 grams	8 grams

POPPY SEED PASTA

- ½ pound whole-wheat noodles
- 3 tablespoons safflower oil
- 1 teaspoon lemon juice
- 2 tablespoons poppy seeds

Cook noodles until tender, then drain. Heat safflower oil and lemon juice in a small saucepan. Pour over noodles and toss. Sprinkle with poppy seeds and serve. Makes 2 servings.

VARIATIONS
Precontest: Reduce safflower oil to 1 tablespoon.
Bulking up: Stir in 2 tablespoons sour cream.

	Calories	Protein	Carbohydrate	Fat
Maintenance	318	11 grams	40 grams	13 grams
Precontest	256	11 grams	40 grams	7 grams
Bulking up	379	12 grams	41 grams	19 grams

BARLEY CASSEROLE

- 2 tablespoons safflower oil
- 1 clove garlic, minced
- 3 green onions, chopped
- ½ cup chopped green pepper
- ½ cup chopped red pepper
- ½ cup pearl barley
- 2 cups beef broth
- 1 cup fresh corn kernels
- 1 teaspoon mixed herbs

Preheat oven to 350°. In a flameproof casserole, heat oil and sauté the garlic and onion until tender. Add the green and red pepper and barley, and sauté until the barley is golden. Add the chicken broth, corn, and mixed herbs. Bring to a boil, then cover and bake in oven for 1 hour. Makes 3 servings.

VARIATIONS
Precontest: Omit the safflower oil and spray the casserole with a nonstick vegetable coating.
Bulking up: Sprinkle casserole with ¼ cup grated cheddar cheese.

	Calories	Protein	Carbohydrate	Fat
Maintenance	204	6 grams	30 grams	8 grams
Precontest	143	6 grams	30 grams	1 gram
Bulking up	239	8 grams	30 grams	10 grams

VEGETABLES COOKED IN FOIL

When cooking vegetables in foil, always use a selection of vegetables that have similar cooking times. For example, green peppers, mushrooms, and tomatoes cook quickly, while carrots, brussels sprouts, and cauliflower take a little longer.

½ green pepper, cut into strips
½ cup stemmed mushrooms
6 cherry tomatoes or 1 medium tomato, quartered
3 green onions, trimmed
1 teaspoon lemon juice
½ teaspoon basil

Preheat oven to 375°. Cut a piece of heavy-duty aluminum foil large enough to enclose vegetables. Arrange vegetables in a single layer, and sprinkle with lemon juice and basil. Fold foil over the vegetables and crimp the edges to seal. Bake for 15–20 minutes. Makes 1 serving.

VARIATIONS

Precontest: No change.
Bulking up: Add ¼ cup red kidney beans to foil package and sprinkle vegetables with 1 tablespoon Parmesan cheese.

	Calories	Protein	Carbo-hydrate	Fat
Maintenance	70	3 grams	10 grams	trace
Precontest	70	3 grams	10 grams	trace
Bulking up	150	8 grams	20 grams	2 grams

BAKED SWEET POTATOES

1 large sweet potato, scrubbed and patted dry
1 teaspoon peanut oil
1 teaspoon sesame seeds

Rub sweet potato with peanut oil. Wrap in foil and bake for 30 minutes at 350°. Remove from oven, prick with a fork in two or three places, then return to oven to bake for a further 40 minutes. When done, split down the center and sprinkle with sesame seeds. Makes 1 serving.

VARIATIONS

Precontest: Omit peanut oil.
Bulking up: Heat ½ teaspoon honey and 1 teaspoon peanut oil with the sesame seeds and drizzle down the center of the baked potato.

	Calories	Protein	Carbo-hydrate	Fat
Maintenance	223	3 grams	37 grams	8 grams
Precontest	173	3 grams	37 grams	2 grams
Bulking up	283	3 grams	40 grams	14 grams

STUFFED TOMATOES

2 large tomatoes
1 tablespoon safflower oil
1 clove garlic, minced
¼ cup chopped onion
1 stalk celery, chopped
½ cup canned red kidney beans, drained
1 teaspoon chili powder

Preheat oven to 325°. Slice the tops off the tomatoes and scoop out the pulp. Set pulp aside. Heat oil in a skillet; add the garlic, onion, celery, and tomato pulp and sauté for 5 minutes. Add kidney beans and chili powder. Stuff the tomatoes with the mixture and bake for 20–25 minutes. Makes 2 servings.

VARIATIONS

Precontest: Omit safflower oil and use a nonstick vegetable spray coating in its place.
Bulking up: Sprinkle with ¼ cup grated cheddar cheese before baking.

	Calories	Protein	Carbo-hydrate	Fat
Maintenance	170	5 grams	20 grams	7 grams
Precontest	108	5 grams	20 grams	.5 gram
Bulking up	226	9 grams	20 grams	12 grams

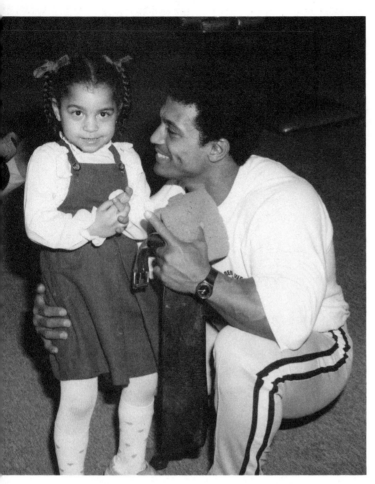

Mohamed Makkawy with his daughter Susie.

STEAMED VEGETABLE PLATTER

This recipe utilizes a variety of herbs that enhance the flavor of each vegetable. Steamed vegetables can also be served chilled with one of the dips in the chapter on snacks.

2 small carrots, peeled and quartered
½ cup cauliflower flowerets
½ cup broccoli flowerets
½ cup green beans
1 tablespoon olive oil
1 tablespoon lemon juice
¼ teaspoon each of thyme, marjoram, dill, and basil

Arrange vegetables in groups in a steamer. Sprinkle carrots with thyme, broccoli with marjoram, cauliflower with dill, and green beans with basil.

Cover and steam over boiling water for 4–5 minutes or until the vegetables are crisp tender. Heat olive oil and lemon juice in a small saucepan and drizzle over vegetables. Makes 1–2 servings.

VARIATIONS
Precontest: Use 1 small zucchini, halved and quartered; ½ green pepper, cut into strips; 6 large mushrooms; and ½ cup cauliflower flowerets in place of the vegetables listed above. Omit olive oil, and drizzle vegetables with lemon juice.
Bulking up: Add a large potato, peeled and cut into julienne strips.

	Calories	Protein	Carbo-hydrate	Fat
Maintenance	215	5.9 grams	19.7 grams	14.6 grams
Precontest	57	4.3 grams	11.5 grams	.4 gram
Bulking up	291	8.0 grams	36.8 grams	14.8 grams

ROASTED VEGETABLES

1 ripe tomato, peeled, cored, and sliced
1 onion, peeled and cut into wedges
½ cup zucchini chunks
¼ cup fava beans
1 teaspoon dried marjoram
1 garlic clove, minced
1 tablespoon olive oil
1 teaspoon vinegar

Preheat oven to 400°. Spray a shallow baking dish with a nonstick vegetable coating. Spread the tomato slices on the bottom of the baking dish and arrange onions, zucchini, and fava beans on top. Sprinkle with marjoram and garlic and drizzle with olive oil and vinegar. Bake for 30 minutes, stir, then continue baking a further 20–30 minutes. Makes 1 serving.

VARIATIONS
Precontest: Omit olive oil and fava beans.
Bulking up: Add a peeled, sliced potato to vegetable mixture.

	Calories	Protein	Carbo-hydrate	Fat
Maintenance	295	10 grams	36 grams	14 grams
Precontest	105	4 grams	24 grams	—
Bulking up	375	12 grams	54 grams	14 grams

SESAME BROCCOLI

1 cup broccoli flowerets
1 teaspoon safflower oil
2 teaspoons lemon juice
½ teaspoon ginger
2 teaspoons sesame seeds

Steam broccoli until tender crisp. Heat safflower oil, lemon juice, and ginger in a small saucepan and pour over broccoli. Sprinkle with sesame seeds. Makes 1 serving.

VARIATIONS

Precontest: Omit safflower oil.
Bulking up: Add 2 ounces tofu, cut into cubes, to safflower oil and sauté for 2–3 minutes; then add lemon juice, ginger, and sesame. Toss with broccoli.

	Calories	Protein	Carbo-hydrate	Fat
Maintenance	168	7 grams	11 grams	10 grams
Precontest	118	7 grams	11 grams	4 grams
Bulking up	299	18 grams	20 grams	16 grams

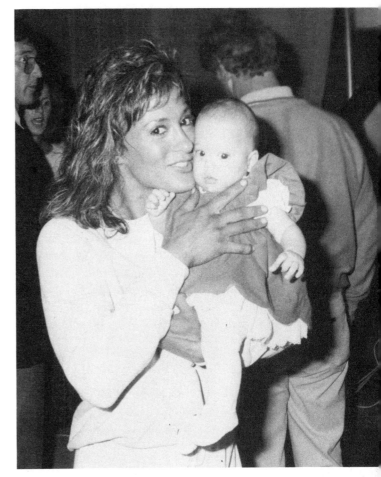

World pro champ Lori Bowen shows off her baby.

GREEN BEANS

2 cups green beans
1 tablespoon safflower oil
¼ cup chopped celery
1 clove garlic, minced

Wash beans and remove the ends. Cut into 1-inch lengths. Cook in boiling water to cover for 15–20 minutes or until tender crisp. Meanwhile, in a small saucepan, heat the safflower oil and add the celery and garlic. Sauté for about 10 minutes or until celery has softened. Drain the beans and add to pan with celery. Sauté for 2–3 minutes. Makes 2 servings.

VARIATIONS

Precontest: Reduce safflower oil to 1 teaspoon.
Bulking up: Add 2 tablespoons slivered almonds.

	Calories	Protein	Carbo-hydrate	Fat
Maintenance	100	2 grams	8 grams	7 grams
Precontest	63	2 grams	8 grams	5 grams
Bulking up	153	4 grams	10 grams	12 grams

RATATOUILLE

Ratatouille is a pleasant blend of vegetables that can be served hot as an accompaniment to grilled meat or cold as a salad. It takes considerable time to prepare, so make it on one of your nontraining days, and you'll have enough to use through the week in such recipes as Pasta Ratatouille. It also makes a delicious filling for an omelette.

4 tablespoons safflower oil
1 Spanish onion, sliced

5 carrots, peeled and cut into julienne strips
3 cloves garlic, minced
1 eggplant, peeled and cubed
2 zucchini, sliced and cut into julienne strips
1 28-ounce can of tomatoes, drained
1 teaspoon basil
1 teaspoon thyme
  Pepper to taste

Heat 2 tablespoons safflower oil in a large casserole and add the Spanish onion, carrots, and minced garlic. Sauté until onion is soft. Meanwhile heat the remaining 2 tablespoons of oil in another pan, add the eggplant and zucchini, and cook until they are slightly browned. Add browned eggplant and zucchini to casserole containing the onion and carrot mixture. Add tomatoes, basil, thyme, and pepper to taste, and simmer, covered, over low heat for 1 hour. Makes 6–8 servings.

VARIATIONS
Precontest: Reduce safflower oil to 1 tablespoon.
Bulking up: Sprinkle each serving with 1 tablespoon Parmesan cheese.

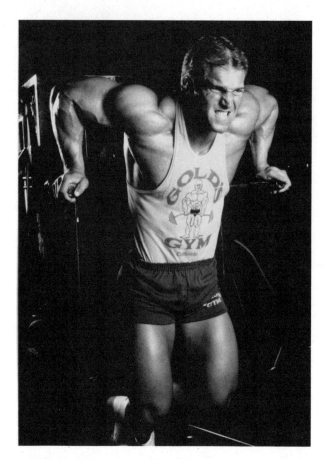

ABOVE AND FACING PAGE: *Gary Strydom.*

	Calories	Protein	Carbo-hydrate	Fat
Maintenance	180	6 grams	18 grams	9 grams
Precontest	134	6 grams	18 grams	2 grams
Bulking up	203	8 grams	18 grams	9 grams

LIMA BEANS IN TOMATO SAUCE

¾ cup frozen lima beans
1 tablespoon safflower oil
2 tablespoons chopped onion
¼ cup chopped green pepper
1 ounce ham, diced
½ cup tomato sauce
½ cup canned tomatoes
1 teaspoon vinegar
½ teaspoon honey

Cover lima beans with cold water and simmer for 5–6 minutes. Drain and set aside. Heat safflower oil in a small skillet, add onion and green pepper, and cook until onion is clear. Add lima beans and heat through, stirring frequently. Now add the ham, tomato sauce, and canned tomatoes; cover and simmer for 15 minutes. Remove the cover and add the vinegar and honey. Simmer until most of the juice is absorbed. Makes 3 servings.

VARIATIONS
Precontest: Omit safflower oil and use a nonstick vegetable coating in its place. Omit the tomato sauce.
Bulking up: Preheat oven to 350°. Place cooked lima beans and tomato sauce in a small casserole and cover with ¼ cup grated cheddar cheese. Bake for an additional 10 minutes.

	Calories	Protein	Carbo-hydrate	Fat
Maintenance	200	7 grams	20 grams	11 grams
Precontest	107	6 grams	16 grams	6 grams
Bulking up	241	9 grams	20 grams	13 grams

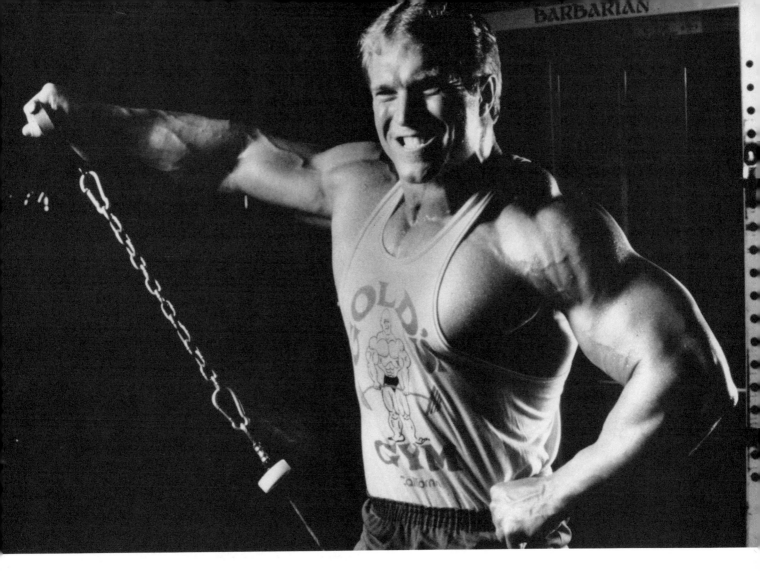

SPAGHETTI SQUASH

If you're dieting, spaghetti squash makes a great substitute for pasta in dishes like spaghetti with clam sauce. It's also delicious when topped with ratatouille and Parmesan cheese.

½ spaghetti squash
1 tablespoon safflower oil
1 teaspoon lemon juice
2 teaspoons chopped parsley

Remove seeds from squash and place in boiling water to cover. Boil gently for about 15 minutes. Remove from water and, using a fork, scrape out the pulp in spaghetti-like strands. Heat oil and lemon juice in a small saucepan and pour over squash. Toss to coat. Sprinkle with parsley. Makes 2 servings.

VARIATIONS
Precontest: Omit safflower oil.
Bulking up: Sprinkle each serving with 1 tablespoon of Parmesan cheese.

	Calories	Protein	Carbo-hydrate	Fat
Maintenance	87	6 grams	2 grams	7 grams
Precontest	25	6 grams	2 grams	trace
Bulking up	110	7 grams	2 grams	9 grams

SPINACH SAUTÉ

4 cups raw spinach
1 tablespoon safflower oil
1 clove garlic, minced
½ teaspoon lemon juice
½ teaspoon chervil

Remove stems from spinach and wash well. Drain but do not pat dry. Heat safflower oil in a skillet and add garlic. Sauté for 1–2 minutes, stirring. Add lemon juice, chervil, and spinach and stir until wilted. Makes 2 servings.

VARIATIONS
Precontest: Reduce safflower oil to 1 teaspoon.
Bulking up: Garnish with a quartered hard-boiled egg.

	Calories	Protein	Carbo-hydrate	Fat
Maintenance	90	4 grams	5 grams	7 grams
Precontest	54	4 grams	5 grams	3 grams
Bulking up	137	7 grams	5 grams	10 grams

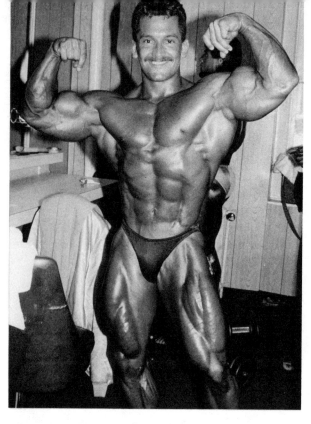

Lee LaBrada.

BASIC BAKED POTATO

Baked potatoes are a favorite carb-up food, used prior to competition.

Preheat oven to 425°. Wash and dry a baking potato. Wrap in foil and pierce in several places. Bake for about 1 hour or until potato is tender when pierced with a fork. Makes 1 serving.

VARIATIONS
Precontest: No change.
Bulking up: Serve with 1 tablespoon sour cream.

BAKED POTATO SLICES

1 baking potato, scrubbed
1 tablespoon safflower oil
2 tablespoons sesame seeds

Preheat broiler to 425°. Slice potatoes very thin. Spread on a baking sheet and brush with ½ tablespoon of safflower oil, then sprinkle with 1 tablespoon sesame seeds. Place under broiler for 3–4 minutes (until browned). Remove from oven and turn. Brush with remaining oil and sprinkle with remaining sesame seeds. Return to broiler until browned and crisp. Makes 1 serving.

VARIATIONS
Precontest: Spray baking sheet with a nonstick vegetable coating; omit safflower oil.
Bulking up: Serve with 1 tablespoon sour cream.

	Calories	Protein	Carbo-hydrate	Fat
Maintenance	90	3 grams	21 grams	trace
Precontest	90	3 grams	21 grams	trace
Bulking up	115	3 grams	22 grams	2 grams

	Calories	Protein	Carbo-hydrate	Fat
Maintenance	324	6 grams	24 grams	24 grams
Precontest	199	6 grams	24 grams	10 grams
Bulking up	439	6 grams	24 grams	26 grams

DESSERTS

CARROT CAKE

1 cup safflower oil
½ cup honey
¼ cup raisins
1 tablespoon grated lemon peel
2 cups grated carrots
½ cup chopped walnuts
2 cups whole-wheat flour
2 tablespoons baking soda
1 teaspoon cinnamon
1 teaspoon nutmeg
½ teaspoon allspice

Preheat oven to 350°. In a large bowl, combine the oil, honey, raisins, lemon peel, and carrots. In another bowl, combine the walnuts, flour, baking soda, and spices. Make a well in the center of the dry ingredients and stir in the wet ingredients. Spray an 8-inch square pan with a nonstick vegetable coating and bake for about 45 minutes. Yields an 8-inch cake (12 slices).

VARIATIONS
Precontest: Omit walnuts from recipe.
Bulking up: Add frosting: Mix together in a bowl ½ pound cream cheese, ¼ cup honey, 1 teaspoon vanilla, and juice of one lemon. Beat until smooth.

	Calories	Protein	Carbo-hydrate	Fat
Maintenance	235	4 grams	30 grams	12 grams
Precontest	208	3 grams	30 grams	10 grams
Bulking up	326	6 grams	35 grams	19 grams

FRESH FRUIT SALAD

1 cup fresh pineapple, cut into chunks
2 bananas, peeled and sliced into chunks
2 oranges, peeled and cut into segments
1 apple, cored and diced
1 cup seedless green grapes
Juice of ½ lemon
¼ cup fresh orange juice
2 tablespoons honey

Combine pineapple, bananas, oranges, apples, and grapes in a glass bowl. Squeeze lemon juice over fruit. Heat the orange juice and honey in a small saucepan, and pour over fruit. Chill and serve. Makes 4 servings.

VARIATIONS
Precontest: Omit honey and use a sugar substitute in its place.
Bulking up: Sprinkle salad with ¼ cup grated coconut before serving.

	Calories	Protein	Carbo-hydrate	Fat
Maintenance	205	2 grams	51 grams	1 gram
Precontest	173	2 grams	43 grams	1 gram
Bulking up	226	2 grams	53 grams	2 grams

STRAWBERRY BANANA PARFAIT

6 ounces plain yogurt
1 teaspoon honey
½ teaspoon vanilla flavoring
6 strawberries, hulled and sliced
½ banana, sliced

Mix together the yogurt, honey, and vanilla flavoring. In a parfait glass, alternate layers of fruit and yogurt. Makes 1 serving.

VARIATIONS
Precontest: Use a skim-milk yogurt and omit the honey.
Bulking up: Add 2 tablespoons granola to layers of fruit.

	Calories	Protein	Carbo-hydrate	Fat
Maintenance	197	7 grams	36 grams	6 grams
Precontest	186	11 grams	40 grams	1 gram
Bulking up	245	8 grams	43 grams	8 grams

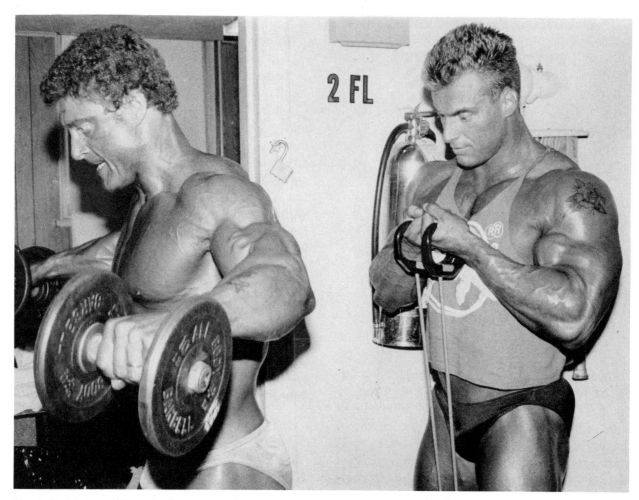

Frank Richards and Berry DeMey warm up backstage in preparation for competition.

BAKED APPLES

2 large Granny Smith apples, cored
1 teaspoon lemon juice
2 tablespoons raisins
1 tablespoon liquid honey
2 tablespoons granola
¼ teaspoon cinnamon
½ cup apple juice, unsweetened

Preheat oven to 350°. Brush cavity of the apples with lemon juice to prevent discoloration. Place apples in a small baking dish. In a small bowl, combine the raisins, honey, granola, and cinnamon. Stuff the apples with this mixture. Pour the apple juice into the baking dish and add ¼ cup boiling water. Bake for 50–60 minutes, basting occasionally with the apple juice. Makes 2 servings.

VARIATIONS
Precontest: Omit honey, and sweeten with a sugar substitute if desired.
Bulking up: Add 2 tablespoons chopped walnuts to the filling before baking.

	Calories	Protein	Carbo-hydrate	Fat
Maintenance	211	1 gram	51 grams	2 grams
Precontest	180	1 gram	42 grams	2 grams
Bulking up	260	3 grams	52 grams	6 grams

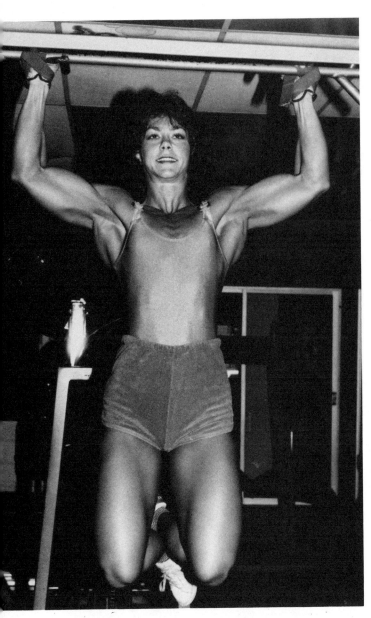

Clare Furr performs wide grip chins.

BROILED FRUIT KEBABS

If you feel like a change from the normal fresh fruit or fruit salad dessert, give this recipe a try. It takes only a few minutes to assemble and is ideally prepared in conjunction with any broiled main course. It also makes a great snack.

   Juice of 1 lemon
   Juice of 1 lime
1 tablespoon honey
½ banana, sliced into 1-inch pieces
½ apple, cored and sliced into 4 sections
½ pear, cored and sliced into 4 pieces

Preheat broiler for 10–15 minutes. Heat the lemon juice, lime juice, and honey in a small saucepan over medium heat, stirring until heated through. Set aside. Thread fruit sections onto 2 metal skewers, alternating fruits. Brush with glaze and broil for 5 minutes.

VARIATIONS
Precontest: Substitute ½ cup fresh pineapple (cut into chunks) and 1 small orange (sectioned) for the banana and pear.
Bulking up: Serve with 3 ounces vanilla-flavored yogurt.

	Calories	Protein	Carbo-hydrate	Fat
Maintenance	220	2.5 grams	57 grams	trace
Precontest	165	3.0 grams	43 grams	trace
Bulking up	295	6.5 grams	65 grams	1.5 grams

SNACKS

TUNA DIP

Serve this high-protein dip with steamed or raw vegetables as a snack or a light lunch.

½ cup tuna, drained
3 tablespoons plain yogurt
1 green onion, chopped
1 teaspoon fennel seed
1 teaspoon lemon juice
1 teaspoon capers

Mix tuna, yogurt, green onion, fennel seed, and lemon juice in a food processor or blender. Stir in capers. Chill and serve.

VARIATIONS

Precontest: Use water-packed tuna and omit capers.
Bulking up: Use 3 tablespoons sour cream in place of yogurt.

	Calories	Protein	Carbo-hydrate	Fat
Maintenance	186	24 grams	4 grams	7 grams
Precontest	156	29 grams	4 grams	2 grams
Bulking up	252	25 grams	6 grams	16 grams

COTTAGE CHEESE DIP

¼ cup cottage cheese
2 tablespoons yogurt
1 green onion
1 clove garlic, minced
1 teaspoon lemon juice
½ teaspoon dill

Mix all ingredients in a blender until smooth. Serve with steamed or raw vegetables.

VARIATIONS

Precontest: Use a low-sodium, low-fat cottage cheese.
Bulking up: Use 2 tablespoons sour cream in place of yogurt.

	Calories	Protein	Carbo-hydrate	Fat
Maintenance	78	7 grams	5 grams	3 grams
Precontest	71	9 grams	6 grams	2 grams
Bulking up	115	10 grams	5 grams	8 grams

Hanne Von Aken, Holland.

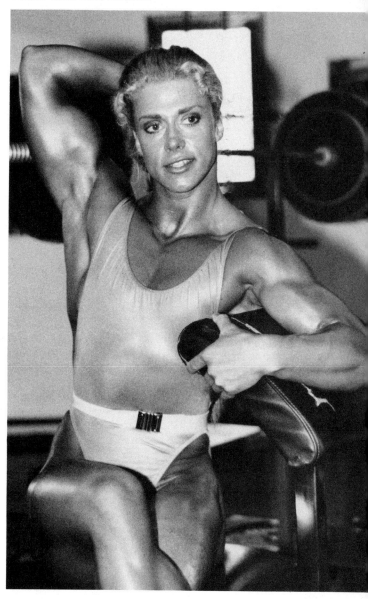

MUSHROOMS STUFFED WITH CRAB MEAT

2 teaspoons safflower oil
1 green onion, finely chopped
½ teaspoon dry mustard
2 ounces crab meat
1 tablespoon milk
2 tablespoons whole-wheat bread crumbs
  Pinch of cayenne pepper
  Lemon juice to taste
6 large mushroom caps

Preheat oven to 450°. Heat safflower oil in a small saucepan. Add green onion, dry mustard, and crab meat and sauté for 2–3 minutes. Add milk, bread crumbs, cayenne pepper, and lemon juice, and sauté for a further 5 minutes. Divide mixture among mushroom caps and bake on a baking sheet for 5 minutes. Makes 1 snack serving.

VARIATIONS
Precontest: Spray pan with a vegetable coating and omit safflower oil.
Bulking up: Sprinkle with ¼ cup grated cheddar cheese before baking.

	Calories	Protein	Carbo-hydrate	Fat
Maintenance	294	18 grams	27 grams	13 grams
Precontest	194	18 grams	27 grams	2 grams
Bulking up	414	26 grams	27 grams	21 grams

CHEDDAR CHEESE MUFFINS

Cheddar cheese muffins make an ideal snack when served with a couple of cherry tomatoes and a stick of celery.

¾ cup all-purpose flour
¾ cup rye flour
2 teaspoons baking powder
1 teaspoon caraway seeds
½ teaspoon baking soda
1¾ cups grated sharp cheddar cheese
⅓ cup safflower oil
1 cup yogurt
1 egg
  Pinch of cayenne pepper

Preheat oven to 400°. Mix together the all-purpose flour, rye flour, baking powder, caraway seeds, baking soda, and cheese. Whisk oil, yogurt, egg, and cayenne. Make a well in the center of the dry ingredients and stir in the yogurt mixture until just combined. Spray muffin tins with a vegetable coating and fill ¾ full. Bake for 25–30 minutes. Makes 12 muffins.

VARIATIONS
Precontest: Reduce safflower oil to ¼ cup and reduce cheese to 1 cup.
Bulking up: Add ⅓ cup chopped walnuts.

	Calories	Protein	Carbo-hydrate	Fat
Maintenance	192	7 grams	11 grams	7 grams
Precontest	148	6 grams	12 grams	4 grams
Bulking up	213	8 grams	12 grams	9 grams

BAKED CHEESE TARTLETS

2 slices whole-wheat bread
1 teaspoon olive oil
1 ounce Gruyère cheese, grated
2 slices of tomato
½ teaspoon basil

Preheat broiler for 10 minutes. Remove crusts from bread and cut into 4-inch rounds. Place bread rounds in tart tins to form tartlets. Brush with olive oil. Fill each tartlet with grated cheese, top with a slice of tomato, and sprinkle with basil. Broil 8 inches from heat for about 3 minutes or until bread is crisp and cheese has melted.

VARIATIONS
Precontest: Omit olive oil.
Bulking up: Use 2 ounces Gruyère cheese and garnish each tartlet with a black olive.

	Calories	Protein	Carbo-hydrate	Fat
Maintenance	279	13 grams	29 grams	15 grams
Precontest	238	5 grams	39 grams	10 grams
Bulking up	431	22 grams	54 grams	24 grams

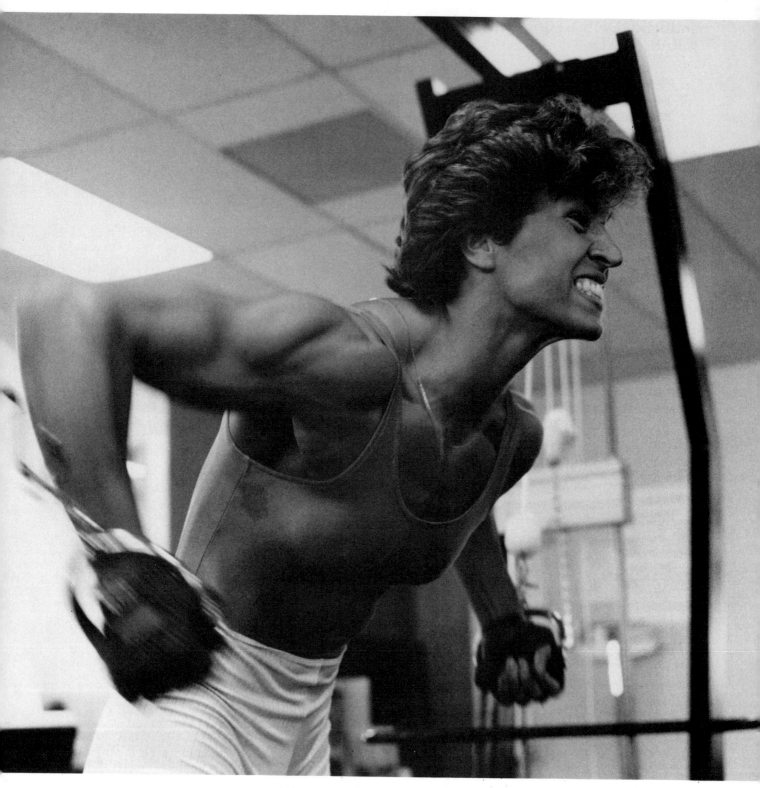

Marjo Selin performs cable crossovers.

CHICKEN LIVER SKEWERS

3 ounces chicken liver
6 cherry tomatoes
6 mushrooms
½ green pepper, cut into chunks

MARINADE

1 tablespoon olive oil
1 teaspoon Worcestershire sauce
1 teaspoon lemon juice
¼ teaspoon oregano

Combine ingredients for marinade and add chicken livers. Refrigerate for 2 hours. Alternate tomatoes, mushrooms, green pepper, and chicken livers on skewers and brush with reserved marinade. Broil for 3 minutes, turn and brush with marinade. Return to broiler for a further 3 minutes. Makes 1 snack serving.

VARIATIONS

Precontest: Omit marinade and sprinkle chicken livers with 1 teaspoon lemon juice before broiling.
Bulking up: Add 1 ounce of cubed ham to skewers.

	Calories	Protein	Carbo-hydrate	Fat
Maintenance	292	20 grams	14 grams	18 grams
Precontest	164	20 grams	13 grams	5 grams
Bulking up	359	25 grams	14 grams	28 grams

STUFFED EGGS

2 hard-boiled eggs
1 ounce canned tuna, drained
1 teaspoon olive oil
½ teaspoon thyme
    Leaf lettuce
2 cherry tomatoes

Halve the hard-boiled eggs (see below) lengthwise and scoop out the yolks. Mash the egg yolks with the tuna, adding in the olive oil and thyme. Spoon into egg whites and serve on a bed of lettuce, garnished with cherry tomatoes. Makes 1 snack serving.

VARIATIONS

Precontest: Use only 1 egg yolk and make sure to use a water-packed tuna.
Bulking up: Top each filled egg with an anchovy fillet.

	Calories	Protein	Carbo-hydrate	Fat
Maintenance	216	19 grams	3 grams	14 grams
Precontest	149	17 grams	3 grams	6 grams
Bulking up	244	22 grams	3 grams	16 grams

TO HARD-BOIL EGGS

Place eggs in cold water to cover in a heavy saucepan. Bring water to boiling over high heat. Reduce heat to medium and simmer for 9 minutes for large eggs. Remove saucepan from heat and pour off the boiling water. Run cold water over the eggs until water is completely cold. Let eggs stand for about 3 minutes. Tap each egg gently to break shell, and peel.

PITA PIZZA

1 whole-wheat pita round
1 tablespoon tomato sauce
½ clove garlic, minced
½ teaspoon oregano
2 ounces grated mozzarella cheese
1 tablespoon chopped green pepper
1 tablespoon chopped mushrooms
1 tablespoon chopped tomato

Preheat broiler for 10 minutes. Spread tomato sauce over whole-wheat pita. Sprinkle with garlic and oregano. Layer with mozzarella cheese, green pepper, mushrooms, and tomatoes. Place on a baking sheet and broil for 5 minutes. Makes 1 snack serving.

VARIATIONS

Precontest: Use 1 ounce of skim milk mozzarella in place of regular mozzarella

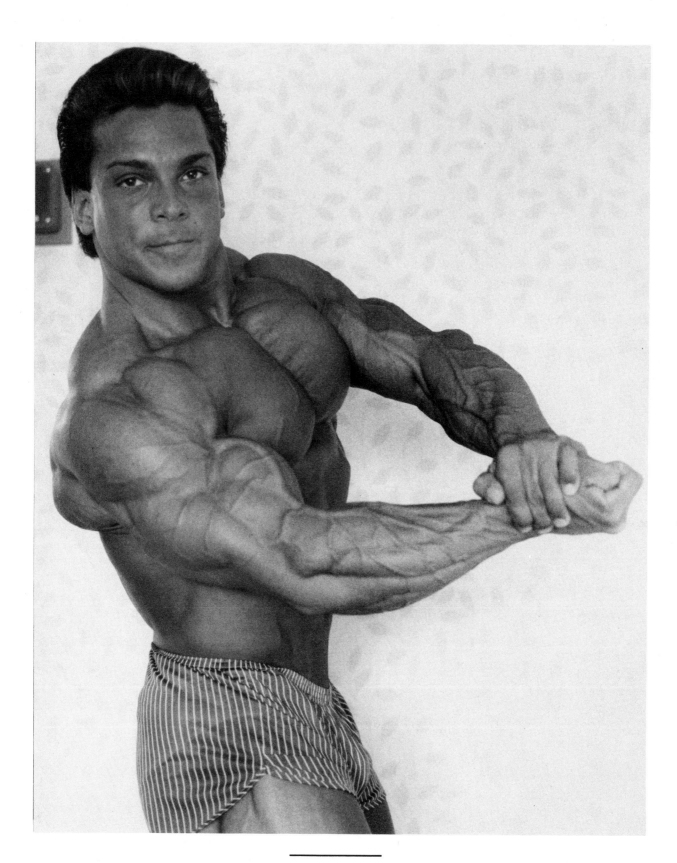

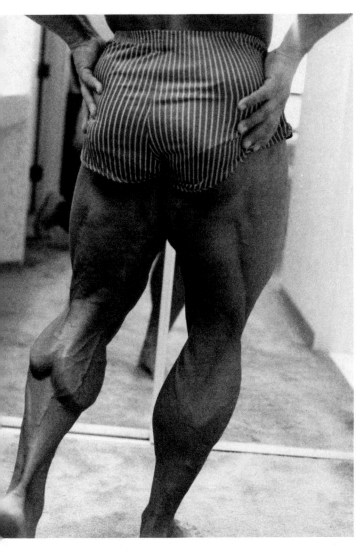

Rich Gaspari.

Bulking up: Add ¼ cup cooked ground beef before layering vegetables.

	Calories	Protein	Carbo-hydrate	Fat
Maintenance	316	18 grams	30 grams	14 grams
Precontest	235	13 grams	29 grams	6 grams
Bulking up	366	23 grams	30 grams	17 grams

HERBED POPCORN

2 cups popped, unsalted popcorn
2 tablespoons safflower oil
¼ teaspoon basil
¼ teaspoon oregano
½ teaspoon lemon zest (optional)

Heat safflower oil, herbs, and lemon zest over medium-high heat until heated through. Pour over popcorn and toss. Makes 2 servings.

VARIATIONS
Precontest: Omit safflower oil.
Bulking up: Add 2 tablespoons of Parmesan cheese and toss.

	Calories	Protein	Carbo-hydrate	Fat
Maintenance	164	1 gram	5 grams	16 grams
Precontest	40	1 gram	5 grams	2 grams
Bulking up	187	3 grams	5 grams	17 grams

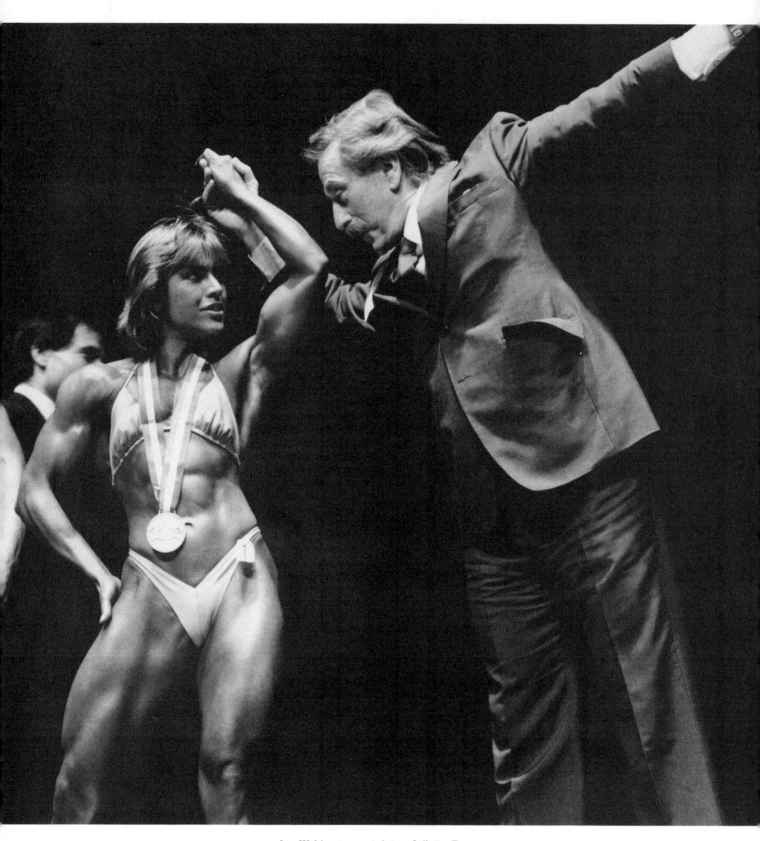

Joe Weider congratulates Juliette Bergman.

Conclusion

This is as far as we go together. As I explained at the beginning of this book, millions of words have been written about nutrition. You can make it as simple or as complicated as you want.

Your success as a bodybuilder depends on nutrition, genetics, drive, training persistence, and recuperation. This book deals principally with nutrition, which is undoubtedly the key to healthy muscle building and ultimate physical perfection.

It has been my observation as publisher of *MuscleMag International* that nutritional knowledge has become a *vital* factor in winning competitions. Gone are the days when bodybuilders could eat instinctively and expect to reach their best contest condition. Now you have to apply nutritional science, and this is particularly true during those last two weeks prior to appearing on stage. You *must* use the proper scientific formulas for ripping up your muscles and peaking perfectly on the day you are judged.

Without applying the knowledge in this book you simply can't peak out. You won't win.

Good-bye and good luck. Perhaps we'll meet again through the pages of *MuscleMag International.* My thoughts and best wishes for success are with you. I envy your chances!

Index